HEALTH CARE AND GENDER

HEALTH CARE
and
GENDER

Charlotte F. Muller

RUSSELL SAGE FOUNDATION / NEW YORK

The Russell Sage Foundation

The Russell Sage Foundation, one of the oldest of America's general purpose foundations, was established in 1907 by Mrs. Margaret Olivia Sage for "the improvement of social and living conditions in the United States." The foundation seeks to fulfill this mandate by fostering the development and dissemination of knowledge about the political, social, and economic problems of America. It conducts research in the social sciences and public policy and publishes books and pamphlets that derive from this research.

The Board of Trustees is responsible for oversight and the general policies of the Foundation, while administrative direction of the program and staff is vested in the President, assisted by the officers and staff. The President bears final responsibility for the decision to publish a manuscript as a Russell Sage Foundation book. In reaching a judgment on the competence, accuracy, and objectivity of each study, the President is advised by the staff and selected expert readers. The conclusions and interpretations in Russell Sage Foundation publications are those of the authors and not of the Foundation, its Trustees, or its staff. Publication by the Foundation, therefore, does not imply endorsement of the contents of the study.

Library of Congress Cataloging-in-Publication Data

Muller, Charlotte Feldman, 1921–
    Health care and gender / Charlotte Muller.
        p.   cm.
    Includes bibliographical references.
    ISBN 0-87154-610-8
    1. Women—Medical care. 2. Men—Medical care. I. Title.
    [DNLM: 1. Delivery of Health Care—United States. 2. Health Policy—United States. 3. Insurance, Health—United States. 4. Women's Health Services—United States.   W 84 AA1 M95h]
    RA564.85.M85   1990   90-8383
    362.1′082—dc20
    DNLM/DLC

The paper used in this publication meets the minimum requirements of American National Standard for Information Sciences—Permanence of Paper for Printed Library Materials, ANSI Z39.48-1984.

10 9 8 7 6 5 4 3 2 1

Contents

List of Tables *vii*

Acknowledgments *ix*

Introduction *xi*

PART ONE / INSIDE THE SYSTEM

CHAPTER ONE

Health Care Utilization by Men and Women 3

CHAPTER TWO

Treatment Issues 23

PART TWO / CONCERNING SOME MAJOR GROUPS

CHAPTER THREE

Health Care, the Workplace, and Gender:
Health Needs 57

CHAPTER FOUR

Health Care, the Workplace, and Gender:
Insurance and Financing Issues 73

CHAPTER FIVE

The Elderly 103

CHAPTER SIX

Medicaid: The Lower Tier of Health Care for Women 147

v

PART THREE / FERTILITY-RELATED SERVICES

CHAPTER SEVEN

Reproductive Care   *171*

PART FOUR / SUMMING UP AND LOOKING AHEAD

CHAPTER EIGHT

How the Issues have Changed   *219*

Name Index   *241*
Subject Index   *247*

List of Tables

CHAPTER ONE

Self-assessed Health, by Sex 5

Smoking and Alcohol Use, by Sex 6

Visits to Different Specialties, by Sex 8

Table 1.1 Most Frequent Principal Diagnoses in Visits to Obstetrician-Gynecologists, 1980–1981 14

Table 1.2 Principal Reason for Visit, Three Specialties, January 1980–December 1981 15

Table 1.3 Percentage with Physician Contact Within Last Year, by Age and Sex, 1986 18

Table 1.4 Number of Physician Contacts per Person per Year, by Place of Contact, Sex, and Age, 1986 19

CHAPTER THREE

Per Capita Direct Costs of Health Care, by Employment Status and Sex 69

CHAPTER FOUR

Table 4.1 Percentage of Those Who Worked During Year in Full-time and Part-time Employment 78

Table 4.2 Full-time and Part-time Workers, by Occupation, 1985 80

Table 4.3 Prevalence of Selected Reported Chronic Conditions, by Sex, for Working-age Population, 1986 93

Table 4.4   Measures of Illness, by Sex, for Working-age Adults, 1986   *94*

CHAPTER FIVE

Preventive Services, by Sex   *116*

Use of Minor Tranquilizers, by Sex   *119*

Persons Served per 1,000 Aged Medicare Enrollees, 1984   *128*

CHAPTER SIX

Table 6.1   Medicaid and Non-Medicaid Population, by Age and Sex, 1980   *152*

Table 6.2   Female-headed Family Household Receiving Medicaid, by Income Level, 1984   *153*

Table 6.3   Medicaid as a Source of Payment, by Type of Service and Sex, 1977   *154*

Acknowledgments

MANY PEOPLE HAVE GIVEN valuable help to the author by providing information, guidance to sources, criticism and comments on portions of this book, and, very important, interest and encouragement. I acknowledge with thanks the help of the following:

Trude Berkowitz
Bernice Bernstein
Rachel Boaz
John Brown
Ronald Brown
Kathleen Christensen
Mark Cronin
Cynthia Fuchs
  Epstein
Marianne C. Fahs
Leonard R. Freifelder
Norma Frey
Estelle Giammusso
Richard Hausknecht
Eugenia Herbst

Thomas Hodgson
Grace M. Kaufman
Robert Kaufman
Joel Kleinman
Mary Grace Kovar
Linda Lamel
Judith Lorber
Michele Marcus
Diane Meier
P. Ellen Parsons
Maria Pego
Jon Piano
Judith Pilson
Bernard Pisani
Paul Placek

William Pratt
Carol Raphael
Cordelia Reimers
Concha Robertson
Beverly Rosignolo
William Shankman
Clyde Schechter
Carl Schoenberg
John L. Shurtleff
Miriam Smith
Jeanne Mager
  Stellman
James Vinicombe
Leon Warshaw

The staffs of the Levy Library at Mount Sinai Medical Center and the Teaneck Public Library helped check references.

Bob Lehrer, DiAnn Pierce, and the staff at Lawrence Letter Service provided essential manuscript production service.

At the Russell Sage Foundation, special thanks are due to Alida Brill, who encouraged me to develop a plan for this book; to Marshall Robinson for helpful discussions at the start; to Peter de Janosi, vice president, for friendly advice and assistance through the project; and to Priscilla Lewis for editorial guidance.

Introduction

RECOGNITION OF GENDER INEQUALITY in the United States as a civil rights issue brought about changes in the law that have affected many lives. Aided by affirmative action and changes in social attitudes, women have gained a footing in many "public sphere" activities previously denied to them. It would be surprising if health care, a major social institution and industry, had been immune from invidious distinctions based on gender before the women's movement took shape. But such distinctions, once awareness of them develops, do present a challenge to both the humanistic and the scientific values of the health professions. If women are to fulfill their individual goals, the health care system must respect these goals and respond to changes in gender roles. Whether the response is sufficient will be indicated by how much women's health benefits from their journeys through the system, whether they avoid excessive economic burdens, and whether, by control of their fertility, they become more able to pursue their personal life goals.

The system's adjustment is complicated by many surrounding changes (e.g., health technology and population trends) to which the health economy is continually responding and by financial restraints, competition, and new forms of organization that affect the conduct of health service activities.

The present volume examines different facets of the interaction of gender with health care and is intended to provide background for interpreting contemporary policy issues. It is also intended as a stimulus to scholarship, because unresolved questions, newly arising questions, and unexplored aspects of gender in health care provide a rich research agenda.

The discussion is set in the current period that has followed the women's movement of the 1960s and 1970s. Following an examination of statistics on various aspects of utilization of health care by women and men presented in Chapter 1, the discussion turns to treatment issues. Many of the interconnections of gender with health care are indirect, depending on how gender roles influence individual ability to pay, needs of the elderly, and so forth. The question of whether and how gender influences actual treatment once a person has entered the system has many aspects, among them communication problems, quality of life concepts, and risks as perceived by the practitioner. These are set forth in Chapter 2.

Working-age adults are the focus of Chapters 3 and 4. Chapter 3 presents health comparisons by gender. Women have more acute illness and need more services, even excluding conditions of pregnancy. Their specific chronic conditions differ from those of men, but the patterns for both sexes shift with aging; and chronic problems, including killer diseases and causes of discomfort and disability, become more prevalent after age 65. Thus financing of care is an important concern. Financial protection against costs of health care, as explained in Chapter 4, is influenced by gender role factors that have placed more men than women in the primary labor market, by insurance customs regarding family coverage that may not fit current household types, and by differences in wage supplements across industries.

For the elderly, health-related phenomena are experienced through the filter of gender because of women's greater life expectancy, spousal age differences at the time of marriage, and the precariousness of pension rights and other economic resources of aged women. Gender aspects of the health care needs of the elderly, including aid for functional impairments, utilization patterns, and policy issues are discussed in Chapter 5. The intricacies of Medicaid, the federal–state program largely serving the poor, single-parent families, discussed in Chapter 6, show what a "less eligible" status with respect to health care has meant, in terms of geographical variations in conditions of eligibility and extent of benefits, for women with insufficient earned income to enter mainstream medical markets.

No discussion of gender and health care can omit fertility-related services: some, such as pregnancy and delivery services, are specific to women and, thus, provide a measure of whether the system is meeting women's needs. Others, such as contraception and infertility treatment, involve both men and women and may give rise to gender equity questions. Reproductive care is one of the most complicated areas of health care because of new and changing technological powers over conception, pregnancy, and birth and the ethical and attitudinal conflicts they stimulate. These conflicts, in conjunction with the high cost of services, may affect access to innovative services. Yet many problems of distributional equity remain for services that are routine for the well-financed. At the same time, scientific controversies surround the choice process in reproductive medicine, affecting system efficiency and chances of individual benefit. These matters are discussed in Chapter 7.

A final chapter contains a summing up of the overall implications of gender in health care. Reforms in the system are suggested that would address women's situational problems interfering with timely and equitable care. In many areas, research is a very useful means of monitoring the performance of the system (including the effects of both new programs and retrenchments), as well as a means of analyzing causes of problems and, thus, moving closer to appropriate solutions. Research and reform stimulate each other, to help society toward greater equity and, thus, toward a better match of deployment of health care resources with human need.

Changes in health care come at a rapid pace and from many sources: control of environmental hazards and emergence of new ones, maturing of cohorts exposed to different economic and political contexts, new legislation intended to either expand or to shrink certain services, medical discoveries, and others. Data are therefore also subject to change, and it has not been possible, nor indeed was it my intention, to secure late-breaking statistical news on each topic under review in this book. I have tried to stay reasonably close to the present, of course. But the emphasis in this book is on the economic and social relationships, roles, and motivations, including those within the health care system, that are likely to generate fairly stable statistical patterns associated with gender—and that have equity implications. The interactions of various traditions and roles with scientific progress and financing arrangements are seen as recreating fresh potential sources of inequities that need consistent attention from society and alert inquiry from researchers. Data are used to assess and illustrate situations and, in many cases, provide a baseline from which to evaluate both progress and the shifting importance of specific problems. The discussions in the book may give scholars, analysts, and policymakers interested in health care more insights into gender issues and those interested in gender equity a firmer appreciation of health care system issues.

It should be added that, in some subject areas, the aging of data and the absence of recent data can be traced to a spurt of interest in women's issues that faded away late in the 1970s and that needs renewal. These cases, particularly the dates shown for the statistics, carry the message of recent neglect by the government's data systems—and of the persistence of reasons for withholding belief that gender problems in health care, too, will fade away.

PART ONE

INSIDE THE SYSTEM

CHAPTER ONE

Health Care Utilization by Men and Women

COMPARISON OF THE RELATIONS of the two sexes with the health care system in statistical terms shows that, generally, women have a more active connection with health care providers. Since women also report more illnesses and have extra reproductive needs, study of patterns of use by sex may seem to be unimportant for health care policy or for gender equity. However, this impression does not hold up. First, unmet need (no care) is not precluded; it may exist and should be assessed. Second, although need measured in terms of illness rates may seem to provide a rational base for use patterns, need for treatment of illness may result from failure to identify, organize, and deliver preventive services.

Patterns of use change in response to many factors that may affect sex comparisons. New methods of prevention and treatment of diseases of one sex are developed; changes in employment status result in physical examinations at hiring. Certain conditions are added to the dictionary of "diseases" qualifying for medical attention rather than being interpreted as flaws in personal behavior or perceptions. Cost pressures on hospitals affect discharge policies, and regulation of physicians' charging practices modifies their behavior. The subjects reviewed in the following pages will acquaint the reader with some of the major dimensions of interest in considering the experience of the two sexes in seeking health care and will supply a background to the discussion of treatment issues in the next chapter.

Measures discussed in this chapter include having a regular source of care, probability of physician contact during a year, number of visits, expense, source of payment, content of visits, use of women doctors, and hospital use. Women are only slightly more likely than men to have a regular source of care, but women who do not have one are in worse health than men without a regular source. Women are less likely to report excellent or very good health, they are more likely to see a doctor in a given year, and they make more visits. They are more often told by the doctor to return for care. Incurring more expense than men, women meet more of the charges with Medicaid or out of pocket and less with private insurance.

Women's visits are over half the visits in all major specialties except pediatrics. Their use of general and family practitioners (GFPs) is different from men's: a larger share of women's visits are visits for non-illness care and return visits for old problems. But content of visits is more affected by the doctor's specialty than the patient's gender, and it appears to be based on the type of problem that led to the visit, regardless of sex. The likelihood of any patient's seeing a woman doctor also varies by specialty. Women doctors tend to attract women patients, particularly young females with genitourinary conditions.

Women use hospitals more than men, with and without deliveries included, but the percentage of cases with surgery is similar to men's. The percentage of cases that are female varies among broad diagnostic categories. Discharges for exclusively female reproductive conditions far outnumber those for exclusively male prostate conditions. The hospitalized patients of certain medical and surgical specialists are primarily male.

There is a general impression that women use physician services more often than men; in particular, women are thought to be more attuned to care of their health and more likely to seek preventive services. National data support the perception that men and women differ in the overall rate of visits to physicians and in the rate of visits for prevention, which is, to a large extent, associated with women's reproductive needs. Yet, as described later, women's general health is not necessarily better, and they do not necessarily get more nonreproductive preventive care.

Although women have generally been thought to be more likely to seek care early in response to symptoms, their care-seeking behavior does not necessarily result in superior outcomes. Waldron (1983) reports that, for certain serious diseases (for example, cancer and ischemic heart disease), the stage of disease at which women's cases were discovered was no earlier than for men; hence, prognosis was not different for the two sexes. Her review of pertinent studies casts doubt on the likelihood that women are more sensitive to cardiac symptoms and, thus, more often seek timely care. In an electrocardiogram (ECG) study of a general population, the proportion with myocardial infarction that had been previously unrecognized was no less for women than for men. Improved outcome for women with angina, compared with men, was related to differences in pathophysiology, rather than in care-seeking behavior. (The response of providers to women with cardiac symptoms or test findings should also be considered, and this is discussed in chapter 2.)

Since employment, insurance, family responsibilities, and other contextual factors, as well as health status and behavioral responses to illness, influence use of health care services, simple gender comparisons of use may be misleading. Service use by men and women may be more similar once various contextual elements are taken into account. Thus, study of occupations where substantial numbers of both sexes are employed shows that the degree of sex difference in use of hospital care and physician care varies considerably among occupations. Furthermore, variation within one sex may be substantial: utilization by employed women differs from that by homemakers for several reasons including health status, pregnancy, and insurance (Muller, 1986a, 1986b).

UTILIZATION OF PHYSICIANS

Health Levels

Sex differences in general health are not remarkable. The self-reported health status of women in 1985 was slightly lower than that of men, as shown by the following age-adjusted figures:

Self-assessed Health, by Sex

Self-assessed Health	Male (percent)	Female (percent)
Excellent	42.7	37.9
Very good	26.0	27.7
Good	21.3	24.0
Fair or poor	9.5	9.9

Source: National Center for Health Statistics, *Health, United States, 1986 and Prevention Profile.* (Hyattsville, MD, 1986), table 39.

The proportion of persons reporting excellent or very good health in each age group between 18 and 64 years is only a little less for women than for men (differences are 5–6 percentage points). After age 65, there is even less sex difference (Dawson and Adams, 1987, table 70).

For all ages, males are no more likely than females to have limitations in their major activity because of health problems (9.5 percent) (Dawson and Adams, table 67), but the males have more at ages 65–69, and the females have more at ages 70+. More men have definitely elevated blood pressure or a borderline elevation, but women are a bit more likely to be overweight and to have excessive serum cholesterol levels (National Center for Health Statistics, 1986a, tables 44–47). Fewer women 20 years of age and older smoke, and those who do smoke fewer cigarettes per day than men (tables 40–41), but in the college population more women than men are daily smokers (Johnston, O'Malley, and Bachman, 1986). The sex difference in heavy use of alcohol (1+ ounces of ethanol daily) is much greater than the smoking difference.

Smoking and Alcohol Use, by Sex

Smoking and Alcohol Use	Male (percent)	Female (percent)
Current smoker	32.7	28.3
Among smokers: 25+ cigarettes daily	32.8	20.6
"Heavier" use of alcohol	14	3.0

Source: L.D. Johnston et al., *Drug Use among American High School Students, College Students, and Other Young Adults.* (Washington, DC: National Institute on Drug Abuse, 1986).

Regular Source of Care

Women are only a little more likely than men to have regular sources of care, whether single or multiple; to have a single regular source of care; and to have a particular doctor as that source. A single regular source is reported by 87.4 percent of women, versus 82.7 percent of men, in the analysis of 1978 data from the National Health Interview Survey (Bloom and Jack, 1985).

But the reasons for not having a regular source show differences in the circumstances of the two sexes. When people who had no regular source of care were asked why this was so, more of the males than of the females said they had not needed a doctor (65.6 percent versus 53.5 percent). The women were more apt to say that they could not find the right doctor, or that they had recently moved, or that their previous doctor was no longer available. Not being able to find the right doctor was more frequent for those with Medicaid (for both sexes); those who gave this reason had the most illness and disability of all those without a regular source and more than those with a regular doctor. Those who said they did not need care were healthier than those with a regular doctor. Thus, among those without a regular source, the women tended to be in worse condition than the men.

Contacts with Doctors

Females were more likely than males to have consulted a doctor in the last year (81.4 percent versus 70.3 percent), according to data from the 1986 National Health Interview Survey (Dawson and Adams, 1987, table 72). Under 18, the sex difference is small. This survey also shows that females of all ages made 3.4 office visits per person per year; males, 2.5 visits (table 71). Therefore, the sex difference is greater for the number of visits (females 36 percent higher) than for the percentage with any contact (16 percent higher) or the percentage having a regular source (6 percent higher). The female rate of office visits per person per year rises continually with age throughout life, but the male rate dips to 1.7 visits at 18–44 years and rises thereafter. At 18–44 years, the female rate of 3.3 visits is 1.94 times the male rate. Women also use the telephone to consult with physicians 80 percent more often than men. As these consultations are counted as "visits," this contributes to their having more doctor visits per person at all places of service than men: 6.2 versus 4.6 visits. Women have more visits to general and family practitioners and internists (IMs) than do men. The visits of women are less likely to be first visits and more likely to end in the doctor's recommending a return visit, but the differences are small.

Expense

National Medical Care Expenditure Survey (NMCES) data for 1977 (National Center for Health Services Research, 1983) provide information on gender differences in expenses. Mean charges per visit were very similar for the two sexes, but the expense per person, counting only those with visits, was higher for females ($148 versus $132), and the aggregate charges amounted to $454 million for females, versus $318 million for males, the amount for females being 1.43 times as high as for males. Females were more likely than males to use family and Medicaid as sources of payment, whereas males covered a higher share of cost from private insurance,[1] the Veterans Administration, and workers' compensation sources. Accordingly, a higher proportion of females had out-of-pocket expenses of $100 or more, and, for those with out-of-pocket expenses, the amount was higher for females ($230 versus $175). Thus, females' extra use occurred despite their having less private insurance, and some was only possible because of a public program for the poor.

---

[1]However, these data antedate the Pregnancy Discrimination Act of 1978 (PDA) mandating equal treatment of maternity in group health insurance.

Women may have unmet needs even though they have a higher utilization rate and greater expense than men. Strong evidence of this comes from nonreceipt of early prenatal care by many of the economically and socially disadvantaged. Moreover, because the NMCES sex comparisons did not have an age breakdown, female minors covered by parents' policies were merged with adult females, and the economic problems that some women have in meeting health care costs are not sharply revealed. More current data will become available from a new national survey by the Agency for Health Care Policy and Research. This will be welcome because of the many changes in health care since 1977 data were gathered.

Utilization by Physician Specialty

The distribution of ambulatory care for each sex by specialty is shown in data on office visits per person per year from the 1981 National Ambulatory Medical Care Survey. The figures were used to compute the sex ratio of visits per person to different specialties.

Visits to Different Specialties, by Sex

	Visits		
Specialty	Male	Female	F/M
General and family practice	.71	.93	1.31
Internal medicine	.28	.35	1.25
Obstetrics/gynecology	—	.42	—
Pediatrics	.34	.32	.94
General surgery	.13	.15	1.15

Source: National Center for Health Statistics, *Health, United States, 1984.* (Hyattsville, MD, 1984), 99.

All specialties together, including those omitted from the table, account for 2.19 visits for males and 2.95 for females. The five specialties shown account for 1.46 and 2.17 visits, respectively. According to 1977 figures, five specialties account for 80.4 percent of visits by women age 15+: general and family practice, obstetrics-gynecology, internal medicine, general surgery, and ophthalmology. Seven other specialties account for another 14 percent, and "all other", for 5.3 percent (Cypress, 1980b, p. 42). Only one-sixth of women's visits are to obstetrician-gynecologists, the specialty that has an almost exclusively female clientele, but the dollar value of deliveries and related in-hospital services is not reflected in the number of visits. Moreover, the interventions of this specialty may have particular importance for women, both physically and psychologically.

The care received by women and men at general and family practitioners' and internists' offices can be compared using 1980–1981 data from the National Ambulatory Medical Care Survey (NAMCS). Together these two specialties account for 525,882,000 visits, of which 72.6 percent were visits to GFPs. The visit rate to IMs is 36.8 per 100 for women and 27.6 for men; to GFPs it is 99.5 and 70.9, respectively. Hence the female/male ratio is similar for the two specialties. The ratio exceeds one for all ages over 15 for both specialties but declines with age (Cypress, 1984a, p. 27; 1983, p. 24). Women and men have similar major reasons for the visits in the two specialty groups, except that a larger share of women's visits to GFPs, compared with men's (16.5 percent and 10.7 percent), is for nonillness care, whereas acute problems make up a larger share of men's visits (51.2 percent versus 45.5 percent).

Female patients of generalists are more likely than males to be "old" (established) patients with old problems (58 percent versus 53 percent), but for internist visits there is virtually no sex difference in prior visit status. Similarly, the proportion told to return at a specified time is higher for women among those seeing a GFP, but there is less sex difference for IMs. Patients seeing an internist are more often given a return appointment and are less likely to have no planned follow-up at all.

For both sexes, going to an IM, rather than to a GFP, makes more likely the use of laboratory tests, general examinations, X rays, ECGs, and other diagnostic services. However, men are more likely to have an ECG. The IM visits are longer for both sexes, consistent with the fact that IMs are more apt to include, not only diagnostic services, but also medical and diet counseling and prescribing of three or four medications in one visit. Although some sex differences exist, the content of the care seems to be more affected by the specialty visited than by the gender of the patient. Thus, the functional requirements of the condition as perceived by specialists with a given training, rather than any cultural biases, determine what is done. (However, there could still be sex differences in the way a procedure is carried out. For example, the content of counseling could vary from patient to patient.)

Sex of Physician

Feminist writings on medicine in the early 1970s describe it as a field dominated by men both numerically and in terms of the relationship with the patient. In their critical analysis of both the doctor–patient relationship and treatments administered, these writings range over several different situations: those in which male doctors enjoyed a collective monopoly over services required by women (obstetrics-gynecology), those in which alleged social labeling and other cultural factors resulted in a large proportion of women in the clientele of a specialty (psychiatry), and those in which, although the clientele was mixed in gender, the treatment was less adequate medically and psychologically when the client was a woman. With the increase in the number of women in medicine and physicians' growing awareness of patient alienation, changes could be expected.

In 1983 there were about 70,000 women physicians, who numbered 15.5 percent of all physicians, according to the American Medical Association (Roback et al. 1984). The ratio of females to all physicians in obstetrics-gynecology (1 in 6) was similar to that for medicine in general. Fifty-four percent of women obstetrician-gynecologists were under 35, compared with 44 percent for all specialists, showing that the growth of the female minority in obstetrics-gynecology is relatively new. Women accounted for 14 percent or more of physicians in internal medicine, pediatrics, psychiatry, anesthesiology, and pathology. Among five specialties with the highest proportions of physicians under 35 (internal medicine, family practice, general surgery, diagnostic radiology, and obstetrics-gynecology), women were least likely to be found in general surgery (4.4 percent). Thus, patients of either sex, while more likely to encounter male than female physicians, were quite unlikely to have their general surgery performed by female doctors. This was also true for ophthalmology, where only 6.8 percent of physicians were female, and orthopedics, with 1.4 percent female. Other smaller surgical specialties had few females; thoracic, colon and rectal, and urological surgery all having only 1 percent female practitioners. However, many patients seeking physical medicine and rehabilitation services might encounter female practitioners, who made up 27.7 percent of this specialty.

The male doctor–female patient situation in obstetrics-gynecology helped create a client group subjected to certain ritual subordination, and certain assumptions in clinical decision making gathered force from, and helped reinforce, social expectations concerning gender power relations. But, eventually, a collective sense of grievance about many of the specialty's practices developed and was articulated by women's groups. Obstetrics-gynecology became a target for the critiques of feminists, and, eventually, some customary practices were modified, a change supported by many female consumers (Chapter 7 on reproductive care discusses this further). Modifications also occurred outside obstetrics-gynecology, notably in breast cancer therapy, as described in Chapter 2, Treatment Issues.

The relationship of various aspects of utilization to the physician's sex is shown in NAMCS data for 1977. The caseload (children and adults) of female doctors was 72 percent female, compared with 60 percent for male physicians, and this difference held for all age groups of patients. For male doctors, 36 percent of visits were by patients over 50; for female doctors, only 25 percent. This is because visits to pediatricians accounted for 20 percent of all visits to women doctors, whereas internal medicine, the specialty with the highest concentration of elderly patients, was the second most often visited specialty for male physicians. Male physicians, except for dermatologists, saw more patients each week than did female physicians. The men were in specialties with shorter visits and had longer work weeks. Additionally, women doctors tended to be younger and, therefore, to have new patients receiving a comprehensive workup on their first visit (Cypress, 1980a). When office care was classified by the patient's principal reason for the visit, the "symptom" module accounted for a larger share of visits to female than to male doctors in GFP and IM, obstetrics-gynecology, pediatrics, and psychiatry. For men doctors in GFP and IM, the "disease" module was proportionately larger, reflecting elderly patients with prior diagnoses like hypertension and heart disease. The women doctors saw more genitourinary cases; young females may have sought women doctors to care for such conditions (Cypress, 1980a). Female doctors were more likely than male doctors to check blood pressure during visits for genitourinary symptoms (61.7 percent versus 35.4 percent) and to give their female patients with such symptoms a Pap smear test. This could have occurred because the women doctors, whether by reason of their age or their sex, had a different perception of prior probabilities (risk factors). A better quality of care is suggested. With the increase in the number of women in medicine in the 1980s, more current information is needed on utilization and visit content by sex of doctor.

PREVENTION

A split between prevention and treatment occurred in the United States some decades ago. Pioneer advocates of a complete and comprehensive health care program for all saw early treatment as an integral part of prevention of damage to health. However, because health leaders sought to define a noncompetitive role for public health departments that would not be opposed by private physicians, certain immunizations and examinations were separated out as preventive services (Muller, 1986c). Later, possibilities for prevention via services that could be provided and billed by private physicians emerged, owing partly to the shift of health risks to noncontagious diseases (that were, in many cases, asymptomatic in early stages) and partly to the development of effective screening technologies.

For the public, using preventive services became identified with prudence and personal control over one's future. Advocacy of annual physical examinations became conventional wisdom, and an offshoot, multiphasic screening, had a good run of popularity in the 1950s and 1960s. More recently, the worth of these medical activities in terms of health yield for a general population has been questioned, and the focus of professional interest has shifted to specific screening services that can be shown to be useful, especially for defined risk groups. (Going beyond utility, demonstrating that a measure is cost-effective assures its attractiveness to rational policymakers. Cost-effectiveness means an acceptably low net cost, after considering cost of disease averted, per year of life saved, adjusted for quality of life. It is a more demanding standard than merely showing that treatable cases were detected.)

Traditionally, women have been praised for their foresight in using preventive services, although the compliment was somewhat offset by a perception of women as more prone to bring trivial complaints to physicians, to see themselves as ill, and to overuse illness care. Some feminist writers have asserted, to refute a long-standing depreciation, that women are more alert than men to the rhythms and signals of their bodies, through exposure to menstruation, pregnancy, and birth, and more attuned to care of their own bodies through household roles as caregivers for others.

What do national data indicate? The National Ambulatory Medical Care Survey used eight different "modules" to classify data on the patient's principal reason for a visit. The proportion of visits to GFPs accounted for by the diagnostic, screening, and preventive module (in the judgment of the physician) is 19.9 percent for women, versus 11.8 percent for men. A small sex difference in the opposite direction is found in visits to internists. As visits by both sexes to IMs are only 27.4 percent of the total for IMs and GFPs combined, women, overall, tend to make more visits for preventive purposes to these two specialties than do men. In addition, 61.9 percent of the 109,035,000 visits made to obstetrician-gynecologists are in the preventive module. The combined visits for the three specialties show that 13.7 percent of men's visits and 30.2 percent of women's visits are in the preventive module, but the visits to obstetrician-gynecologists account for over half (52.8 percent) of the preventive visits of women to these three specialties.

Patients' specific reasons for visits to obstetrician-gynecologists have been analyzed. Over half (51.7 percent) were accounted for by the following preventive purposes: normal pregnancy (36.2 percent), gynecological examination (9.1 percent), contraceptive management (3.3 percent), and postpartum care (3.1 percent) (Cypress, 1983, 1984a, 1984b).

Thus, although women obtained more preventive, diagnostic, and screening services than men, these were chiefly pregnancy-related services and family-planning visits. However, the possibility of receiving regular Pap tests because of such visits is important because of the test's effectiveness in detecting cervical cancer in a pre-invasive phase.

The size of the sex difference depends on what is counted. Women are more likely to obtain medical examinations voluntarily than men, whereas men are more likely to get them because they are required for employment, military service, insurance, or sports (U.S. Department of Health and Human Services (DHHS), 1985]. These required examinations are reported, under the module classification of the National Ambulatory Medical Care Survey, in the administrative module, not in the diagnostic, screening, and preventive module. The female/male ratio of percentage of visits with diagnostic or screening content is 2.58 when only the diagnostic and screening module is considered, but it drops to 1.41 when the administrative module is included. In other words, men and women become more similar in regard to preventive visits made when the administrative examinations are counted. Furthermore, although only 12.3 percent of men's visits are in the screening plus the administrative module, compared with 17.3 percent of women's visits; yet, since women have more return visits than men, the sex difference in percentage of *persons* having diagnostic and screening examinations in a given year is less than the sex difference in percentage of *visits* for these purposes. The proportion seeing a doctor for a general checkup during the year is 44.4 percent for women, versus 33.8 percent for men.

The sex difference in the frequency of administrative examinations is larger than can be accounted for by the percentage of the two sexes in the labor force, but type of employment and military service of men are partial explanations.

When examinations (general checkups) for both sexes are analyzed, the male visits were more likely to include vision and hearing tests, chest X rays, ECGs, blood tests, rectal examinations, and urinalyses. Thus, the female excess is reduced, removed, or even reversed when specific screening services are considered (U.S. Department of Health and Human Services, 1985).

To the sociologist focusing on models of individual behavior that may be influenced by social demands and expectations, it is discretionary or voluntary use that is perhaps more interesting. To those concerned with the extent of deficits in health services, both obligatory and discretionary utilization are significant. Because the proportion of general examinations that include certain specific tests is greater for men than for women, chances of finding treatable conditions should be greater. But

TABLE 1.1

Most Frequent Principal Diagnoses in Visits to Obstetrician-Gynecologists, 1980–1981

	All Ages	Under 25[a]	25–44[b]	45 and Over[c]
Normal pregnancy	36.2	46.1	38.1	
Gynecological exam	9.1	7.4	10.3	12.2
Inflammatory disease of cervix, vagina and vulva	3.9	3.9	3.8	
Follow-up exam after surgery	3.6	2.1	3.8	6.9
Contraceptive management	3.3	3.9	3.6	
Postpartum care and exam	3.1	3.9	3.3	
Disorders of menstruation	3.0	2.8		
General medical exam		1.9	3.2	4.3
Menopausal and postmenopausal disorders	1.9	13.2		13.2
Candidiasis	1.5	*1.1	1.6	

Source: Beulah K. Cypress, *Patterns of Ambulatory Care in Obstetrics and Gynecology: The National Ambulatory Medical Care Survey.* (Hyattsville, MD: National Center for Health Statistics, 1984), 33.

[a]Other frequent diagnosis: pain and other symptoms.
[b]Other frequent diagnoses: pain, infertility, inflammatory disease of ovary, and others.
[c]Other frequent diagnoses: essential hypertension; inflammatory disease of ovary, fallopian tube, and others; uterine biomyoma; and genital prolapse.
* This figure does not meet standards of reliability.

employment-related examinations may be used simply to screen out insurance risks, rather than to aid examinees in caring for their health. Thus, in both voluntary and required examinations, health is not improved unless findings are acted upon. Furthermore, the effectiveness of different services in actually preventing disease may vary, and this affects the significance of the sex differences. Screening efficacy is affected by the quality of examinations and laboratory work. It has been reported that many physicians are poorly trained in breast examinations (Bassett, 1985), and Pap tests are said to be less accurately analyzed when there are many repeat normals in the laboratory work flow (testing of low-risk women), when laboratory volume is too small (Miller, 1985), and when supervision is lax. Despite these difficulties, there is consensus that periodic screening by cervical cytology is efficacious in preventing disease progression and death, and it is cost-effective (Miller, 1985).

The efficacy of mammography in certain age and risk groups in preventing deaths from breast cancer is also supported by the literature. For several other conditions that may be asymptomatic, gathering information at preventive examinations may assist in detection and control. Le-

TABLE 1.2
Principal Reason for Visit, Three Specialties, January 1980–December 1981

	Internists		General and Family Practitioners		Obstetrician-Gynecologists
	Male Patients	Female Patients	Male Patients	Female Patients	All Patients (Females = 99.0%)
Symptom module	51.5	57.2	58.6	57.5	23.5
Disease module	13.7	12.6	9.3	7.8	3.9
Diagnostic, screening, and preventive module	18.7	17.2	11.8	19.9	61.9
Treatment module	7.9	7.3	7.3	7.5	7.2
Injuries and adverse effects module	1.7	1.3	6.9	3.4	0.4
Test results module	0.9	0.8	0.6	0.6	1.1
Administrative module	2.7	1.2	3.9	3.9	0.3*
Other	2.9	2.4	1.6	1.6	1.7
Number of visits (in thousands)	59,374	84,798	152,265	229,445	109,035

Sources: Beulah K. Cypress, *Patterns of Ambulatory Care in Internal Medicine: The National Ambulatory Medical Care Survey, United States, January 1980–December 1981.* (Hyattsville, MD: National Center for Health Statistics, 1984a), 28; Beulah K. Cypress, *Patterns of Ambulatory Care in General and Family Practice: The National Ambulatory Medical Care Survey, United States, January 1980–December 1981.* (Hyattsville, MD: National Center for Health Statistics, 1983), 25; Beulah K. Cypress, *Patterns of Ambulatory Care in Obstetrics and Gynecology: The National Ambulatory Medical Care Survey, United States, January 1980–December 1981.* (Hyattsville, MD: National Center for Health Statistics, 1984b), 29.

* This figure does not meet standards of reliability.

verage may be gained for blood pressure (both sexes) but not for endometrial cancer (female). (Tests for early lung cancer, mostly male, have been tried but are not in general use.)

Statistics show both increases and gaps in the use of screening tests for breast and cervical cancer. The American Cancer Society survey for 1987 showed that 81 percent of women had ever had a breast examination, and 87 percent had ever had a Pap smear, and 62 percent of women age 50+ had ever had a mammogram. The figure for the first two of these was not much higher than in 1980; mammography, however, had jumped from 43 percent in 1980 (Gluck, Wagner, and Duffy, 1989). These proportions were all higher than the proportions for both sexes (in relevant ages) who had ever had proctosigmoidoscopy (43 percent for men and 42 percent for women) or rectal examinations (53 percent for men and 58 percent for women). It should be kept in mind that the proportions who receive these tests within the last 1–3 years are considerably lower than the proportions who "ever hàd" them. Because government programs—Medicaid, community health centers, and family-planning centers—are credited with the wider diffusion of these preventive services, the adequacy of screening is dependent on the political ideology and priorities underlying future federal budgets. Congress in 1989 dropped a new mammography benefit under Medicare before it was implemented, but a few weeks later voted to add Pap test screening to Medicare.

Hospital Use and Physician Work Loads

Based on 1984 figures, women use hospitals slightly more than men (National Center for Health Statistics, 1985). They have more discharges, somewhat offset by shorter stays. Their discharge rate, including deliveries, is 19 percent higher. If deliveries are set aside, the female rate is still 15 percent greater. The male length of stay is 7.0 days, compared with 6.3 days for females, but, if deliveries are excluded, the average lengths are similar. (One condition, fracture of the neck of the femur—179,000 females and 64,000 males—had the longest stays of any diagnostic category, averaging 15.8 days.) Female discharges as a proportion of all discharges, and deliveries as a proportion of all discharges, are similar in all sizes of hospitals. However, statistics on hospitalizations may change because of rapid shifts in the hospital service market. Hospital use in the United States dropped substantially after the federal government introduced a prospective payment system to control costs. Discharges fell 17 percent from 1983 to 1987 (Kozak, 1989). In particular, surgery of short duration and with other characteristics favorable to use of outpatient settings moved out of the hospital, but cardiovascular operations increased.

Forty-eight percent of female inpatients and 41 percent of male inpatients had surgical procedures. Women received 21.6 million surgical procedures (including 1.5 million episiotomies); men, 14.4 million. The sex difference was less for nonsurgical diagnostic procedures, such as endoscopies and computerized axial tomography scans, and surgical procedures combined, with 58 percent of female patients and 53 percent of male patients having had one or more (Graves, 1986, table F).

For both sexes, heart disease and malignancies were the most common first-listed diagnoses. Surgical services, including cardiac catheterization and open-heart surgery, have been used increasingly for heart ailments in recent years, as mentioned. Most heart surgery patients were males in

1984, but this was less true for pacemaker insertion and removal. Hernia repairs and endoscopies of the urinary system were most often done in males, but herniorrhaphies are now shifting to outpatient locations. The relative use of hospitals by the two sexes is similar to the sex ratio in ambulatory care.

The 1983 report from the National Hospital Discharge Survey provides further detail on gender differences in diagnoses and procedures (Kozak and Moien, 1985). Based on first-listed diagnoses, stays for injuries and poisonings tend to be male more often than female. To a lesser degree, this is true for mental disorders, chiefly because of alcoholism admissions of men. The female excess is most marked for genitourinary and endocrine conditions.

Among all specific diagnoses with a total for either males or females of 100,000 or more in 1983, and not exclusive to one sex, the lowest female/male ratio was .11 for inguinal hernia. Other low ratios (under 1.0) were found for alcohol dependence, calculus (stone) of the kidney and ureter, and acute appendicitis. Myocardial infarction and other heart conditions, intervertebral disc disorders, and airway obstruction also had a majority of male cases. Conditions for which the female/male ratio was higher than 1.0 included kidney infections and acquired foot deformities; a group of disorders of the digestive system, the gallbladder, and fluid and electrolyte balance; urinary tract infection; and fracture of the neck of the femur. Cataracts, bone disorders, and affective psychoses also had more female cases. Exclusively female conditions, involving the breast, the genital tract, and disorders of menstruation, aggregated 1,662,000 discharges, or four times as many as the all-male conditions, chiefly hyperplasia and malignant neoplasm of the prostate.

Since surgical treatment is used in certain of these conditions, statistics on procedures follow the gender distribution of the diagnoses. Patients seeking surgeons to perform hernia repair, lung resection, diagnosis of lesions of the heart, and open-heart surgery tend to be male, as do those seeking medical specialists for care of obstructive pulmonary disease and kidney stones and internists and psychiatrists for care of alcohol dependence.

Individual physicians have work loads of mixed gender both in and out of the hospital. The sex ratio for a given doctor's work load depends on what conditions that doctor treats and the size of the market for the procedures he or she performs; the general surgeon or even the abdominal or chest surgeon does not rely on a single procedure for a livelihood, and subspecialty lines are not absolute. The same is true for medical specialists. Since even urologists who treat prostate conditions have female patients, obstetrics-gynecology stands out as the single field with a female clientele. In this field, all issues concerning professional and institutional practices affecting patient welfare become gender issues, whether or not the motivations for provider behavior are related to attitudes concerning gender.

However, in any of the other fields, decisions as to discharge timing, choice of therapies, and so forth may be affected by patient gender insofar as there are sex differences in support networks, learned assertiveness in dealing with doctors, and financial resources, and insofar as gender relations in the culture have shaped practitioner attitudes. But the free space for any gender influence on care decisions may depend on the cohesion of doctor agreement as to indications for particular actions and as to the superiority of particular treatment modes. If there is lack of consensus, it is less likely that the actions taken will be impervious to the interaction of personalities formed by the culture and to the social milieu itself.

TABLE 1.3
Percentage with Physician Contact Within Last Year,
by Age and Sex, 1986

	Interval Less than 1 Year (%)
MALE	
All ages	70.3
Under 18	78.8
18–44	62.2
45–64	70.3
65+	81.0
FEMALE	
All ages	81.4
Under 18	81.5
18–44	80.8
45–64	79.3
65+	86.3

Source: Deborah A. Dawson and Patricia F. Adams, *Current Estimates from the National Health Interview Survey: United States, 1986.* (Hyattsville, MD: National Center for Health Statistics, 1987), table 72.

TABLE 1.4
Number of Physician Contacts per Person per Year,
by Place of Contact, Sex, and Age, 1986

Sex and Age	Place of Contact				
	All Places	Telephone	Office	Hospital	Other
MALE					
All ages	4.5	0.5	2.5	0.8	0.7
Under 18	4.2	0.6	2.4	0.7	0.5
18–44	3.4	0.3	1.7	0.7	0.7
45–64	5.4	0.5	3.1	1.1	0.6
65+	8.4	0.7	4.6	1.2	1.8
FEMALE					
All ages	6.2	0.9	3.0	0.8	1.0
Under 18	4.2	0.8	2.4	0.4	0.6
18–44	5.7	0.7	3.3	0.7	0.9
45–64	7.6	1.0	4.1	1.3	1.2
65+	9.5	1.2	5.0	1.0	2.3

Source: Deborah A. Dawson and Patricia F. Adams, *Current Estimates from the National Health Interview Survey: United States, 1986.* (Hyattsville, MD: National Center for Health Statistics, 1987), table 71.

References

Bassett, Alan A. "Physical Examination of the Breast." In *Screening for Cancer,* edited by A. B. Miller. Orlando, FL: Academic Press, 1985

Bloom, Barbara, and Susan S. Jack. *Persons with and without a Regular Source of Medical Care: United States.* Series 10, No. 151. DHHS Pub. No. (PHS) 85-1579. Hyattsville, MD: National Center for Health Statistics, September 1985.

Cypress, Beulah K. *Characteristics of Visits to Female and Male Physicians: The National Ambulatory Medical Care Survey, United States, 1977.* Series 13, No. 49. DHHS Pub. No. (PHS) 80-1710. Hyattsville, MD: National Center for Health Statistics, June 1980a.

———. *Office Visits by Women: The National Ambulatory Medical Care Survey, United States, 1977.* Series 13, No. 45. DHEW Pub. No. (PHS) 80-1796. Hyattsville, MD: National Center for Health Statistics, March 1980b.

———. *Patterns of Ambulatory Care in General and Family Practice: The National Ambulatory Medical Care Survey, United States, January 1980–December 1981.* Series 13, No. 73. DHHS Pub. No. (PHS) 83-1734. Hyattsville, MD: National Center for Health Statistics, September 1983.

————. *Patterns of Ambulatory Care in Internal Medicine: The National Ambulatory Medical Care Survey, United States, January 1980–December 1981.* Series 13, No. 80. DHHS Pub. No. (PHS) 84-1741. Hyattsville, MD: National Center for Health Statistics, September 1984a.

————. *Patterns of Ambulatory Care in Obstetrics and Gynecology: The National Ambulatory Medical Care Survey, United States, January 1980–December 1981.* Series 13, No. 76. DHHS Pub. No. (PHS) 84-1737. Hyattsville, MD: National Center for Health Statistics, 1984b.

Dawson, Deborah A., and Patricia F. Adams. *Current Estimates from the National Health Interview Survey: United States, 1986.* Series 10, No. 164. DHHS Pub. No. (PHS) 87-1592. Hyattsville, MD: National Center for Health Statistics, October 1987.

Gluck, Michael E., Judith L. Wagner, and Brigitte M. Duffy. "The Use of Preventive Services by the Elderly." *Preventive Health Services under Medicare, Paper 2.* Washington, DC: Office of Technology Assessment, January 1989.

Graves, Edmund J. *Utilization of Short-Stay Hospitals, United States, 1984, Annual Summary.* Series 13, No. 84. DHHS Pub. No. (PHS) 86-1745. Hyattsville, MD: National Center for Health Statistics, March 1986.

Johnston, Lloyd D., Patrick M. O'Malley, and Gerald G. Bachman. *Drug Use among American High School Students, College Students, and Other Young Adults: National Trends through 1983.* DHHS Pub. No. (ADM) 86-1450. Washington, DC: National Institute on Drug Abuse, 1986.

Kozak, Lola Jean. *Hospital Inpatient Surgery: United States, 1983–87.* Advance Data No. 169. Hyattsville, MD: National Center for Health Statistics, May 23, 1989.

Kozak, Lola Jean, and Mary Moien. *Detailed Diagnoses and Surgical Procedures for Patients Discharged from Short-Stay Hospitals, United States, 1983.* Series 13, No. 82. DHHS Pub. No. (PHS) 85-1743. Hyattsville, MD: National Center for Health Statistics, 1985.

Miller, Anthony B. "Screening for Cancer of the Cervix." In A. B. Miller, ed., *Screening for Cancer.* Orlando, FL: Academic Press, 1985.

Muller, Charlotte. "Health and Health Care of Employed Women and Homemakers: Family Factors." *Women & Health,* vol. 11, no. 1 (Spring 1986a): 7–26.

————. "Health and Health Care of Employed Adults: Occupation and Gender." *Women & Health,* vol. 11, no. 1 (Spring 1986b): 27–46.

————. "A Review of Twenty Years of Utilization Research." *Health Services Research,* June 1986c.

National Center for Health Services Research. *Contacts with Physicians in Ambulatory Settings: Rates of Use, Expenditures, and Sources of Payment.* National Health Care Expenditures Study. Data Preview 16, DHHS Pub. No. (PHS) 83-3361. Rockville, MD, 1983.

————. *Health, United States, 1984.* DHHS Pub. No. (PHS) 85-1232. Hyattsville, MD, December 1984.

National Center for Health Statistics. *1984 Summary: National Hospital Discharge Survey.* Advance Data No. 112. Hyattsville, MD, September 1985.

————. Division of Health Interview Statistics. *Current Estimates from the National Health Interview Survey: United States, 1983.* Series 10, No. 154. DHHS Pub. No. (PHS) 86-1582. Hyattsville, MD, June 1986a.

————. *Health, United States, 1986 and Prevention Profile.* DHHS Pub. No. (PHS) 87-1232. Hyattsville, MD, 1986b.

Roback, Gene, Lillian Randolph, Diane Mead, and Thomas Pasko. *Physician Characteristics and Distribution in the U.S.* 1984 ed. Chicago: American Medical Association, 1984.

U.S. Department of Health and Human Services, Public Health Service. *Health Status of Minorities and Low Income Groups.* DHHS Pub. No. (HRSA) HRS-P-DV 85-1. Washington, DC: Government Printing Office, 1985.

Waldron, Ingrid. "Sex Differences in Illness Incidence, Prognosis and Mortality: Issues and Evidence." *Soc. Sci. Med.,* vol. 17, no. 16 (1983): 1107–1123.

CHAPTER TWO

Treatment Issues

HEALTH EXPERIENCES OF WOMEN and men have both similarities and differences, according to Verbrugge (1986). In her analysis, based on Detroit data, the two sexes have the same daily symptoms of ill health. Similar conditions cause acute and chronic disability and activity limitation in both sexes, appear in the health care they receive, and become causes of death. With aging, the types of conditions responsible for ill health and use of services become even more alike, as injuries (male) and reproductive disorders (female) give way to chronic illness (both sexes). Sex differences are found, however, in the rates of these health measures. Women have higher rates of daily symptoms, most acute conditions, and physician visits; men have higher rates of the leading fatal chronic conditions, limitations, and hospital use and mortality for the leading causes of death. Verbrugge describes women as having more frequent but less serious sickness.

Her analysis may be interpreted as implying that the quantity of physician and hospital care utilized by the two sexes is a natural reflection of their health care needs. However, unmet needs for diagnostic, treatment, and preventive services can exist even though the quantity of services used is greater for the most frequent conditions (or for the sex with more conditions) and even if mortality for a condition is lower for women. For example, use of mammography, the one imaging technique applicable to a major cancer site that has an impact on prognosis (Hall, 1986), is far less widespread than recommended by cancer experts. In addition, figures on numbers of persons seeing doctors or on quantities of service used do not necessarily tell whether appropriate treatments were provided.

Comparison of the experiences of men and women in the health care system has been stimulated by concern that, because of the historical position of women in society, they may be subject to differential and discriminatory treatment. The women's movement has described a number of scenarios of unsatisfactory and unequal treatment, many of which have been accepted as fair criticism by members of the medical profession and, indeed, have contributed to changes in the conduct of medical practice. In these scenarios either under- or overtreatment of women's illnesses occurs, or an inferior or undesirable form of treatment is substituted for another, better, one when a patient is female rather than male. An example is a tendency to misinterpret women's presenting problems as psychological and treat them with tranquilizers. Another flaw in women's treatment, according to critics of traditional practices, is infusion of gender biases in the doctor–patient relationship, degrading in itself and a block to appropriate clinical decisions.

Interestingly, suspicion, consciousness, and allegation of unequal treatment have coexisted with generally favorable mortality rates for women, compared with men, the reasons for which are not fully understood. Both biological and social factors have been considered. "[G]enetic differences have been held at least partially responsible for lower infant mortality rates among females and for women's greater longevity; and possibly for the male's greater susceptibility to many cancers of nongenital origin" (Nathanson and Lorenz, 1982, p. 50). However, differences among countries in the size of the sex differential in adult mortality are difficult to account for genetically, according to these authors. While a relation between hormonal factors and illness has been postulated, there is conflicting evidence as to a possible protective effect of estrogens against cardiovascular disease and as to either positive or negative effects of female hormones on other major causes of death among women.

Recognition that a biological advantage of women is far from a full explanation of sex differences in health indices, and that health levels and use of care vary within each sex, directs one's attention to the influences of individual history (including past exposure to harmful environments), personal habits, and medical care on mortality. Thus, some part of the sex gap in death rates is attributed to differences in voluntary (albeit socially conditioned) behavior involving risk taking (e.g., smoking by men).[1] Hence, the mortality gap can be narrowed by a change in behavior of either sex. The part that is due to involuntary exposure risk through

---

[1]Half of the sex differential in past mortality rates is attributed to men's higher smoking rates (Waldron, 1986).

work[2] may also be affected by more continuous labor force participation and changing occupational distribution of women.

Differential treatment remains a social concern, despite women's longevity advantage. This is due in part to an interest in preventing avoidable iatrogenic or producer-generated mortality for either sex (e.g., from inadequate investigation of symptoms and from harmful drugs and devices), plus a belief that women are more at risk of this than men. But much of the concern is based on criteria other than mortality; specifically, preservation of quality of life and reduction of morbidity. In addition, there is interest in maintaining older women's functional levels against the assault of chronic disease. Men's higher mortality, plus the age difference of bride and bridegroom, leads to the survival of older women as widows. If they acquire disabilities, they may lack familial sources of help with daily needs, and they often have restricted means of paying for purchased help (see chapter 5.)

In this chapter I shall discuss themes that have a direct or indirect connection with gender differences in treatment. They include aspects of the doctor–patient relationship, the consideration given to quality of life, and methods of measuring indirect costs. Following these, the treatment of men and women patients with the same condition, differences between decisions of male and female practitioners, and the appropriateness of care for certain conditions restricted to one sex will be discussed.

The documentation of the actual prevalence of any form of inappropriate treatment by sex has rarely been provided in a research mode. Rather, the case has rested on norms presented and attitudes revealed in medical textbooks, experiences reported by women as patients, and the gleam of recognition shown by many listeners or readers.

It has been difficult to present direct and exact gender comparisons because many of the abuses complained of were in situations limited to women, such as gynecological surgery. Also, for a study to be objective, patients ought to be comparable as to severity of illness and other factors. (This has been a problem for many evaluations of treatments not involving gender issues.) Changes in medical practices, such as the preferred type of surgery for breast cancer, have often followed scientific demonstrations, suggesting that health system practices respond to reason alone. Yet, when medical authors have recommended that previously

---

[2]Neoclassical economics would regard assumption of risk as voluntary in a free market, but many workers are not aware of health risks, and many have limited choice in real-life markets.

accepted approaches be reconsidered, they have sometimes acknowledged that changes in women's position in society have been influential in focusing interest on, and improving analysis of, women's problems. This has been mentioned in recent literature rejecting the previous skepticism that trivialized premenstrual syndrome (PMS) as an imagined or psychosomatic problem (see page 42).

The adaptations made by the health care system that have addressed shortcomings experienced by women have had varied purposes. They have aimed to retain and develop markets against competition, including that of facilities sponsored by women's groups; to comply with laws; to validate an ethical professional or institutional identity; and to assure community support. Hospitals, for example, have begun to design and operate women's health centers with a range of inpatient and outpatient services targeted to both younger and older groups and with hours convenient to employed women.

Yet, despite adaptive changes, gender issues continue to arise with changing health needs, treatment opportunities, and a lag of evaluation behind innovation. For example, women as patients with eating disorders may be exploited by some providers claiming that a given treatment method is efficacious. Such exploitation can continue because a scientific consensus on treatment has not been achieved, while awareness of the problem has grown.

Furthermore, geographical and class diffusion of new behavior patterns in a personal service industry is a complex process. It is made more so by commitment of both capital and professional learning time to existing modes of treatment and by multiple payer sources with different reimbursement rules. Hence, at any given time, some of the population tends not to share equally in the benefits of health system changes. Additionally, health care is delivered in the context of social controversy over employment equity, fertility management, family roles, and so forth. It is questionable whether the system, no matter how technological and functional its processes, can ever be perfectly immune to social biases. Economic weakness of certain groups of women interferes with choice and makes their treatment especially vulnerable to cost control or cost shifting.

Patient rights issues raised by women have improved the system's responsiveness to all consumers, exemplified by fuller implementation of informed consent. Nevertheless, the system has been shown to contain many subjective influences on decision making that belie its supposed objectivity and have dysfunctional consequences for users of both sexes. Some of them may also result in gender biases.

COMMUNICATION

Physicians' deficiencies in ability to communicate with patients are now acknowledged by medical leaders and are regarded as a serious problem in attaining good medical care. Physicians may fail to use open-ended questions that let the patient contribute types of information that they may not have thought of in going through the standard protocol used in reaching clinical decisions. With conscientious, but rigid, adherence to learned methods of gathering a data base, physicians may show little interest in what a patient has just said, thereby cutting off the flow of information, as well as impairing the patient's sense of control. They tend to underestimate how much information the patient wants and overestimate the time they have spent in giving explanations (Coleman, 1988).

These behavioral tendencies may be worse when male practitioners see female patients. If women are undervalued as informants, appropriate treatment decisions are hindered. Physicians who believe that women are more likely than men to complain of physical pain with a given problem may not accept women's reported pain, or their immediate reaction to pain in words or gestures, as an important clue to the diagnosis, and severity may be underrated.

In addition to physical pain, painful feelings and psychologically harmful events in the patient's history are also part of the doctor's data base. Specific past events or current complaints that are now increasingly regarded as credible were otherwise interpreted in previous times, in line with Freudian theory about sexual fantasies and social attitudes about women's reliability as reporters. Reports of childhood sexual abuse, spouse battering (National Institute of Mental Health, 1983), date rape, and so forth lead to quite different provider responsibilities for treatment if the information supplied by patients is not automatically discounted. Obstetrician-gynecologists are now being informed that battering is the major cause of injury to women, is never excusable, and may continue during pregnancy (Chez, 1988). Criminal charges, civil suits, and community shelters are among the remedial actions discussed.

Recently, there has been more conceptualization of psychologically abusive dating relationships in adolescence that may be accompanied by violence and that are damaging to maturation. A relationship is abusive if the girl is afraid to make the boy angry, needs his permission to engage in activity, fears he might hurt her, and so on (Samson, 1989). The lack of understanding and of support services until now is said to be embedded in society's image of women as caring and forgiving, men as powerful and in charge.

The behavior of patients, not only the attitudes of physicians, affects what happens during receipt of care. A patient who has been conditioned by her upbringing not to interrupt or question (once considered standard etiquette for females) may not have much influence on the physician's decision making. A patient may have a more expressive style than the physician expects, which influences how the information she provides is received. (The disparity of style is intensified when patients are members of ethnic minorities and doctors are not.) Various studies of the doctor–patient encounter as a psychosocial phenomenon suggest a difference based on the gender pairing involved. Although the connection with the actual clinical decision is not usually pursued by the researcher and would require more complex research designs, achieving successful two-way communication is conducive to more appropriate choices of treatment.

The analysis of encounters is illustrated by two studies in which the sex of the participants was considered. The first, a study of the interaction of male physicians with men and women patients, showed that, even if questions are asked, the patient may not receive useful answers. The women asked more questions initiating explanations and more questions after an explanation, but they were less likely to receive responses that were at as high a technical level as their questions. The physicians may have been influenced by stereotypical perceptions, in that they were more likely to consider the illness as psychologically caused if the patient was female. The authors suggest that the doctors, thinking in this fashion, interpreted requests for information as a sign of dependence rather than as an interest in finding out how to get well (Wallen et al., 1979). It is also possible, however, that the physicians were affected by a stereotype about women patients' level of understanding, despite the quality of their questions.

In the second study, interruptions in conversation between physicians and patients were interpreted as indicators of the exercise of dominance (West, 1984). They are also direct control devices that a doctor may use to cut off discussion on the patient's condition and that determine the focus of the decision process. Studying male and female doctors at a family practice center in the South, West found that men physicians were twice as likely to interrupt patients as the reverse. But when the doctor was female, the patients interrupted twice as frequently as the physician. West suggests that the incomplete acceptance of the doctor's authority is due to gender having primacy over professional status in the patient's perspective.

Zambrana, Mogul, and Scrimshaw (1987) explored gender differences and level-of-training differences in attitudes of obstetricians toward their patients during childbirth. The residents were more concerned than the senior physicians (attendings) with whether patients were compliant. Among the residents, women doctors did not use more psychosocial or humanitarian descriptors of patients, and, in fact, attached more importance than the men doctors to having quiet, controllable patients. The author offers two possible reasons for these results: either the women doctors were "turning away from other women" (resisting their identification with parturient patients) "in order to survive" in the professional and institutional system, or women patients felt more free to express their discomforts and complaints in the presence of women physicians. Thus, the increase in the number of women obstetricians may not solve the traditional problems of conflicting expectations in the doctor–patient relationship nor relieve the strains caused by professional dominance.

Whether the growth in the number of women physicians in various specialties will affect the conduct of encounters may depend not only on whether they adopt an egalitarian style and find it functional, but also on whether competition leads male physicians to do the same. The many trends in the organization and financing of medical practice that coexist with the increase in women physicians make prediction concerning communication style and medical decisions difficult. For example, clinical decision making may be less an autonomous act of the physician, regardless of gender, and more a performance within bureaucratic rules in structures such as large health maintenance organizations (HMOs). If a relative value scale giving more weight to cognitive skills is adopted for paying physicians (it will soon begin for Medicare under new legislation), it will alter incentives of all physicians, including fee-for-service practitioners, to do different types of procedures.

When the patient goes for help, does sex play a role in the vigor with which symptoms are followed up by the physicians? Armitage, Schneiderman, and Bass (1979) studied the response of male physicians to five common complaints in male and female adults: back pain, headache, dizziness, chest pain, and fatigue. The sample comprised fifty-two married couples who were served by nine male physicians in a group practice in the San Diego area. Age, education, and socioeconomic level of subjects were fairly homogeneous. All physicians did significantly more extensive workups for the men. The authors comment that, although the women had been seen more often than the men and the physicians might have had a greater stock of information to go on, the data could also support the proposition that male physicians take illness more seriously when the patient is male. If men as a group have a greater risk of heart disease, does this rationalize a less thorough investigation of a woman presenting with chest pain? Decision theory applied to medicine supports more extensive study of patients in a higher-risk group as rational behavior. A complication in evaluating a sex difference in cardiovascular testing, it has been argued, is the possibility that the testing is overutilized today, so that the group with a lower rate of use is actually better off, avoiding side effects, unnecessary surgery based on false-positive test results, and expense. In other words, it is argued, if chest pain in women were in fact less fully studied, women as a class might benefit by avoiding the risks of excessive use of technology. But this is not a reliable gain for an individual, and the situation could not be considered acceptable for those whose problems were missed and who could have been helped.

In any case, the Armitage et al. study findings were challenged by a later study. Greer et al. (1986) studied male and female physicians in an HMO (ten of each sex) to examine further the hypothesis that women patients are taken less seriously than men when the physician is a male. The sample patients were one hundred married couples, five from each of the twenty physicians. The complaints were chosen to be common, "not directly related to sexual organs or functions," and entitled to a workup because of their potential seriousness. In fact, they were the same as those in the Armitage et al. study. Indices were created to measure the extent of the history, physical examination, and laboratory procedures initiated by the doctor and to compare the items with a standardized criteria list for each condition.

There were no significant differences between male and female patients in either the content or the extent of care provided. Nor was there any difference in the workups by male and female physicians. Finally, there was no interaction effect that would suggest that male and female doctors worked up their male and female patients differently.

Since the results differed from the findings of the previous study by Armitage et al. showing a difference by sex of patient, the authors discuss possible reasons why their findings did not agree. Both studies had white, middle-class, suburban patients and board-certified family doctors practicing in well-regarded groups, but the Greer study doctors were younger and the patients older. Because of this, the authors suggest that more of the women patients may have passed a critical age at which doctors sense the need for an enhanced workup and/or that sexism may have diminished in younger cohorts of doctors.

Since both men and women had more extensive workups in the study by Greer et al. than in the earlier study, a difference in the method of reimbursement (prepayment versus fee-for-service) was rejected by them as a possible explanation of their findings of no sex differences. It is conceivable that physicians joining HMOs differ in attitudes, whether related to this choice alone or also to their ages, from their fee-for-service colleagues. But further research is necessary to elucidate these possible influences.

QUALITY OF LIFE

Practitioners who do not accept patients' quality of life as a treatment goal or who place a lower valuation on certain states of life than their patients do affect adversely the care their patients receive.

Undervaluation of the quality of life of a patient may predispose to more minimal treatment, as well as to excessively radical surgery or surgery on shaky indications. Some surgeons may hesitate to perform orthopedic surgery in patients with pathological fractures and a limited prognosis due to bone cancer. Gersh et al. (1985) note physicians' reluctance to do bypass surgery on patients over 65, although there was marked benefit from surgery in the highest-risk quartile of the patients in the study reported on. The authors comment that "subtle conditions" enter into the clinical judgment as to who is to receive a specific therapy and that the consideration of physiological age as part of the clinical evaluation has subjective aspects. Willingness to do any type of surgery on patients over 85, where the time horizon is limited, involves accepting a quality-of-life goal. This affects women because they predominate in the oldest age group.

Kassirer (1983) notes that physicians' choices are greatly influenced by the desire to avoid life-threatening consequences of an action, even if the risk is very low, and that this may conflict with maximizing the patient's quality of life. He proposes reasons for this tendency of physicians. They may not trust patients to make a good decision and may even interpret resistance to their professional opinion as evidence of the patient's irrationality. They may resist allocating their limited time to full explanations; they may have insufficient command of the data the patient is likely to request; or they may lack an aptitude for communicating medical facts to the patient. Finally, they may wish to protect patients from anxiety and, indeed, place a therapeutic value on a paternalistic relationship.

Whenever consensus among physicians as to preferred treatments is lacking, personal outlooks of practitioners may have more influence on decision making. For example, the role of radiotherapy in treatment of breast cancer patients after mastectomy remains controversial. It is claimed that many of the published studies have flawed designs; possibly for this reason, most studies showed no improvement in outcome through radiotherapy (Prosnitz et al., 1983). There is consensus that chemotherapy after breast surgery is beneficial for premenopausal women whose cancer has spread to the lymph nodes, but there have been problems in selecting the right combinations and doses to derive practical benefit from this therapy (General Accounting Office, 1988, 1989). Since such controversy appears to be a permanent feature of modern medicine, the leeway for personal outlooks will remain.

Undervaluation of the importance of body integrity as part of the quality of life was one of the most challenging charges of feminist critics against the medical profession. The performance of unnecessary surgery (e.g., hysterectomies) or overly extensive surgery (e.g., the radical mastectomy introduced by Halsted) was attributed to physicians' indifference to the body integrity of women or even to a predisposition to impairing it as a means of behavior control. The sorry history of the mutilative gynecological surgery performed in the nineteenth century and surviving mutilation rituals in other cultures were cited to support these contentions.

In the case of mastectomy, medical opinion changed in the 1970s, after demonstration that more limited surgery did not reduce survival. The clinical trials displacing radical mastectomy from its preferred place among clinicians reversed seventy-five years of consensus (Weitzman et al., 1987). The Halsted method was the standard treatment for most of the twentieth century, although it produced a long scar and caused restricted shoulder motion and other uncomfortable effects. It was replaced with less-disfiguring and less-disabling procedures for early-stage breast cancer (Willis, 1986). The modified radical mastectomy and, later, the simple mastectomy, procedures of less extensive scope, became common and were shown to generate ten-year survival rates as good as those for the Halsted operation. Additionally, segmental mastectomy or lumpectomy plus radiation were shown to have better five-year disease-free survival than total (simple) mastectomy (Fisher et al., 1985).

These developments gave women in the 1980s much more choice than they had in 1970. The diffusion of the change was, however, irregular, and the likelihood of a woman's having access to the most up-to-date treatment remained dependent on her geographical location and her command of resources. New York State passed a law in 1985 to protect women with breast cancer from undergoing the most invasive procedures simply because a surgeon failed to inform them of all their options, an action generally understood to be an essential part of informed consent. The New York law (L. 1985, ch. 203), as well as the laws of several other states, requires that a breast cancer patient be informed of all alternative treatments. When biopsy is followed by surgery or other treatments, a distinct occasion can be provided for consent to the second step, which may include choosing a different setting, a different and more specialized surgeon, and an individualized set and sequence of therapies.[3] If, as Nancy Reagan did, a woman chooses a more radical type of surgery, it is presumably a voluntary and informed choice.

Such laws are a recognition that quality of life could be endangered for women with a serious disease unless they are empowered as consumers. Among male conditions, prostate surgery, although not affecting physical appearance, is similar in that data on risks and outcomes suggest that men might make different choices if they had more information (see page 41). In addition, circumcision of male infants, a ritual in the Jewish faith and widely accepted as a hygienic practice, is currently being debated. Although opponents claim that pain in infants has been underestimated, medical experts agree that pain is short-lived and complications are rare, but are divided as to the extent of health benefit in the long run (Schoen, 1990; Poland, 1990).

GENDER AND MEASUREMENT OF INDIRECT COSTS OF ILLNESS

Measurement of the socioeconomic costs of illness in a way that emphasizes men's activities may promote application of more resources to treatment for conditions principally affecting men or, within a given condition, for men, rather than women, patients. Such emphasis also may orient the approaches and services provided in a program open to all to the needs of men. Measurements that draw heavily on valuation of lost work time of higher-salaried employees and that give limited weight to those with lower earnings or less lifetime labor force participation contain a tendency to sex bias.

The identification of morbidity with male morbidity helps perpetuate a bias in provider attitudes and in planning. For example, the title of a journal article refers to the effects of antihypertensive therapy on the quality of life, although only the quality of life of male patients is considered (Croog et al., 1986). Similarly, a government-financed report entitled "Morbidity Costs: National Estimates and Economic Determinants" is exclusively concerned with males of working age (Salkever, 1985).

Russell (1986) notes that the evidence for the value of exercise to health is derived from the study of middle-aged men. Research studies often use only male subjects for practical reasons: if the incidence of the disease is higher in males, it is easier to accumulate large enough samples to test treatments for efficacy and derive publishable results (Smith et al.,

---

[3]It has been suggested that the importance of two steps will be less if lumpectomy becomes widely used.

1982). Even if women are included in a study sample, they are often omitted from the analysis of economic effects of treatment (i.e., return to work).

An extensive report on 1980 costs of alcohol and drug abuse and mental illness in those under 65, supported by the Alcohol, Drug Abuse, and Mental Health Administration, was completed in 1984. Because of the measures used, it indicates a lower lost value per capita for women problem drinkers than for men, based on both lower wages for employed women and low valuation for homemakers. Thus, men make up 68.4 percent of problem drinkers under 65, but their lost productivity is valued at 76.1 percent of the total loss (Harwood et al., 1984, table III-18). For mental illness, men make up 42 percent of those with complete work disability, but their lost employment is valued at 53.6 percent of the total employment value lost (table III-26). For partial disability due to mental illness, males are 48.1 percent of the disabled, but 58.1 percent of the lost value is due to them (table III-25).

Recently a new sensitivity to measurement biases was shown in a NCHSR report on costs of illness, in which the implications of using current earnings to show the impact of disease are discussed. Specifically, when the human-capital approach is used, "market-determined earnings reflect both market and social imperfections" and "the lost output of working-age white men tends to be higher than that of women, minorities, and older or younger people in the work force" (Parsons et al., 1986 p. 5).

A related problem is the value placed on homemaker services. When, as was done in early studies of economic costs of illness, domestic workers' wages were used, the measured social losses due to women's illnesses were small relative to men's. An alternative method, evaluation of lost output of homemakers based on the market price of services purchased (or purchasable) to replace those that the women had been providing, results in values that are lower than annual earnings of women working full-time year-round and lower than men's earnings. In fact, output values for women at home were only 37.6 percent of men's earnings at ages 45–49, when men's earnings are at their peak (Rice, 1983).

A study of the indirect costs of schizophrenia, done in the early 1980s, departed from assuming domestic roles for women by using an opportunity-cost concept to measure lost production of ill homemakers, based on the assumption that women who are well and choose to be homemakers are giving up the average wage earned by their age-sex-ethnic group (Muller and Caton, 1983).

With the increasing labor force participation of women, valuations based on loss of paid employment will be less likely to result in a focus on male morbidity, but the sex wage gap would have to be closed to equalize fully the evaluations of indirect costs of equal amounts of male and female morbidity. In any case, survival of women into old age, when they are not economically active, will continue to depress the statistical impact of illness on women measured in economic terms. This situation is complex because investment in their health at appropriate points in the life cycle could reduce disability at later ages and increase older women's capacity for paid work. This expectation is supported by findings (cited in chapter 5) that activity limitations due to chronic disease are a cause of retirement of older women.

Undertreatment as a gender problem, influenced by perceptions of the indirect costs of illness, may infiltrate into treatment decisions in individual cases and into professionwide treatment norms. In addition, social-program priorities for conditions confined to women may be low, whereas, based on indirect costs, more ambitious treatment goals are set up in conditions for which men are frequently treated.

Yet women's increased labor force activity should stimulate attention to economic and other losses incurred by conditions affecting women. Washington, Arno, and Brooks (1987) analyze the direct and indirect costs of pelvic inflammatory disease (PID), a condition affecting over one million women annually, and of ectopic pregnancy and infertility, which are often associated with PID. Emotional stress caused by PID is also noted. Although not directly measured, it is inferred from incidence data and appreciation of the serious physical health effects of PID. The cost for women age 15–44 is estimated to reach $3.5 billion per year in 1990. The analysis is used to advocate prevention and control programs including alerting physicians to "maintain a high index of suspicion" for the varied clinical presentations of PID. This type of article reflects a newer consciousness.

DISEASES OF BOTH SEXES

Underutilization of available and proven therapies for serious disease is a problem for both sexes. The General Accounting Office has presented to Congress information indicating underuse of chemotherapy for six types of cancer and, for rectal cancer, underuse of adjuvant radiotherapy, in patients for whom these treatments were deemed clearly appropriate. Controlled trials, done, in many cases, ten or more years ago, had shown that these treatments extend patient survival. Yet substantial percentages of patients did not receive state-of-the-art treatment. The worst rate was for colon cancer: 94 percent of the patients meeting the criteria for being suitable candidates for these treatments did not receive them (General

Accounting Office, 1988). The gender ratio of the incidence of these conditions varies, but clearly both sexes were affected.

Doubilet and Abrams (1984) believe that a superior treatment for peripheral vascular disease (not sex-specific) is underutilized. They suggest that triage to vascular surgeons limits patients to procedures with which these practitioners are more familiar. The physician is biased against change if the old method appears to work and is not trained to do (or accept) a careful quantitative analysis of benefits, risks, and costs of alternatives. Physicians also have a financial incentive to practice self-referral rather than pass the patient on to a radiologist for nonsurgical care.

Gallbladder disease is common to both sexes but is more prevalent in women. The criteria for managing it are agreed on; however, there is a problem in diagnosis in the following case. A patient has symptoms that are due to depression but that are confused with those of gallbladder disease. A physician recommends surgery, and, when the operation is done, gallstones are found, apparently confirming the diagnosis. In such a case, inappropriate treatment would have been given on the basis of a misdiagnosis. (Neither the surgery nor the surgical scar adds to quality of life.) This tends to be a woman's problem for epidemiologic reasons, since the prevalence of depression is higher in women (Schechter, 1988).

Heart disease is a condition common to both sexes but more frequent in men. Differential access to appropriate treatment for heart disease would have serious consequences. A report from the Framingham research project on cardiovascular disease indicates a rather high proportion of myocardial infarctions (MIs) that either were silent (asymptomatic) or caused atypical symptoms and were picked up only on routine biennial ECGs (Kannel and Abbott, 1984). The rate was higher in women and older men. These unrecognized MIs were as likely as recognized ones to cause death, heart failure, or stroke, but the women who had recognized MIs had higher cardiovascular mortality, evidently because of more than one episode per person. Different interpretations of ECG changes for women and men are believed to be necessary when patients have symptoms, because the changes in persons with unrecognized MIs were "more non-specific" in women. Neither patient nor doctor had considered an MI as the explanation for the symptoms experienced.

In a study of patients with suspected or proven ischemic heart disease, the question of possible sex bias in decisions to refer for catheterization and coronary artery bypass surgery was explored. The study was conducted at Bronx hospital sites by Albert Einstein College of Medicine researchers (Tobin et al., 1987).

After nuclear medicine exercise studies were done, 64 percent of the men with abnormal results were referred for catheterization but only 31

percent of the women; only 4 percent of the women with abnormal ra-
dionuclide scans were referred, versus 40 percent of the men. After a
multiple logistic regression analysis controlling for age and other factors,
the probability of referral was found to be six and a half times more for
men than for women. This is a difference far in excess of what could be
expected from sex differences in prevalence of coronary artery disease.
The authors state that the results cannot be explained by gender-related
differences in test efficacy, nor by history or symptoms. They acknowledge that the higher operative mortality rate for women, based on the
documented smaller size of the heart and blood vessel diameter, would
make surgeons feel they were reasonable in avoiding surgery. However,
the findings of a higher risk of death for women during surgery shown in
the previous studies were, in the authors' view, influenced by delaying
surgery in women until they were older and sicker than the men included in these studies. Long-range survival is not worse for women, if adjustment is made for mortality during surgery. The authors conclude:
"We raise a question that has hitherto been neglected: Should there be a
difference?" (p. 24)

Data on all patients with coronary artery bypass surgery at Mt. Sinai
Medical Center in New York City in 1984 show that the severity of
disease, as measured by the number of grafts performed per case, was no
different for men and women, but the women (who numbered under
one-fourth of the cases) were four and a half years older (64.1 versus
59.6 years). One cannot conclude that the women were less likely to be
promptly diagnosed and, therefore, that intervention did not occur until
their disease had progressed (Mt. Sinai, 1987). Their greater age at the
time of surgery could have been due to occurrence of heart disease as a
complication of diabetes. This suggests that it would be worthwhile to
analyze the reasons for the age difference between men and women. Data
on outcomes for cases of equal severity would also be relevant.

The decline in death rates from coronary artery disease since 1970, at
a time when availability of cardiac care resources increased and more
active treatments were used, suggests the importance of medical care for
survival, although this is still being debated (Sagan, 1987). However, the
rate of decline in heart disease deaths for women, and for black men,
slowed after 1975 (Kovar et al., 1988).

Women have a higher cumulative mortality within eighteen months
after a myocardial infarction than men, especially black women (36 percent versus 21 percent) (Toffler et al., 1987). Many of these deaths occur
in the hospital. The National Hospital Discharge Survey shows that,
since 1970, women admitted with a myocardial infarction have had a

higher hospital fatality rate than men within each ten-year age group between 45 and 74, especially in the groups under 65.

How effective is bypass surgery in treating heart disease? In a meta-analysis reviewing ninety-one studies of coronary artery bypass graft (CABG) surgery, it was found that those in which subjects were not randomly assigned to surgical or medical treatment groups greatly overestimated the benefits from CABG. Randomized clinical trials showed only a 6 percent reduction in mortality, compared to a medical regimen. This probably was an underestimate, because patients with the worst prognosis tended to shift over to surgery during the study, thus biasing the reported benefits of surgery downward (a more reasonable estimate would be a 10 percent drop in mortality). CABG was shown by randomized clinical trials to give considerable relief from angina, thereby increasing quality of life (National Center for Health Services Research and Health Care Technology Assessment, 1989).

Whether raising the rate of CABG surgery for women candidates is in their best interest depends on whether the procedure is the treatment of choice. A recent study shows that a second-opinion program for CABG affords "a significant and safe option," namely, a shift to medical therapy in selected cases. However, being based on a small sample of self-selected patients, the study cannot be extrapolated to the general population (Graboys et al., 1987). Thus, we don't really know the "right" rate of bypass surgery for either sex, and the right rate will change as alternative treatments (e.g., percutaneous transluminal coronary angioplasty) establish their place (Gruentzig et al., 1987). But, at any given time, the separation of valid clinical considerations from differential treatment by reason of gender presents a research and policy issue, because sex differences in prevalence may cause treatments to be tailored to the majority.

It appears from the information on heart disease treatment that cognitive factors may play a major role in producing different clinical decisions for the two sexes even when attitudinal distinctions related to gender are subdued. Conditions that occur in both sexes but have a low incidence in women may be handled differently in women because their infrequency alters the outlook and ability of the physician. The physician may fail to conceive that the patient's symptoms could have a particular explanation. The disease may present itself somewhat differently in women, thereby increasing the need to pursue the investigation with appropriate questions and tests. But, even if tests are done, the results can still be interpreted in different ways. The physician who lacks experience with the condition in women is less familiar with the clinical course and outcomes. If surgery is an option, the physician may be reluctant to use it, for risks are evaluated on the basis of a smaller sample and, hence, the standard error of the estimates, that is to say, the uncertainty faced by the physician, is increased.

The same problem could arise for men patients. If health risks for women and men change because of life-style changes, such as women's increased participation in high-tension work situations, clinicians will gradually become aware of changing incidence patterns of certain conditions. Variations in their perceptivity and readiness to respond may be expected.

Hysterectomy

The propriety of clinical decisions related to hysterectomy has been much questioned. Although less common now than in the mid-1970s, it is still the most frequently performed major surgery in the United States, and its incidence in younger women is increasing. The rate in the United States is double that in England and Wales, although women's health has not been shown to be worse in those countries. Interarea variation is great and is unexplained by population or disease patterns. Researchers from the Centers for Disease Control found that one in every seven of the 3.5 million hysterectomies performed in the 1970s was questionable, even by conservative criteria; yet many of the patients incurred at least one complication requiring further care (Levin, 1986). Whether the performance rate persists because patients do not receive adequate explanations of benefits and risks, because of the permanent birth control produced as a side effect, or for other reasons, is undetermined. Several recent studies may, however, be pertinent.

In a traditional medical environment, women are more likely to be in a subordinate relationship with a physician, especially an older female patient with an older male physician (West, 1984). In such relationships, decisions tend to be made by the doctor and not to be based on full sharing of information. Patients may have high expectations of treatment and little knowledge of risks and failure.

Objectively, the probabilities of benefits from hysterectomy for women in different age and risk groups vary. Sandberg et al. (1985) found improvement in quality of life and life expectancy through prevention of reproductive tract cancer when elective hysterectomy was done for certain indications between the ages of thirty and sixty. However, surgical mortality rates affect the probability of net gain for a given age group. The mortality rate is worse if the surgical care rendered is below current standards and if women at high risk of mortality are inappropriately selected for surgery. Both of these factors appear to be preventable by giving more adequate information to prospective patients, including providers' performance records, by guidelines of third-party payers, or by other means.

Roos (1984), studying surgery in Manitoba, found that certain doctors were far more likely to perform or recommend hysterectomies than others. These doctors drew their surgical patients from their own caseloads of primary-care patients but did not profit from the surgery, since patients have open access to specialists and care is free. To explain the difference in rates, therefore, Roos suggests that the "hysterectomy-prone" doctors were biased toward a particular type of treatment. Patients may also be biased in this way; hysterectomy for medical reasons results in sterilization without conflicting with Catholic doctrine, and the areas of high rates had an ethnic composition associated with Catholic church membership.

Feminist critiques of a health care system characterized by professional dominance and a majority of male doctors have predicted that there would be fewer abuses when women physicians cared for women patients. A report from the Italian-speaking part of Switzerland found that women gynecologists performed only one-half as many hysterectomies as their male counterparts (Domenighetti, Luraschi, and Marazzi, 1985), and the data showed no significant difference in the number of years of practice. The authors surmise that women practitioners identify more easily with their women patients' reluctance to lose the organ that represents womanhood to them and, thus, go by "more restrictive" indications for operating, but they also speculate that women who are most resistant to the surgery or think it is unnecessary seek out women doctors in the first place. The study does not have data on the necessity of the procedure in each case or the ultimate health results of doing it or not doing it. To resolve questions about physician gender and treatment choices, studies that dig deeper into selection bias and that augment process analysis with outcome studies would be helpful.

Interarea Variation: Prostatectomy

Surgery rates vary substantially, not only among physicians, but also among institutions and areas. This is thought to be more frequent when professionals disagree as to the best treatment for a given condition (Wennberg, 1984). Wennberg, in an analysis of thirty hospital market areas in Maine, found one procedure exclusive to men, transurethral prostatectomy, to have very high variation between areas, and inguinal hernia, usually a male procedure, to have low variation. But there was very high variation for six operations exclusive to women and high variation for two more including hysterectomy. The difference in variation is in accord with the degree of consensus, since the research on herniorrhaphy, for example, is said to be definitive, but that on hysterectomy is not (Luft, 1983). Whether performance of unnecessary surgery or omission of necessary surgery is implied by interareal variation has often been discussed but not resolved. Thus, the possibility of an inappropriate decision as to surgery depends on where one lives and what operation is involved, but further information is needed to determine whether too much or too little surgery is being received. Case review, rather than analysis of rate variation alone, is ultimately needed.

Not only the rate of performance, but also the risk attached to surgery may vary among areas. A study by Wennberg et al. (1987) reveals the variation in risk for men undergoing prostatectomy depending on where they have the surgery done. The study was conducted on records of 4,570 men aged 65 and over from the computerized records of Medicare for the state of Maine and of the Manitoba Health Insurance system. Important patient characteristics were controlled for, and men with a history of prostatic or bladder cancer were excluded. It was found that the risk of dying within three months of surgery was far higher in hospitals of less than 150 beds than in hospitals of 300 beds or more, the death rate being 1.8 times greater in the smaller hospitals. But some of the small hospitals did not have worse mortality rates than the teaching hospitals. Variance in death rates among individual hospitals was greatest for transurethral (rather than suprapubic) procedures. Since information on patient variables relating to severity of illness was limited, the authors speculate that the differences in outcome between hospitals could be due to "as yet unmeasured differences in illness levels" (Wennberg et al., 1987, p. 936). If so, improvement efforts should focus on criteria used to select candidates for surgery. A substantial number of reoperations occurred, implying that the original surgery failed to resolve the patients' urinary tract symptoms. The important inference from the findings is that it is wrong to regard prostatectomy as a low-risk operation that can be counted on to improve health. Alternative methods for treating prostatic enlargement may reduce future demand for surgery for benign disease (*New York Times*, 9 April 1985), but prostatectomy remains the most common surgery for men over 65.

Newly Perceived Conditions

Several conditions of women not formerly perceived as illness are now understood to call for physician care. (Just what therapy is appropriate is problematic.) Bulimia, a serious and potentially life-threatening eating disorder, has only recently been recognized as both a distinct and a common condition. Concentrated in women, bulimia is often concealed and denied by patients. A similar problem exists for the related disorder of anorexia. Physicians are being informed of the need to be alert to possible physical signs and other clues to bulimia (Mitchell et al., 1987). Varied treatments are used for bulimia and anorexia, but the treatments are described as "among the most unsatisfactory in clinical medicine," and more controlled studies of drug therapy are recommended (Herzog and Copeland, 1985). A recent controlled trial in Edinburgh (Freeman et al., 1988) reports that psychotherapy, especially behavior therapy, is effective for bulimia, and the cost is modest. Physicians need a prepared mind-set to make a diagnosis and to deal with the complex psychological and physical problems of the patients and their families, including evasion of medical treatment. Team resources and collaboration may be required.

Premenstrual syndrome is another condition newly accepted into the medical lexicon. Defining an appropriate place among health conditions for PMS involves avoiding both labeling and neglect. Labeling here means ascribing symptoms or experiences in the menstrual cycle to a medical entity and then identifying individuals as members of an afflicted set. The danger is that both individuals so labeled and women as a group may be badly treated in the labor market and elsewhere. Neglect implies that the discomfort and disability of women who are sufferers are not addressed by the health care system.

Both extremes are stereotypes connected to traditions concerning women. In the first, women are seen as generically frail; the uterus, as governor of other organs, especially the mind. In the nineteenth century, this proposition resulted in medicine's being used as a means of social control, preventing advanced education, active sports, and serious public roles for many women. In the second extreme, women are viewed as having a low threshold for perceiving pain and voicing complaints; thus, their discomfort can be dismissed in good conscience. (The implications of these stereotypes extend to contemporary models of PMS causation emphasizing either emotional or hormonal factors.)

Premenstrual syndrome has been treated enthusiastically by various providers, albeit without a firm scientific basis for the alternative therapies used. However, medical specialists state that a reasonable management program can be followed by responsible practitioners until more is known, implying that the patient will gain from seeking care (Rosenwaks, Benjamin, and Stone, 1987).

Men's subjective perception of discomfort is not usually interpreted within a depreciatory gender stereotype; however, labeling as heart patients has been cited as a problem for employed men. Supervisors may be reluctant to have men on the work team whose tolerance of risks is less than the average, an attitude that incorporates norms for men, as well as insurance concerns.

WOMEN AND MENTAL HEALTH CARE

In the 1970s the women's movement revived a spirit of critical evaluation of psychiatric treatment for women that had been fairly dormant for decades.

Half a century earlier, Freudian thought had used a model of women's psychic development that set up masochistic, narcissistic, and passive norms for women. In this model was found the rationale for assigning to mothers responsibility for such diverse conditions as schizophrenia, homosexuality, and eating disorders. Maternity was interpreted as compensation for psychic inadequacy, rather than as a positive creation; pursuit of worldly goals, as a result of distorted sexuality. Women were judged to have incomplete character formation and to be ruled by emotion (Miller, 1974). But Karen Horney, Clara Thompson, Gregory Zilboorg, and others presented alternative explanations for phenomena that had been attributed to the Freudian model. They sought, moreover, to explain why male theorists felt obliged to keep down women's claims to equality through essentially pejorative psychoanalytic models.

Critics in the more recent period repeated the charge of sex bias in psychological theories and added other points that brought the earlier critique up to date in view of changes in mental health research and care and in society. They noted that scales used to measure stress were not relevant to women's lives; thus, marriage was generally positive for men but could be problematic for women. Scales attuned to critical life events failed to pick up problems such as chronic poverty. The newer writers used community study findings on prevalence of depression in untreated populations to demonstrate that many women needed help for depression and that their apparent distress was not explained by a greater tendency to report symptoms to providers of health care (Carmen, Russo, and Miller, 1981). (In fact, a majority of those afflicted were believed to be without medical attention, for various reasons.)

"[T]he pervasive and destructive effects of gender inequality" were in essence identified as risk factors for emotional illness (Carmen, Russo, and Miller, 1981, p. 1319). For example, competent instrumental behavior was not expected of women, and this trained them to be helpless. "They get fewer rewards, have less control over their rewards, and more often see their rewards accompanied by punishment, producing conflict which interferes with learning" (Radloff, 1980, p. 108). The positive effects of employment in preventing depression and promoting recovery from it were used to combat the idea that traditional female roles had normative value for the psychic health of contemporary women. Analysis of marital status and other social factors as variables influencing the prevalence of depression was used as evidence that sex differences were not simply explained by biological causes (Guttentag, Salasin, and Belle, 1980).

Feminist scholars studying mental health care found that clinicians supplied a passive norm for adult women, adopting social stereotypes of women and, thus, it was argued, prolonging attitudes and behavior that made women more vulnerable to depression (Broverman, Broverman, and Clarkson, 1970). Different norms and interactions have been developed by feminist clinicians and self-help groups (Brody, 1987).

In the mental health community, the Diagnostic and Statistical Manual of Mental Disorders (DSM-III) was published by the American Psychiatric Association in 1980, and it quickly became the standard code. The hope was expressed that use of this manual would eliminate sex differences in diagnosis of mental illness (both presence and type) based solely on applying dissimilar standards to women and men patients, rather than on differences in problems and behavior. It was also hoped that variations in treatment produced by sex-biased diagnoses would be eliminated. (There were similar hopes regarding race bias.) But the actual evidence as to the existence of diagnostic bias based on the sex of the patient or the congruence of the patient's and the psychiatrist's sex was conflicted at the time that research on the question ceased in the early 1980s.

Kaplan argued in 1983 that male-biased assumptions about "healthy" and "crazy" behavior are retained and codified in DSM-III and "thus influenced and will continue to influence diagnosis and treatment patterns" (p. 788). She analyzed these assumptions, specifically in relation to histrionic and dependent personality disorders, noting that "unjust sex role imperatives" faced by women may result in normal reactions that are labeled sickness "in lieu of labeling society as unjust" (p. 789). Men's forms of dependence (relying on others to maintain their houses and take care of their children) are not viewed as illness. Kaplan showed how a masculine stereotype of devotion to work and career, allowing others to assume responsibility for social life, and denial of emotional needs would not be considered ill in DSM-III (Kaplan, 1983).

A study by Loring and Powell (1988) using simulated cases (vignettes) with race and sex varied for different respondents showed that, DSM-III's clear-cut diagnostic criteria notwithstanding, race and sex congruency of psychiatrist and case retained an influence on diagnosis. "Male psychiatrists, when diagnosing white females, are most likely to choose histrionic personality disorders" (p. 14), but the same case in a black female was assigned by them to paranoid personality disorders. Male clinicians tended to evaluate females as having depressive disorders. Choice of medications would be affected by these decisions. The authors acknowledge several limitations in the study, including a substantial nonresponse rate. They warn, however, that the perceptions of the white male majority in the profession influence statistics presented to the public, as well as important treatment decisions for individual patients.

The reevaluation of women's "careers" as patients with emotional problems included the use of tranquilizers and other psychotropic drugs. Although use of these drugs was growing, they were not harmless. They had side effects and carried risks of dependence. Furthermore, they could substitute for focused interventions. A tendency for women in Canada to receive prescriptions for psychotropic drugs more frequently than men was described by Cooperstock in the 1970s. She found that 23.9 percent of women in a southern Ontario insured population in 1973–1974 received one or more prescriptions for all psychotropic drugs, versus 14.5 percent of men. Also, there was a sex difference in the percentage who received such a prescription in both 1970–1971 and 1973–1974 (Cooperstock, 1976). She suggested that, when women sought relief from male physicians, the physicians interpreted distress due to social problems as a symptom of psychological disorders. A campaign launched in Canada to reduce the volume of tranquilizer prescriptions was evidently successful in cutting down the use of mood-modifying drugs, especially for female patients, between 1977 and 1982 (Bass and Pederson, 1986).

The problems of excessive use are both age- and sex-related. According to a study in the United Kingdom among a random sample of 1,020 elderly persons, women were twice as likely as men to use hypnotics (mainly benzodiazepine) at least sometimes (20 percent versus 10 percent), and, for women, the likelihood of use increased with age. Most users of both sexes (73 percent) had been taking such drugs for more than one year (Morgan et al., 1988). Another British study shows that the long-term users of benzodiazepines in a general practice were mainly elderly women who "were experiencing appreciable ill health," including depression. Yet the benzodiazepines "are generally devoid of antidepressant effects." The authors question whether "chronic treatment with tranquilizers was necessarily the best form of management" (Rodrigo, King, and Williams, 1988, p. 605).

Treatment of women for alcoholism has also been viewed critically from a feminist perspective. Although most sufferers from alcoholism are males, alcoholism is a unisex condition. But female cases may be underreported because the condition is associated with being male, and it has tended to be concealed by the family, denied by the patient, and missed by clinicians.[4] Many women drank away from the public gaze, and so their problem was less often recognized. If they were employed, it is said that they were more likely to be discharged than referred for treatment, owing to their replaceability in a sex-typed labor market. Use of a male model of disease genesis affected treatment. Etiology of alcohol abuse in women is currently interpreted as an outgrowth of their experience in female nurturing roles, but for men, different problems, involving power and dependence, have been implicated. Studies based on male subjects were used to set up generic etiologic models and to develop treatments oriented to male stresses (National Institute on Alcohol Abuse and Alcoholism, 1986). A review by the National Institute on Alcohol Abuse and Alcoholism (NIAAA) notes limitations of past research done on women and alcohol. There has been less research on effects of alcohol on adult women than on fetuses, and studies of the effects of alcohol on human sexuality have focused on male ability to perform sexually. In treatment programs, practical services that would have enabled women with family responsibilities to enter treatment were omitted from planning, and traditional sex role values were reported to influence attitudes of personnel in treatment agencies (National Institute on Alcohol Abuse and Alcoholism, 1985).

Thus, there was a shortfall in research, programming, and clinical protocols, according to critics, and (perhaps consequently) in service use by women. However, the NIAAA states its intention to increase research on the relationship of alcohol to women's health and to improve care for women.

Changes in mental health care for women were stimulated by, and reflected in, the development of women's therapy groups (replacing consciousness-raising groups) and female clinicians catering to women patients. Changes have also been encouraged by more assertive attitudes of women, their purchasing power in the market for services, and efforts of government agencies. This does not imply that statistical patterns of use for the two sexes will converge. Women may seek different sources of care and may prefer separatism. But provider competition for the market they represent (given that women are less willing than formerly to accept traditional approaches) is a positive stimulus to aligning mental health care with the demands of equality. Pressure of third parties to set limits

---

[4]Cirrhosis deaths were used to develop statistical rates of incidence and prevalence; reluctance to designate a woman decedent as alcoholic led to underestimation.

on the duration of treatment and, thus, limit their overall financial responsibility has also stimulated a shift away from traditional modes of therapy, most notably long-term, individual psychoanalysis.

HIV Infection

The epidemic of acquired immune deficiency syndrome (AIDS) has involved enormous suffering to the individuals involved and to their close circle. At the same time, health care services for people with AIDS or Human Immunodeficiency Virus (HIV) infection present many problems to society because of the combination of heavy and uncertain costs, the association of incidence with membership in unpopular high-risk groups and with personal behavior, and the poor prognosis. Additionally, some proposed control measures risk violating civil liberties and exposing individuals to job loss and other discriminations. Others have involved departing from long-standing taboos regarding sex and intravenous drug use in the interest of saving lives.

Women with AIDS have some special problems. It appears that they enter treatment later than men and at a later stage, sometimes after tending an ill partner. Whether this is because of sex differences in opportunistic infections that result in detection of HIV-positive status is not known, but doctors may not consider AIDS a possible cause of women's symptoms and may not order tests for them. This may change if cases among women increase. It is argued that, if the sensitivity of tests to the menstrual cycle and previous pregnancies could be ascertained, women could plan more realistically for their care (and that of children dependent on them). As improved treatments for AIDS and its complications are discovered, it will be important to have effective diagnosis and therapies available to all. It has been pointed out that being able to enter clinical trials is an important means of access to promising new drugs and that terms that would assure entry to women, racial minorities (AIDS Action Now! 1989), and low-income groups should be worked out. It has been suggested that guidelines for physicians involved in clinical trials of drugs to prevent complications of AIDS could allow pregnant women a choice rather than precluding their enrollment.

CONCLUSION

The process of obtaining medical care contains rational and functional elements in which the behavior of the parties, the information base of decisions, and the actual decisions are quite standardized, reflecting well-understood body functions and disease processes and well-known diagnostic procedures, treatments, and preventive measures. But these are not all the elements! The process of innovation has created a gap between devising new techniques or therapies and objective evaluations. The diffusion of new knowledge involves, not a simple intuitive acceptance, but market forces, readiness of third parties to pay costs, and other social factors. The relationship between the patient and the practitioner, being a human one, is steeped in a rich and ever-changing brew of social and psychological influences on each of the parties, affecting the range of the possible and the probability of the optimal. That an ascribed social status (gender) could carry over into health care activities should not surprise one, but neither should important shifts in behavior over time be ruled out.

The thread of gender wends its way through this complicated texture, and the exact strength of its influence in the overall pattern is variable and not easy to assess. In certain cases there seems to have been a definite gender bias, in that women's sex-specific conditions were handled in a way that reflected a low valuation of women's time, distress, body image, or quality of life. Also, the generic question of sex bias in measurement of indirect costs of illness, with a broad potential effect on a variety of health policy decisions, has been squarely raised. For sex-shared conditions or symptoms consistent with serious disease, questions have been asked about less appropriate care for women that merit continued investigation in different settings (HMOs versus fee-for-service practice) and for different types of patient samples. Confirmation or disconfirmation of bias and study of the intervening variables that may be influential present a challenge to research design.

There are also cases in which the economic self-interest of practitioners, the lack of autonomy of consumers, and the maldistribution and insufficiency of information, combined with scientific uncertainties, put patients of both sexes at risk of excessive or misdirected ministrations.

The literature of medicine and health care suggests that many of these forces affecting both sexes are self-renewing. Patients may gain more autonomy in general, but, at any given time, those with the socially most threatening or least understood conditions or with needs that are most deeply entwined with the meaning of the good life form a fringe that is especially vulnerable to provider dominance. Providers' self-interest is protean and can take many forms, including struggle of independent practitioners over turf (the right to give routine gynecological care or do plastic facial surgery); counterattack of employed or participating doctors against organizational regulations controlling use of their time and tests allowed; and selection of the most easily handled and rewarding patients. Scientific uncertainty is absolutely predictable, given an ever-changing list of new therapies and other discoveries, and this leaves room for the influence of personal biases and cultural norms on the care process.

There are, however, reasons to believe that gender bias in health care is preventable. Changes in women's lives are bound to have affected their expectations and the attitudes of children about gender. The counterforce is the threat this represents to some part of the male population and to institutions that rely on traditional values or a male mystique for their existence. But these changes have included consolidation of institutions and groups that speak for women and work to influence policy, do battle in the courts, and protect achieved gains.

The economic problems of the health care system seem to me a critical problem for sex equality. With constraints on social resources to be shared, prejudices of all kinds are often rekindled. Also, the client is thrown back on her or his own resources, which disadvantages those in the weakest economic positions such as many of today's single-parent families. In a "tight" health economy, actions that would add years of life but not necessarily save money for the economy are less likely to be approved and are vulnerable to cutbacks.

If the problems of the health economy can be solved, the trend toward fuller recognition of women's claims to equal consideration should enhance the prospects of achieving health care free of sex bias. However, gender equality has a realistic meaning only if it embraces helping disadvantaged women to obtain access to basic care, as well as promotes fairness in the conduct of medical care processes for well-sponsored clients. Gender, in combination with social phenomena of poverty, old age, and reproductive needs, defines a broader terrain for equity efforts.

References

AIDS Action Now! *Testing AIDS.* Publication distributed at the Fifth International Conference on AIDS Research, Toronto, Canada, June 4–9, 1989.

Armitage, K. J., Lawrence J. Schneiderman, and Robert A. Bass. "Response of Physicians to Medical Complaints in Men and Women." *Journal of American Medical Association*, vol. 241, no. 20 (May 18, 1979): 2186–2187.

Bass, Martin J., and Linda L. Pederson. "Is There a Trend away from Tranquilizing Women?" *Canadian Journal of Public Health*, vol. 77 (March/April 1986): 119–122.

Brody, Claire M., ed. *Women's Therapy Groups: Paradigms of Feminist Treatment*. New York: Springer Publishing Company, 1987.

Broverman, Inge K., Donald M. Broverman, and Frank E. Clarkson. "Sex-Role Stereotypes and Clinical Judgments of Mental Health." *Journal of Consulting and Clinical Psychology*, vol. 34, no. 1 (1970): 1–7.

Carmen, Elaine Hilberman, Nancy Felipe Russo, and Jean Baker Miller. "Inequality and Women's Mental Health: An Overview." *American Journal of Psychiatry*, vol. 138, no. 10 (October 1981): 1319–1330.

Chez, Ronald A. "Woman Battering." *American Journal of Obstetrics and Gynecology*, vol. 158, no. 1 (January 1988): 1–4.

Coleman, Daniel. "Physicians May Bungle Key Part of Treatment: The Medical Interview." *New York Times*, 21 January 1988.

Cooperstock, Ruth. "Psychotropic Drug Use among Women." *CMA Journal*, vol. 115 (October 23, 1976): 760–763.

Croog, Sydney H., Sol Levine, Marcia A. Testa, and Byron Brown. "The Effects of Antihypertensive Therapy on the Quality of Life." *New England Journal of Medicine*, vol. 314, no. 26 (June 26, 1986): 1657–1664.

Domenighetti, Gianfranco, Pierangelo Luraschi, and Alfio Marazzi. "Hysterectomy and Sex of the Gynecologist" (Letter). *New England Journal of Medicine*, vol. 313, no. 23 (1985): 1482.

Doubilet, Peter, and Herbert L. Abrams. "The Cost of Underutilization: Percutaneous Transluminal Angioplasty for Peripheral Vascular Disease." *New England Journal of Medicine*, vol. 310, no. 2 (January 12, 1984): 95–102.

Fisher, Bernard, Madeline Bauer, Richard Margolese, Roger Poisson, et al. "Five-Year Results of a Randomized Clinical Trial Comparing Total Mastectomy and Segmental Mastectomy with or without Radiation in the Treatment of Breast Cancer." *New England Journal of Medicine*, vol. 312, no. 11 (March 14, 1985): 665–673.

Freeman, C. P. L., F. Barry, J. Durkel-Turnbull, and A. Henderson. "Controlled Trial of Psychotherapy for Bulimia Nervosa." *British Medical Journal*, vol. 296 (February 20, 1988): 521–525.

General Accounting Office. *The Use of Breakthrough Treatments for Seven Types of Cancer: Cancer Treatment 1975–1985*. Washington, DC, January 1988.

————. *Breast Cancer Patients' Survival*. Washington, DC, February 1989.

Gersh, Bernard J., Richard A. Kronmal, Hartzell V. Schaff, and Robert L. Frye, et al. "Comparison of Coronary Artery Bypass Surgery and Medical Therapy in Patients 65 Years of Age or Older." *New England Journal of Medicine*, vol. 217 (July 25, 1985): 217–224.

Goldwyn, Robert M. "Breast Reconstruction after Mastectomy." *New England Journal of Medicine*, vol. 317, no. 27, (December 31, 1987): 1711–1714.

Graboys, Thomas B., Adrienne Headley, Bernard Lown, Steven Lampert, and Charles M. Blatt. "Results of a Second-Opinion Program for Coronary Artery

Bypass Graft Surgery." *Journal of the American Medical Association,* vol. 258, no. 2 (September 25, 1987): 1611–1614.

Greer, Steven, Vivian Dickerson, Lawrence J. Schneiderman, et al. "Responses of Male and Female Physicians to Medical Complaints in Male and Female Patients." *Journal of Family Practice,* vol. 23, no. 1 (1986): 49–53.

Gruentzig, Andreas R., Spencer B. King III, Maria Schlumpf, and Walter Siegenthaler. "Long-Term Follow-up after Percutaneous Transluminal Coronary Angioplasty." *New England Journal of Medicine,* vol. 316, no. 18 (April 30, 1987): 1127–1132.

Guttentag, Marcia, S. Salasin, and D. Belle, eds. *The Mental Health of Women.* New York: Academic Press, 1980.

Hall, Ferris M. "Screening Mammography: Potential Problems on the Horizon." *New England Journal of Medicine,* vol. 314, no. 1 (January 2, 1986): 53–55.

Harwood, Henrick J., Diane M. Napolitano, Patricia L. Kristiansen, and James J. Collins. *Economic Costs to Society of Alcohol and Drug Abuse and Mental Illness: 1980.* Research Triangle Park, NC: Research Triangle Institute, 1984.

Herzog, David B., and Paul M. Copeland. "Eating Disorders." *New England Journal of Medicine,* vol. 313, no. 5 (August 1, 1985): 295–302.

Kannel, William B., and Robert D. Abbott. "Incidence and Prognosis of Unrecognized Myocardial Infarction: An Update on the Framingham Study." *New England Journal of Medicine,* vol. 311, no. 18 (November 1, 1984): 1144–1147.

Kaplan, Marci. "A Woman's View of DSM-III." *American Psychologist* (July 1983): 786–792.

Kassirer, Jerome P. "Adding Insult to Injury: Usurping Patients' Prerogatives." *New England Journal of Medicine,* vol. 308, no. 15 (April 14, 1983): 898–901.

Kovar, Mary Grace, John Gary Collins, and James DeLozier. "Trends in the Availability and Use of Medical Care for Coronary Heart Disease and Related Diseases." In *Trends in Coronary Heart Disease Mortality: The Influence of Medical Care,* edited by Millicent W. Higgins and Russell V. Luepker. New York: Oxford University Press, 1988, 31–43.

Levin, Arthur A. "Hysterectomy." *The Fund Reporter* (Consumer Commission on the Accreditation of Health Services) (January/February 1986): 3.

Loring, Marti, and Brian Powell. "Gender, Race, and DSM-III: A Study of the Objectivity of Psychiatric Diagnostic Behavior." *Journal of Health and Social Behavior,* vol. 29 (March 1988): 1–22.

Luft, Harold S. "Economic Incentives and Clinical Decisions." In *The New Health Care for Profit,* edited by Bradford H. Gray. Washington, DC: National Academy Press, 1983, 103–123.

Miller, J. B., ed. *Psychoanalysis and Women: Contributions to New Theory and Therapy.* New York: Brunner/Mazel, 1974.

Mitchell, James E., Harold C. Seim, Eduardo Colon, and Claire Pomeroy. "Medical Complications and Medical Management of Bulimia." *Annals of Internal Medicine*, 107 (1987): 71–77.

Morgan, Kevin, Helen Dallosso, Shah Ebrahim, Tom Arie, and Peter H. Fentem. "Prevalence, Frequency, and Duration of Hypnotic Drug Use among the Elderly Living at Home." *British Medical Journal*, vol. 296 (February 27, 1988): 601–602.

Mount Sinai School of Medicine. Table on Coronary Bypass Operations for 1984 (unpublished). Prepared in 1987.

Muller, Charlotte, and Carol C. Caton. "Economic Costs of Schizophrenia: A Post-discharge Study." *Medical Care*, vol. 21, no. 1 (1983): 92–104.

Nathanson, Constance A., and Gerda Lorenz. "Women and Health: The Social Dimensions of Biomedical Data." In *Women in the Middle Years*, edited by Janet Zollinger Giele. New York: Wiley, 1982, 37–88.

National Center for Health Services Research and Health Care Technology Assessment. *Research Activities*, no. 115, March 1989.

National Institute of Mental Health. *Plain Talk about Wife Abuse*. Plain Talk Series, edited by Ruth Kay. Rockville, MD, 1983.

National Institute on Alcohol Abuse and Alcoholism. "Sex-Related Alcohol Effects." *Alcohol Resources: Update, June 1985*. Rockville, MD, 1985.

————. *Women and Alcohol: Health-related Issues*. Research Monograph No. 16. Pub. No. (ADM) 86–1139. Rockville, MD, 1986.

New York Times, 9 April 1985.

Parsons, P. Ellen, Richard Lichtenstein, S. E. Berke, Hilary A. Murt, et al. *Costs of Illness: United States, 1980*. NCHSR, NMCUES, Series C, Analytical Report No. 3. DHHS Pub. No. 86-20403. Hyattsville, MD: National Center for Health Statistics, April 1986.

Poland, Ronald L. "The Question of Routine Neonatal Circumcision." *New England Journal of Medicine*, vol. 322, no. 18 (May 3, 1990): 1312–1315.

Prosnitz, Leonard R., Daniel S. Kapp, and Joseph B. Weissberg. "Radiotherapy." *New England Journal of Medicine*, vol. 309, no. 13 (September 29, 1983): 771–777.

Radloff, Lenore Sawyer, "Risk Factors for Depression: What Do We Learn From Them?" In *Mental Health of Women*, edited by M. Guttentag et al. New York: Academic Press, 1980.

Rice Dorothy P. "Sex Differences in Mortality and Morbidity: Some Aspects of the Economic Burden." In *Sex Differentials in Mortality*, edited by A. D. Lopez and L. T. Ruzicka. Selection of the papers presented in Canberra, Australia, 1–7 December 1981. Canberra, Australia: Australian National University, 1983.

Rodrigo, E. K., M. B. King, and P. Williams. "Health of Long-term Benzodiazepine Users." *British Medical Journal*, vol. 296 (February 27, 1988): 603–608.

Roos, Noralou P. "Hysterectomies in One Canadian Province: A New Look at Risks and Benefits." *American Journal of Public Health*, vol. 74, no. 1 (1984): 39–46.

Rosenwaks, Zev, Fred Benjamin, and Martin L. Stone, eds. *Gynecology, Principles and Practice*. New York: Macmillan Publishing Co., 1987.

Russell, Louise B. *Is Prevention Better Than Cure?* Studies in Social Economics. Washington, DC: Brookings Institution, 1986.

Sagan, Leonard A. *The Health of Nations: True Causes of Sickness and Well-Being*. New York: Basic Books, 1987.

Salkever, David H. *Morbidity Costs: National Estimates and Economic Determinants*. DHHS Pub. No. 86-3393. Rockville, MD: National Center for Health Services Research, October 1985.

Samson, Suzanne. "Concern Grows on Teen-Age Dating Abuse." *New York Times*, 11 June 1989.

Sandberg, S. I., B. A. Barnes, M. C. Weinstein, et al. "Elective Hysterectomy: Benefits, Risks, and Costs." *Medical Care*, vol. 23, no. 9 (1985): 1067–1085.

Sawyer, Lenore. "Risk Factors for Depression: What Do We Learn From Them?" In *The Mental Health of Women*, edited by M. Guttentag, S. Salasen, and D. Belle. New York: Academic Press, 1980, 92–108.

Schechter, Clyde. Interview, May 2, 1988.

Schoen, Edgar J. "The Status of Circumcision of Newborns." *New England Journal of Medicine*, vol. 322, no. 18 (May 3, 1990): 1308–1312.

Smith, Hugh C., LaVon N. Hammes, Sudhir Gupta, Ronald E. Vlietstra, et al. "Employment Status after Coronary Bypass Surgery." *Circulation*, 65, supp. II (1982): 120–125.

Tobin, Jonathan N., Sylvia Wassertheil-Smoller, John P. Wexler, Richard M. Steingart, et al. "Sex Bias in Considering Coronary Bypass Surgery." *Annals of Internal Medicine*, vol. 107 (July 1987): 19–25.

Toffler, Geoffrey H., Peter H. Stone, James E. Muller, Stefan N. Willich, et al. "Effects of Gender and Race on Prognosis after Myocardial Infarction: Adverse Prognosis for Women, Particularly Black Women." *Journal of American College of Cardiology*, vol. 9, no. 3 (March 1987): 473–482.

U.S. Congress. Office of Technology Assessment. *Breast Cancer Screening for Medicare Beneficiaries: Effectiveness, Costs to Medicare and Medical Resources Required*. Washington, DC: Government Printing Office, November 1987.

Verbrugge, Lois M. "From Sneeze to Adieux: Stages of Health for American Men and Women." *Social Science Medicine*, vol. 22, no. 11 (1986): 1195–1212.

Waldron, Ingrid. "The Contribution of Smoking to Sex Differences in Mortality." *Public Health Reports*, vol. 101, no. 2 (March/April 1986): 163–173.

Wallen, Jacqueline, Howard Waitzkin, and John D. Stoeckle. "Physician Stereotypes about Female Health and Illness: A Study of Patient's Sex and the Informative Process during Medical Interviews." *Women & Health*, vol. 4, no. 2 (1979): 135–146.

Washington, A. Eugene, Peter S. Arno, and Marie A. Brooks. "The Economic Cost of Pelvic Inflammatory Disease." *Journal of the American Medical Association*, vol. 255, no. 13 (April 4, 1987): 1735–1738.

Weitzman, Sigmund, Irene Kuter, and Hank F. Pizer. *Confronting Breast Cancer: New Options in Detection and Treatment*. New York: Random House, Vintage Books, 1987.

Wennberg, John E. *Small Area Variation in Hospitalized Case Mix for DRGs in Maine, Massachusetts, and Iowa*. Hyattsville, MD: National Center for Health Services Research and Health Care Technology Assessment, 1984.

Wennberg, John E., Noralou Roos, Loredo Sola, Alice Schori, et al. "Use of Claims Data Systems to Evaluate Health Care Outcomes, Mortality, and Reoperation Following Prostatectomy." *Journal of the American Medical Association*, vol. 257, no. 7 (February 20, 1987): 933–936.

West, Candace. "When the Doctor Is a 'Lady': Power, Status, and Gender in Physician-Patient Encounters." *Symbolic Interaction*, vol. 7, no. 1 (1984): 87–106.

Willis, Judith. "Progress against Breast Cancer." In *Women's Health*. PHS Pub. No. (FDA) 86-1127. Rockville, MD: Government Printing Office. 1986.

Zambrana, Ruth E., Wendy Mogel, and Susan C. M. Scrimshaw. "Gender and Level of Training Differences in Obstetricians' Attitudes towards Patients in Childbirth." *Women & Health*, vol. 12, no. 1 (1987): 5–24.

PART TWO

CONCERNING SOME MAJOR GROUPS

CHAPTER THREE

Health Care, the Workplace, and Gender: Health Needs

IN THE NEXT TWO chapters the interaction between gender and health needs and health care for the working-age population will be explored. Chapter 3 focuses on health needs of working-age men and women and the relation of work to health. Chapter 4 discusses insurance and financing issues for employed adults and special vulnerabilities that are gender specific.

Trends in women's labor force participation, the control of fertility, and the sex wage gap are a background to understanding women's problems in regard to health care. Sex differences and similarities with respect to acute and chronic illness, mortality risks, and prevention opportunities provide a perspective on the need for care. Certain health problems of women that were previously ignored or dismissed as trivial (or psychosomatic) are now receiving attention. Environments in which women work present important risks to health, and reproductive health hazards have become an issue for both men and women. Generally, occupational hazards to health are probably understated for both sexes.

Insurance is important as a means of meeting health care costs, and it influences access to needed care. Both the numbers of persons covered and the benefits provided count. Sex differences in the rate of coverage are influenced by marital status, part-time work, and occupation. Quality of benefits depends on the size of employer contributions. Cost-control methods currently used by employers may have more burdensome effects on low-income employees, who are often female, or on those filling caregiver roles in the family. Maternity coverage has been improved by legislation barring differential benefits for pregnancy as discriminatory, but abortion, although included in contracts under maternity coverage, is often paid for out of the employee's pocket.

In important ways, the financing structure is in disequilibrium. Adaptation of employer policies to family responsibilities of two-earner couples will require changes in health care and related benefits. Coverage of women through an employed husband, which may have been appropriate when women were not regular members of the labor force, loses its rationale as women cease to spend their time exclusively as homemakers and as single women function as heads of households. At the same time, the expansion of peripheral, or contingent, employment with few or no benefits makes it less logical to rely on the workplace to assure individual protection against health care costs. Furthermore, the uncertain fortunes of the economy and the irrationality of some health care system features create continuing threats to personal security against the risks of health care costs, especially if this protection is derived from individual employers.

WOMEN IN THE PAID LABOR FORCE

Today, two-thirds of women under sixty-five are in the U.S. labor force, and, consequently, the health care of employed women is a significant concern for women in general. The wage level of women is a major determinant of their ability to buy health care, and low wages and lack of insurance often go together. Women's access to care through their employment is shaped by sex differences in the type of job held and the fringe benefits accompanying the job.

Since women tend more and more to combine work with motherhood, their reproductive functions, including fertility control, need to be taken into account in health benefit programs. Limitations in the amount of benefits may deter or delay use of prenatal care, and office visits for family planning may not be covered. Maternity leave provisions may affect entitlement to health benefits. Other wage supplements, where they exist, such as retirement programs, paid parental leave for child care, and day-care facilities, free resources of low- and moderate-income workers for use in the purchase of health care.

Women's current pattern of economic activity is the result of trends in occupation, education, and family life. Before 1900, many women were driven by economic necessity to obtain either domestic work or factory jobs. In the twentieth century, the development of clerical and service jobs with light physical demands attracted many younger women to paid employment. (While there are some biological sex differences in strength, affecting ability to do given jobs, some of women's physical limitations were socially created by norms regarding exercise and dress; others were imagined as parts of stereotypes; and still others were simply due to the fact that machines and tools were designed for the physiques of men.) Clerical and white-collar work done by women used skills developed by formal education, that is, by off-the-job, rather than on-the-job, training, which did not depreciate with age or with extended absence from the labor force (Goldin, 1989).

In the decades after World War II, many married women entered or returned to the labor force after their children had passed into their teenage years, trends that the United States shared with other industrial countries (NBER Digest, 1985). Another related trend was marital breakup. The divorce rate has been close to one-half the marriage rate in recent years (National Center for Health Statistics, 1987). The increase in divorce and separation brought many women into the work force, and the ability of women to support themselves became a factor in higher rates of divorce.

As with divorce, fertility changes affected women's labor force participation and were in turn affected by it. Unwanted childbearing (especially for married women) declined (Pratt and Horn, 1985). Smaller families and fewer unplanned births were made possible by legal and other changes allowing access to technologically up-to-date contraception, sterilization, and abortion services. More married women were thus able to enter the labor force and have continuous work careers.

Delayed childbearing and families with two working parents added to the female labor force, which now includes many currently married women with young children. The trend of rising real wages due to productivity growth made staying at home a less attractive economic choice. The impairment of real income of families by inflation drew many women into the labor force in the 1970s (*New York Times*, 19 June 1985). Educational levels of women rose after World War II, stimulating their interest in professional and managerial careers and encouraging a political demand for affirmative action. Today the percentage of women of working age in the labor force is over three-quarters that of men, compared with one-fifth in 1890 and one-third in 1940 (Bergmann, 1986).

As a result of these trends, the current cross-section of employed women represents a mix as regards planned and completed fertility, occupational levels, earning potential, marital status, and age. The type of health care they need and the specifics of equity issues in the workplace will reflect this diversity.

Review of the history of the U.S. economy shows that a female/male wage ratio of 58 percent persisted for decades after 1885, despite many changes in job structure. Today, wages of women working full-time are less than two-thirds of those of men working similar hours.

The reasons for the sex gap are disputed. Explanations based on sex differences in individuals' voluntary investment in human capital are unsatisfactory because other factors are ignored. Earnings are affected by parental decisions to invest in their sons' or daughters' education. Returns on their education (i.e., human capital) received by women have been lower than for men. Many women have left the labor market because of their husbands' career needs or perceived lack of opportunity for themselves or are crowded in sex-typed jobs. According to Bergmann, discrimination has been an important factor in the gap (1986). Even though over two decades have passed since the enactment of civil rights legislation, sex discrimination in the workplace has been acknowledged as a continuing issue by the Council of Economic Advisers (Silk, 1987), and cases continue to be adjudicated (American Civil Liberties Union, 1987).

Younger cohorts of women in the labor force have a narrower sex-based wage differential than do older women, but current progress can be overstated if wages of younger women are compared with those of younger men. Women's age-earning profile has tended to peak early, while men's has continued to rise with length of career (Goldin, 1989). Thus, men have more increases with the passage of time, owing to promotions (Brandwein, 1987). Furthermore, progressive narrowing of the sex wage gap might be interrupted by economic recessions or by ups and downs in the vigor with which equal opportunity laws are enforced and the disposition of the Supreme Court to interpret them narrowly or broadly. (Today, narrow interpretation is favored, and vigor is down.) These factors affect the ability of women to pay residual out-of-pocket health care costs under insurance and the costs of uncovered services. Also affected is ability to pay for a health-promoting pattern of foods and other consumer goods and services.

HEALTH OF WORKING-AGE ADULTS

General Health

The National Health Interview Survey of 1986 provides information on ill health based on a national probability sample. Findings for the age groups 18–44 and 45–64 indicate the health status of men and women of working age. Except for data on work injuries and on illness or injury days lost from work, the figures embrace nonworkers and workers. The pattern revealed, however, is similar to that shown in an analysis restricted to men and women in the labor force using National Health Interview Survey data for 1983–1985, not broken down by age group (Collins and Thornberry, 1989).

Women in both the younger and older age groups have 1.4 times as many acute conditions (a term that includes "delivery and other conditions of pregnancy") as men (National Center for Health Statistics, 1986, table 21). Pregnancy is included in acute conditions, but it accounts for only 4 percent of the 205.6 acute conditions per 100 women per year at ages 18–44. Thus, the sex comparison suggests that women have more need of physician services for acute illness. In addition, the acute conditions of women are slightly more likely to be medically attended (table 12). Women, moreover, are more likely to have seen a doctor within the past year (table 72) and have a higher rate of office visits for all purposes: acute and chronic conditions, plus prevention other than prenatal care (table 71). The sex differences in use of doctors are greater for the 18–44 age group, owing largely to fertility-related services. But the sex difference in restricted activity days (RAD) from acute illness is greater for the 45–64 age group, largely because these days increase with age only for women (table 17). The sex difference for bed days is even stronger (table 27).

Currently employed women have more work-loss days (WLD) than men, again, the difference being greater for older adults (table 37), but there is less gender difference in WLD than in total RAD, as I found in my analysis of the National Health Interview Survey of the mid-1970s. Working women appear to hold down their absences from work when ill and restrict their activities on their nonworking days to deal with illness (Muller, 1986).

For both sexes the prevalence of some activity limitation due to chronic conditions and, a more severe impairment, of limitation in major activity increases greatly after age 45. In contrast with acute illness, the rates for the two sexes are similar: 17.3 percent of each sex have a limitation in major activities at ages 45–64 (National Center for Health Statistics, 1986, table 67). If all types of disability days due to acute and chronic conditions are counted, women's rates, like men's, increase monotonically with age, but the rates for women are consistently higher at ages 18–64 (table 69).

The pattern for self-reported health status resembles that for limitations: the proportion of both men and women reporting excellent health declines noticeably after age 45, and more men than women report being in excellent health at ages 18–64. However, the two sexes are similar at all ages in the proportions with fair or poor health (table 70).

The distribution of chronic conditions varies by sex. From 18 to 64 years, women have higher prevalence rates (cases per 1,000 persons) for arthritis, migraine, chronic sinusitis and bronchitis, dermatitis, and diabetes. Men have higher rates for impairments of the lower extremities, vision, and hearing. Male and female rates are similar for ulcer. Certain patterns shift after age 45. Women have higher rates of prevalence for high blood pressure (a reversal of the sex difference at younger ages), but men show higher rates for heart disease, back impairment, hemorrhoids (all reversals of the female excess at younger ages), and frequent indigestion (National Center for Health Statistics, 1986, table 58).

The prevalence pattern of chronic conditions suggests that, although the body systems that cause limitation in activities and poor health after age forty-five may vary by sex, there is a shared need for regular health care. Both life-threatening conditions and conditions potentially causing serious discomfort and disability become more prevalent after that age. A diversity of health services are needed for prevention or control of these conditions (e.g., vision and hearing services, diabetic regimens, and blood pressure control).

The death rate for adults 25–64 in 1985 was 444 per 100,000. The Public Health Service announced the goal of reducing this to 400 by the year 1990 (U.S. Department of Health and Human Services, 1987, p. 19). Rates of death from heart disease and stroke in 1984 were well below those reported in 1970; these conditions accounted for 32.5 percent of deaths. Cancer had as high a death rate in 1985 as in 1950 and, consequently, became the leading cause of death for this age group in 1983 (30.2 percent).

For men under sixty-five, several measures for control of cancer at the major sites (lung, prostate, colon and rectum, and bladder) are currently available. They include changing smoking behavior, screening for colon and rectal cancer (sigmoidoscopy and testing for occult blood), changing the diet (e.g., increasing fiber intake), and reducing exposure to occupational carcinogens. Gemson (1987) points to the decline of lung cancer among white males as evidence of the efficacy of prevention and the desirability of funding and promoting preventive efforts by physicians and communitywide programs. Effective protection of the work environment would supplement what the health care system could contribute.

For women of the same ages, cancer rates for their major sites (breast, lung, cervix, and corpus uteri) could also be improved by known interventions. These include screening and appropriate treatment for breast cancer (surgery, chemotherapy, radiation) and smoking reversal to change the trend of increased lung cancer deaths among women (from 10 per 100,000 in 1969 to about 25 in 1984). Wide use of Pap smear tests is needed to maintain and accelerate the decline in cervical cancer death rates since 1969 (U.S. Department of Health and Human Services, 1987, p. 39). Useful screening methods for breast cancer include mammography, self-examination, and clinical examination of breasts. However, most women in the age groups at risk are not undergoing regular screening.

Many risk factors for heart disease in both sexes can be controlled by preventive measures, which include (1) screening and control of hypertension, (2) cessation of smoking, (3) identification and treatment of cholesterol abnormalities, and (4) engaging in regular physical activities. However, many individuals, when surveyed, do not give correct answers to questions on needs for physical activity and other vital elements of a healthy life-style (U.S. Department of Health and Human Services, 1987, p. 44) and, therefore, would need some form of health education to protect their health. Contact with physicians who are prepared to help patients minimize risk factors is essential to control of major causes of death for older adults.

Fatal diseases understandably attract the most concern. Yet the health care system can do much to control nonfatal conditions interfering with well-being and activity. Unfortunately, certain health needs of women have been unrecognized or trivialized until recently. Stereotypes about women, low ranking of their life goals, and other forms of gender bias have contributed to this. Other health needs have emerged as women's activities have changed. There is growing awareness of both old and new needs, including reliable control of fertility; alleviation of premenstrual syndrome; reconstruction of the breast(s) after mastectomy; and control of eating disorders, obesity, alcohol abuse, depression, and spouse battering—a wide range, indeed.

Retrospective analysis shows 20 percent to 40 percent of women as having moderately severe premenstrual symptoms. A description of premenstrual tension, supported by estrogen measurements, was published in 1931, but clinicians considered PMS to be psychosomatic and gave it little attention. Later they changed their appraisal, as better methods of study developed—and as society became more sensitive to women's health issues. Much remains unknown about etiology, criteria for diagnosis, and modes of treatment. So-called empiric therapies, based on predominant symptoms, can be offered by physicians, but as treatment success is measured subjectively, alternative healers and self-help have had their appeal (Rosenwaks, Benjamin, and Stone, 1987). Clinics based on estrogen therapy flourished for a while.

Alcoholism is not sex-specific but is often seen as a problem of men. Men are indeed more likely to be heavy drinkers than women (U.S. Department of Commerce, 1986b, table 1973), and alcohol problems are among the five leading causes of hospitalization for men in age groups 15–44 and 45–64 (table 154). Men are heavier users than women of general hospitals, community mental health centers, and (for whites) outpatient psychiatric services for treatment of alcohol-related disorders (U.S. Department of Health and Human Services, 1985). Alcoholism treatment is often based on male experience and role problems, thus limiting its utility to women clients. Furthermore, treatment facilities may not be useful to women unless they are adapted to the needs of families for which women patients are responsible; child care, transportation, and availability of services on an evening and weekend basis could improve participation in programs. For those who have a dual addiction to alcohol and drugs, a longer treatment period needs to be covered by insurance (National Institute on Alcohol Abuse and Alcoholism, 1981).

Much is known about health problems that can lead to serious disease if not checked, and certain preventive measures involving personal health care services have been shown to be effective. Based on this knowledge, access to medical care is rightfully regarded as a basic need for the working-age population of men and women. This belief is enhanced by the prospect of developing effective treatments for disease conditions that are as yet untamed. The proportions with fair or poor health and with activity limitations due to chronic disease are similar for men and women, but women have a greater burden of acute illness. Gender differences in ability to pay out-of-pocket expenses become a risk factor for delay or omission of desirable health services. The coverage of specific, scientifically well-supported cancer screening services and the elimination of obstacles to regular preventive visits are essential to bringing important diseases under control. Hence, the quality of benefits, not just having some insurance, is important. Moreover, benefits should not omit services used mainly or solely by one sex; superficially gender-neutral packages result in neglect of needs and of opportunities to improve health.

Work and Health

Occupational disease and injury are risks of work. Work injuries account for 35.4 percent of all injuries reported by men and 21.5 percent of those reported by women (National Center for Health Statistics, 1986, table 51). Men have a much higher rate of work injuries than women, as shown in episodes and lost days: 8.5 episodes per 100 currently employed men per year, versus 3.9 for women (table 51), and 133.2 RAD per 100 persons per year, versus 42.9 for women (table 53).

Because injury events are more easily observed than illness, we know more about injuries at work than we do about illnesses to which occupation is a major contributor. For example, only a small percentage of cancer is definitely attributed to occupational factors, but this may be the result of epidemiological research problems. So-called latency of disease means that risks of newly introduced substances or other agents are not appreciated, and data on the number of persons exposed are fragmentary. Multiple simultaneous exposures; worker mobility, which results in a sequence of exposures to different agents; and interaction with smoking and other factors have not been addressed in epidemiological research (Selikoff, 1981). An additional practical problem is that management consent is needed to obtain information as to workers' exposure (Last, 1987).

Epidemiological research in spontaneous abortion and congenital malformation related to occupation is described as a particularly difficult and demanding field of study (Lindbohm, Taskinen, and Hemminki, 1985). Women who are not aware that they were exposed or who have had good pregnancy outcomes tend to have low response rates on surveys. Women may not recognize an early miscarriage. Medical records are used as a data source, but their utility depends on people's access to care and whether those who knew they were exposed used more care. If the study is retrospective, neither the timing nor the amount of exposure during the critical period for fetal development can be ascertained. Lindbohm et al. note, however, that at least some of the limitations of past studies result in understating the true association of occupational exposure with congenital malformations, spontaneous abortions, and other adverse outcomes. Environments have been declared safe when only very large risks have been excluded from them (Lindbohm et al., 1985).[1]

Rosenberg and colleagues report similar problems in identifying the proportion of all reproductive impairments of both sexes resulting from occupational exposures. For example, the response rates from exposed men in most studies of sperm quality are only 40 percent, and those of controls are even less. Sample size must be very large to detect rare events. Total reproductive impairment due to occupational causes is very probably understated (Rosenberg, Feldbaum, and Marshall, 1987).

---

[1]VDT users have been found to have a high miscarriage rate by Kaiser-Permanente in a recent study, confirming a number of reports of pregnancy damage, but the biological mechanisms involved are not well understood. (Additional studies of VDT are needed that have sufficient numbers to control for specific occupation and that will prospectively record exposure and pregnancy outcomes over a period of time) (Bureau of National Affairs, 1989).

Men have been more subject to injury and certain devastating illnesses, such as pneumoconiosis and mesothelioma, at the workplace
than women because of the sex segregation of occupations and because
being in the labor force was the social norm for men. However, the labor
force participation of women is becoming more similar to that of men
(Passanante and Nathanson, 1987), and, if women enter traditionally
male occupations, their degree of exposure will resemble that of men.
Furthermore, for new entrants into an occupation, inexperience increases
the risk of injury, particularly if protective equipment and clothing are
not designed for a smaller body size. (This could be a transitional problem, ceasing when women are expected by management and accepted in
the work unit.)

Risks to women are not confined to male occupations. Many health
risks have been identified in occupations where women are concentrated.
They include chemicals found in schools, airplanes, and offices; contami-
nation of air conditioners; eye and muscle effects of video display terminals (Marriott and Stuckly, 1986); and radiation in health facilities. Anesthesia gases breathed in by operating room nurses have been identified as
a risk factor for poor reproductive outcomes (Brunt and Hricko, 1983),
but flaws in past studies have caused Tannenbaum and Goldberg (1985)
to conclude that the evidence for this is inadequate. (Surely it is worth
resolving by well-designed research?) Child care workers are exposed to
infections and to toxins in craft materials, and their environments are
minimally regulated. Back injuries among nurses may cause long periods
of disability. Specific job factors in nursing, namely, service areas of
work, frequency of lifting, and job category, have been found to be significant predictors of back injuries and of the length of time required for
recovery (Venning, Walker, and Stitt, 1987; Venning, 1987). These associations strengthen the conclusion that the job environment is indeed a
major cause of the injuries.

Working women tend to report poorer general health than working
men. Adverse job characteristics may play a part in this. A study in Canadian poultry slaughterhouses supports the view that the work situation,
rather than biological or reporting differences, is responsible. Women
had a higher rate of symptoms in certain areas: upper and lower limbs,
back, and nervous system. But when a subsample who had to work while
immobile, at cold temperatures, in humid air, and exposed to drafts was
studied, sex differences in symptoms diminished. For assembly line
workers, where men and women worked under even more homogeneous
conditions, sex differences disappeared entirely (Mergler et al., 1987).
This seems to imply that nonwork factors have little to do with sex
differences in health. Does this conflict with recognition that double

roles of many women add to fatigue and stress? Perhaps the work environment dominates if it is adverse enough. Research that considers both familial and environmental factors would help resolve questions as to their relative importance for health.

So far, employers, in promoting wellness, have focused on employees' personal habits, and the contribution of occupational hazards to ill health has been essentially avoided in the design of wellness programs. Yet medical care to exposed persons may be misdirected if occupational causes of symptoms are not understood, and some medical care would be avoidable if occupational diseases were prevented by redesign of the workplace environment, equipment, and job tasks. This will become an increasingly important issue for women as they commit a larger proportion of their years to the workplace.

Women workers in clerical and service fields typically lack the union protection that has assisted many blue-collar workers in addressing on-the-job hazards to health. Unions, in any event, have lost ground in terms of proportions of workers covered (U.S. Department of Commerce, 1987, table 667), and this limits both sexes in protecting their environmental health interests through unions.

Stress may be a special problem for working women. On-the-job stress arises from a system in which the individual is not valued. The low valuation may be shown in lack of job security, monotony, pressured pace of work, exclusion from decision making, threat of physical violence, or expressed hostility of male co-workers (Brunt and Hricko, 1983). Awareness of persistent occupational health hazards in the physical environment may add to stress. Stress also develops from the interface of work with the family, affecting women who earn wages insufficient for their family needs, have unshared home responsibilities, and perhaps feel social and personal pressure to stay at home.

Unless social and occupational causes of stress are controlled, stress-related illness and the resulting use of general health care and mental health services to treat it will continue.

Men have a shorter life expectancy than women. Whether women's labor force participation will level out the difference is an important question. Much depends on whether women's economic and social gains from working outweigh the spread of risky behavior among women as a means of coping with stresses of work and the nature of the work environment for each sex.

A Wisconsin study of 1974–1978 data shows that, for each major occupational grouping, men have higher age-specific death rates than women and that death rates of men and women within the work force are not more similar than in the general population. The sex differences are also maintained for each marital status grouping. These findings may be explained by men's concentration in more hazardous occupations and their longer exposure to work-related health risks and also by selection of the healthier women into the labor force in past years. If these circumstances change, the sex difference may eventually change too. A change in circumstances could be negative (if working women adopt less healthy personal practices) or positive (if men change their practices to protect their health, and/or if the worst features of the work environment are improved) (Passanante and Nathanson, 1987). Risky behavior seems to have increased among women who work. Working women appear to have more alcohol-related problems and a higher prevalence of smoking than homemakers (National Institute on Alcohol Abuse and Alcoholism, 1986). In a project at ten work sites in Minnesota, women had higher rates of smoking than men, but the occupational variation in smoking prevalence was the same for both. Men were more likely to have quit smoking (Sorenson and Pechacek, 1986). Interestingly, this runs counter to the general belief that women take better care of their health.

Disability from all causes is a problem for all adults of working age but somewhat more so for women. This is shown in 1984–1985 data from the Survey of Income and Program Participation on the percentage with functional limitations among persons 16 to 64. About 16 percent of women, compared with 13 percent of men, had difficulty performing specific activities of daily living, and the percentage of women with a severe limitation was also higher. Severe limitation, which means being unable to perform the activity at all or needing help from another person in order to perform it (U.S. Department of Commerce, 1986a, table B), sharply reduces labor force participation. Women had a higher rate than men (6.1 percent versus 4.4 percent) of disabilities severe enough to prevent a person from working at all (table D).

HEALTH COSTS BY EMPLOYMENT STATUS

Per capita direct costs of health care for working-age adults in 1980 were 28 percent higher for women than for men. Parsons et al. (1986) present cost figures by employment status, from which I have derived a female/male ratio.

For men, being full-time only part of the year or out of the labor force is related to health status, and this explains why the per capita costs are high for these two groups, especially the second. Among adults who are not in the labor force, men spend 54 percent more than women. But for women, poor health status is not necessarily the reason for less labor force participation. Childbirth and child care account for part-time and

Per Capita Direct Costs of Health Care, by Employment Status and Sex

Employment Status	Per Capita Direct Costs (in dollars)		Female/Male Ratio
	Male	Female	%
Full-time full-year	393	494	125.7
Full-time part-year	881	940	106.7
Part-time	581	706	121.5
Unemployed	802	1,076	134.2
Not in labor force	1,557	1,010	64.9
Total	607	778	128.2

part-year employment of many women (this is reflected in costs of pregnancy, as shown later). Part-time work of women has not been found to be associated with poor health (Herold and Waldron, 1985). Many women not in the labor force are full-time homemakers, rather than disabled.

Women in the labor force, who make up 39 percent of the working-age population, account for 39 percent of all direct costs of illness for working-age adults, whereas women outside the labor force, who make up another 13 percent of the working-age population, account for 19 percent of the total expense (Parsons et al., 1986, table J). Their extra spending is largely due to pregnancy-related care. Pregnancy and its complications, representing a mixture of well-person and illness care, cost $5.2 billion in 1980. This was 10.5 percent of all direct costs for men and women combined at ages 17–44,[2] making pregnancy the second leading condition, after injury and poisoning, for that age group.

The five leading diagnostic categories in the total health care bill of working-age adults (17–64) account for 49.9 percent of total direct costs for this age group, or $41.8 billion (Parsons et al., 1986, p. 19). None of these conditions is sex-specific. The first is injury and poisoning (13.5 percent of costs), followed by circulatory problems (10.9 percent), musculoskeletal problems (9.2 percent), genitourinary problems (8.2 percent), and digestive problems (8.1 percent). These diagnoses generate fairly similar aggregate costs for men and women at all ages, except for genitourinary care (men's costs are only 34 percent of those for women).

The direct costs of illness serve as a measure of the financial demands that must be met either out of pocket or through third parties. If there are gaps in population coverage under insurance or if benefits are inadequate, the worker's economic well-being is, and health outcomes may be, adversely affected. Desiring healthy workers, employers nevertheless

---

[2]This may be an underestimate since normal pregnancy was sometimes recorded as "no condition on admission" (Parsons et al., 1986, p. 17).

have a strong incentive to control their premium costs by cost shifting to employees. Thus, there is conflict between the objectives of the different parties, although redeploying health care resources so as to improve health without increasing outlays of either consumers or employers remains an attractive ideal.

References

American Civil Liberties Union. *Civil Liberties.* (Summer 1987).

Bergmann, Barbara, J. *The Economic Emergence of Women.* New York: Basic Books, 1986.

Brandwein, Ruth A. "Time Widens Male–Female Earnings Disparity" (Letter). *New York Times,* 27 September 1987.

Brunt, Melanie, and Andrea Hricko. "Problems Faced by Women Workers." In *Occupational Health: Recognizing and Preventing Work-Related Disease,* edited by Barry S. Levy and David W. Wegman. Boston: Little Brown & Co., 1983, 403–416.

Bureau of National Affairs. *Working Women's Health Concerns: A Gender at Risk?* A BNA Special Report. Washington, DC, 1989.

Collins, John Gary, and Owen T. Thornberry. *Health Characteristics of Workers by Occupation and Sex: United States, 1983–85.* NCHS Advance Data No. 168. Hyattsville MD: U.S. Department of Health and Human Services, Public Health Service, April 25, 1989.

Gemson, Donald H. Letter. *New England Journal of Medicine,* vol. 316, no. 12 (March 19, 1987): 752–753.

Goldin, Claudia. *An Economic History of American Women and Their Families.* National Bureau of Economic Research Monograph. New York: Oxford University Press, 1989.

Herold, Joan, and Ingrid Waldron. "Part-Time Employment and Women's Health." *Journal of Occupational Medicine,* vol. 27, no. 6 (June 1985): 405–412.

Last, John M. *Public Health and Human Ecology.* East Norwalk, CT: Appleton and Lange, 1987.

Lindbohm, Marja-Liisa, Helena Taskinen, and Karl Hemminki. "Reproductive Health of Working Women: Spontaneous Abortions and Congenital Malformations." *Public Health Reviews* (1985): 13, 55–87.

Marriott, Ian A., and Maria A. Stuckly. "Health Aspects of Work with Visual Display Terminals." *Journal of Occupational Medicine,* vol. 28, no. 29 (September 1986): 833–848.

Mergler, Donna, Carole Brabani, Nicole Vezina, and Karen Messing. "The Weaker Sex? Men in Women's Working Conditions Report Similar Health Symptoms." *Journal of Occupational Medicine,* vol. 29, no. 5 (May 1987): 417–421.

Muller, Charlotte. "Health and Health Care of Employed Adults: Occupation and Gender." *Women & Health,* vol. 11, no. 1 (Spring 1986): 27–46.

National Center for Health Statistics. "Births, Marriages, Divorce and Deaths for July 1987." *NCHS Monthly Vital Statistics Report,* vol. 36, no. 7 (October 8, 1987), Hyattsville, MD.

National Institute on Alcohol Abuse and Alcoholism. *Alcohol Health and Research Worlds,* vol. 5, no. 4 (Summer 1981): 37–38. "Women, Health Insurance and Alcoholism," remarks by Sandra S. Steinberger and Helen Drew.

———. *Women and Alcohol: Health-Related Issues.* Research Monograph No. 16. DHHS Pub. No. (ADM) 86-1139. Rockville, MD, 1986.

NBER Digest, National Bureau of Economic Research, March 1985.

New York Times, 19 June 1988, IV, 28:5. "Working Mothers."

Parsons, P. Ellen, Richard Lichtenstein, S. E. Berki, Hilary A. Murt, et al. *Costs of Illness: United States, 1980.* NCHSR, NMCUES Series C, Analytical Report No. 3. DHHS Pub. No. 86-20403. Hyattsville, MD: National Center for Health Statistics, April 1986.

Passanante, M.R.C., and C.A. Nathanson. "Women in the Labor Force: Are Sex Mortality Differentials Changing?" *Journal of Occupational Medicine,* vol. 29, no. 1 (January 1987): 21–28.

Pratt, William F., and Marjorie C. Horn. *Wanted and Unwanted Childbearing: United States 1973–82.* Advance Data No. 108. Hyattsville, MD: National Center for Health Statistics. May 9, 1985.

Rosenberg, Martin J., Paul J. Feldbaum, and Elizabeth G. Marshall. "Occupational Influences on Reproduction: A Review of Recent Literature." *Journal of Occupational Medicine,* vol. 29, no. 7 (July 1987): 584–591.

Rosenwaks, Zev, Fred Benjamin, and Martin L. Stone, eds. *Gynecology, Principles and Practice.* New York: Macmillan Publishing Co., 1987.

Selikoff, Irving J. "Constraints in Estimating Occupational Contributions to Current Cancer Mortality in the United States." In *Banbury Report 9: Quantification of Occupational Cancer.* Cold Spring Harbor, NY: Cold Spring Harbor Laboratory, 1981.

Silk, Leonard. "Women Gain but at a Cost." *New York Times,* 6 February 1987.

Sorenson, Gloria, and Terry Pechacek. "Occupational and Sex Differences in Smoking and Smoking Cessation." *Journal of Occupational Medicine,* vol. 28, no. 5 (May 1986): 360–364.

Tannenbaum, Terry N., and Robert J. Goldberg. "Exposure to Anesthetic Gases and Reproductive Outcome: A Review of the Epidemiologic Literature." *Journal of Occupational Medicine,* vol. 27, no. 9 (September 1985): 659–668.

U.S. Department of Commerce, Bureau of the Census. "Current Population Reports, Household Economic Studies." In *Disability, Functional Limitation, and Health Insurance Coverage: 1984/85.* Series P-70, No. 8. Washington, DC, December, 1986a.

————. *Statistical Abstract of the United States.* 1987 (107th ed.). Washington, DC, 1986b.

————. *Statistical Abstract of the United States.* 1988 (108th ed.). Washington, DC, 1987.

U.S. Department of Health and Human Services, Public Health Service, Human Resources and Services Administration. *Health Status of Minorities and Low Income Groups.* DHHS Pub. No. (HRSA) HRS-P-DV 85-1. Washington, DC: U.S. Government Printing Office, 1985.

————. Public Health Service, Office of Disease Prevention and Health Promotion. *Prevention '86/'87: Federal Programs and Progress.* Washington, DC, 1987.

Venning, P. J. "Time-Off Patterns for Back Injuries in Nurses." In *Trends in Ergonomic/Human Factors IV,* edited by S. S. Asfour. Amsterdam, Holland: Elsevier–North Holland, 1987, 875–882.

Venning, Penelope J., Stephen D. Walker, and Lawrence W. Stitt. "Personal and Job-Related Factors." *Journal of Occupational Health,* vol. 29, no. 10 (October 1987): 820–825.

CHAPTER FOUR

Health Care, the Workplace, and Gender: Insurance and Financing Issues

MANY OF THE HEALTH care coverage problems of employed women are aspects of poverty. The employed poor are often uninsured. They do not have employers who are committed to contributing to group health insurance, and they do not have funds to pay for individual insurance, which is more costly. Yet most do not qualify for Medicaid because their earned income is higher than the low standard of eligibility in many states. Their health problems and need for care have been demonstrated, yet they obtain less care than those with coverage.

A more general, structural problem is related to changes in women's work and family life. Coverage of women for health care through an employed husband was an accepted pattern when women were primarily homemakers, but this became less appropriate as women became permanent members of the labor force and as more women maintained independent households without a spouse. Independent coverage, benefit content and duplication, and cost sharing are issues that affect women differently in different family situations. Employers have expanded their use of peripheral or contingent workers who have few or no benefit entitlements, drawing on a largely female labor supply. It is not feasible to count on workplace arrangements as the social instrument for protecting individuals against health care costs. The socioeconomic structure of health care financing is in disequilibrium, and change is needed to attain equity.

Insurance and Use of Care

Many studies have shown that, if people have any insurance, and if they have more comprehensive insurance, receipt of physicians' services is less dependent on ability to pay (Muller, 1986b). Use of both treatment and prevention services is affected. Pregnant women are more likely to obtain early prenatal care if insured, and the severely disabled use more physician and hospital service if they are insured (Cooney, 1985; Social Security Administration, 1981). Cost-sharing provisions are known to be a deterrent to use of care.

My previous studies analyzing utilization by both working men, compared with women, and working women, compared with homemakers, have shown that having insurance increases both the recency of doctors' visits (seeing the doctor within the past year) and the probability of hospitalization. For working women and homemakers, however, insurance reduced the number of visits for those with visits. Very likely seeing the doctor more promptly (with the aid of insurance) reduced the total number of visits needed to manage an illness (Muller, 1986a).

The effect of insurance on the amount of care received in fee-for-service practice has been studied by Farley (1986b) using NMCES data. Conditions of varying urgency, but specific to women, are among those selected for study. She found the effect to vary with the urgency of the need, as indicated by the type of condition. In the analysis, only persons who made one or more visits for the condition were included; thus, those lacking *any* medical care for a condition were not studied. In hypertension, office visits serve a basically preventive purpose, and having insurance (first-dollar coverage) was found to affect the number of visits. But in gynecological and urinary tract infections, insurance had no effect on treatment, and only health status was significant. In menstrual disorders, conditions that are less well defined and less urgent than infections, insurance did have an effect. Income had a separate effect on visit content (number of tests) and total charge per visit, an indicator of either more services or more complex services, for more serious gynecological conditions and for other severe illnesses (such as heart problems and hernia). Thus, the possession of insurance influences the number of visits in the less urgent situations and perhaps (as in menstrual disorders) in those where patients are not necessarily confident that medicine offers a solution. Without insurance, problems requiring much service would cause an economic burden, and the amount of care received would be dependent on income.

In 1977, women, who made up 45.4 percent of the labor force of 100 million, were also slightly under half of the 13.7 million with no private insurance. But many of the women without private insurance were eligible for Medicaid, a program for persons with low incomes, because they received Aid to Families with Dependent Children (AFDC), and, therefore, women numbered 51.7 percent of those with public insurance during all or part of the year. This meant that women were only 40.6 percent of those uninsured all year. Women's advantage, however, is limited. Medicaid coverage is sometimes held for only part of the year, it is variable across states, and Medicaid eligibles frequently do not have access to mainstream providers.[1] According to Monheit et al. (1985), the employed uninsured generally were not offered coverage through their employment and, therefore, we can conclude that those who obtained Medicaid did so out of necessity, not out of choice.

Employer or union contributions to premiums are the key to group health coverage through the workplace. Overall, in 1980 there were 49.0 million households with one or more workers covered by a group health plan paid at least in part by the employer or the union, and these constituted 57 percent of all households; for householders under 65 years of age, 69 percent had one or more members covered (U.S. Department of Commerce, 1985). Figures on employer or union contributions are available by sex of worker. In 1980, of the 58.4 million males age 15 and over with wage and salary income, 38.2 million had an employer or a union that paid all or some of the cost; and, of the 50.1 million female workers, 24.9 million had an outside contribution. Thus, overall, 65.4 percent of male workers, but only 49.7 percent of female workers, had some employer or union contribution. The entire cost was paid for only 29.6 percent of the men and even less of the women, 22.9 percent.

Almost two-thirds of employed persons are householders or spouses of householders. For these groups, there are sex differences in coverage through employers or unions.

Among male householders (34.6 million men), 77 percent had an employer or a union contribution, but only 55 percent of female householders (over 7 million women) did. Only 49 percent of women who were spouses of householders (25 million women) had sponsored coverage, versus 66 percent of men (1.8 million men). Among other family statuses, percentages with coverage were similar for men and women: about 30 percent for relatives of the householder other than the spouse (about 13 million men and 9.5 million women), which would include young

---

[1]Coverage of pregnant women in Medicaid has been improved by the Medicare Catastrophic Coverage Act of 1988, which mandates coverage for those at or below 100 percent of the poverty level until the end of the month in which the sixty-day postpartum period ends. This does not, however, change the absence of stable coverage over time.

adult children living in the parental home (who might be covered by a parent's policy), and about 66 percent for unrelated individuals, who numbered about 9 million men and 8 million women (U.S. Department of Commerce, 1985). Unrelated individuals of both sexes had a sponsored coverage rate similar to that of male householders.

Perman and Stevens (1989) report that married men have a coverage rate 19 percent higher than married women. They suggest that some married women choose jobs without employer-financed coverage, knowing that their husbands' policies cover them. But another reason for the sex difference may be that the geographical constraints on the job choices of many married women enable their employers to avoid offering coverage without losing their labor supply.

Currently, married employed women often have the protection of a spouse's plan whose benefits are better than those available through their own employer and equal to those of employed men. Yet there is a distinct reduction in their economic independence from their spouses when their direct coverage is inadequate, and this increases the risk of inequality in the marriage relationship.

Single women do not have access to a spouse's benefit package, and many married women may be at risk of losing coverage through divorce because of the current high rates of divorce. The hardship created thereby is intensified by relatively high rates of utilization and low health status among divorced women (Berk and Taylor, 1983). Loss of coverage through divorce is a bigger problem for nonemployed women, only 32 percent of whom have private insurance, compared with 77 percent of those who are employed. Yet, even for those in the labor force, divorced women are more likely to receive Medicaid benefits (usually received by those without private coverage) than married women. Under the Consolidated Omnibus Budget Reconciliation Act of 1985, employers of twenty or more employees are required to offer continuation coverage to employees' former spouses, but the latter must pay the employer's share of the premium as well as the employee's share. This imposes a sizable, sometimes prohibitive, cost on individuals (Equitable HCA Corporation, April 1986). Some states also mandate continued coverage after divorce or separation; in at least one case, Maryland, the employed spouse must pay the entire cost for the divorced spouse and dependent children (Equitable HCA Corporation, June 1987). Thus, the problem caused by having coverage depend on marriage to a member of a group health plan is recognized but not generally resolved.

The government's 1980 figures show the number of workers covered by a group health plan paid at least in part by an employer or a union in relation to each of eight different socioeconomic characteristics: region, metropolitan versus nonmetropolitan residence, age, full- versus part-time work, occupation, industry, race, and relation to the householder. The sex difference is quite persistent, although its size varies across categories, and there are certain exceptions.\First, mining is the one industry in which men and women have employer-sponsored coverage equally often.(Second, the percentage of black males with an employer or a union contribution is low (it is only 46 percent, compared with 56 percent for white males), and, therefore, the sex difference for blacks is only 4 percentage points, whereas for whites it is 16 percentage points. A third exception involves part-time workers, very few of whom, male or female, have other parties picking up some or all of the premium cost. The large restaurant chain, McDonald's, has no health coverage at all for part-time employees but offers a package of benefits for a small nucleus of full-time employees (Warshaw, 1987).

The statistics do not consider occupation and industry effects together. Perman and Stevens do. They argue that it is industry that ultimately makes the difference, but for a special reason. Occupational segregation by sex results in women's being concentrated in industries with less likelihood of coverage, as inferred from lower benefit outlays. Their proof is that the sex gap in proportions covered disappears after controlling for industry, whereas the gap remains after controlling for occupation. The gap is much greater in nondurable manufacturing, retail trade, and service, fields in which over half of all women with jobs in private industry are employed, than in other fields.

Peripheral Workers As a Less-covered Class

Part-time work has long been a feature of labor force activity, but its form has shifted with a decline in part-year (largely seasonal) work and a rise in other forms of partial employment. The overall proportion of part-time employment has risen in recent decades, as shown in table 4.1.

Women are much less likely than men to be year-round, full-time employees. Table 4.2 shows that full-time, full-year employees are two-thirds of all male workers age 15+ but about half of all female workers. The proportion for each sex varies by occupation. In terms of absolute numbers, women who work part-time, part-year, or both are concentrated in nonhousehold service, administrative support, and sales (18,745,000 women); men who work less than full-time are concentrated in precision production, nonhousehold service, and farming (18,037,000 men) (U.S. Department of Commerce, 1986).

For both sexes, there is a sharp drop in the proportion with sponsored health benefits, as one compares full-time with part-time (defined as un-

TABLE 4.1
Percentage of Those Who Worked During Year
in Full-time and Part-time Employment

Type of Employment	Both Sexes	
	1950	1983
Full-time, total	84.5	77.1
50–52 weeks	55.7	56.8
27–49 weeks	17.4	11.1
1–26 weeks	11.6	9.2
Part-time, total	15.5	22.9
50–52 weeks	4.8	8.8
27–49 weeks	3.2	5.3
1–26 weeks	7.5	8.9

Source: U.S. Department of Labor, Bureau of Labor Statistics, *Handbook of Labor Statistics*, 1985.

der 35 hours a week during most of the weeks the person works in the year): from 73.8 percent down to 15.7 percent for men and from 65.7 percent to 16.6 percent for women. But lack of coverage in part-time work affects more women because of their greater probability of being part-time employees.

A category of peripheral employment that often overlaps with part-time work is home-based work. Many women have made themselves available for homework, as a practical means of combining child care with paid work. Hired to meet a firm's peak demands for administrative and clerical work, homeworkers usually become independent contractors, rather than salaried employees, and are excluded from benefit plans. This gives the employer a lean payroll but makes the worker the risk taker for health needs (Christensen, 1986), unless there is an employed spouse with family benefits.

Part-time and temporary employees and homeworkers, many of whom do not have as steady employment as they wish but are not able to collect unemployment insurance, are particularly disadvantaged by their lack of health coverage if they incur health care costs during spells of unemployment and reduced income.

Given the expansion of peripheral labor, it is more difficult to secure a socially desirable floor of benefits for all when coverage is not mandated for part-time and temporary workers or special pools are not established for them. Legislation with such purposes has begun to appear (Equitable HCA Corporation, November 1987). The state of New Hampshire now requires insurers to include part-time workers in group health insurance if they work at least half of the weekly hours of full-time employees and at least fifteen hours per week. But the State Insurance Department has interpreted this to mean that the carrier must offer the coverage to the master policyholder, that is, the employer (Equitable HCA Corporation, June 1987), which does not assure that the employer will, in turn, offer the coverage to part-time employees. A program passed by the state of Washington set up a Basic Health Plan for the uninsured under 65, with a choice of two prepaid "managed care systems" with premiums and copayments based on ability to pay (American Public Health Association, 1987). A provision introduced by Representative Pete Stark in a budget reconciliation bill in 1987 encouraged states to set up risk pools for the uninsured. Employers with twenty or more employees would have to participate or pay an excise tax of 5 percent of payroll. But the pools could charge up to 150 percent of the average premium on standard individual policies issued in the state (Equitable HCA Corporation, November 1987). The risk pool was deleted from the Omnibus Budget Reconciliation Act of 1987 (Equitable HCA Corporation, February 1988), but it was expected to reappear in future bills. Health insurance companies have begun to advocate federal and state laws that will make it easier for employees of smaller firms to become insured and will provide pools to cover persons with expensive illnesses (cancer and AIDS) rather than permitting their exclusion (Freudenheim, 1990).

If the cost of using a contingent labor force increases, employers could shift clerical and light assembly operations to offshore locations, but activities involving one-to-one services are not amenable to a shift to outside the United States. However, substitution of capital-intensive technology for labor is always a possibility; the problem of assuring coverage for contingent workers through the job will not be solved if the job disappears. Only universal coverage not dependent on a particular labor force affiliation would avoid such difficulties.

Quality of Coverage Through Employment

When, in wage determination, whether done unilaterally by employers or through collective bargaining, health insurance is provided as a wage supplement, its value to employees consists not only in nontaxation of services received as personal income but also in the benefit to each employee of pooling risk in a large group in a given year. Fringe benefits financed by employer contributions tend to be better in industries, occupations, and firms where wages and salaries are high. Sex typing of jobs and sex discrimination in employment, where they exist, affect health benefits provided to employed women.

TABLE 4.2
Full-time and Part-time Workers, by Occupation, 1985
(In Thousands)

Occupation Group	All Workers	Year-Round Full-Time	Part-Time or Part-Year or Both	Perce. Year-R Full-?
A. WOMEN				
Executive, administrative, and managerial	4,792	3,534	1,256	73
Professional specialty	7,691	4,331	3,360	56
Technical and related support	1,624	1,010	614	62
Sales	7,864	2,714	5,148	34.
Administrative support including clerical	15,858	9,120	6,738	57
Precision production, craft, and repair	1,323	753	570	56.
Machine operators, assemblers, and inspectors	3,700	1,948	1,752	52.
Transportation and material moving	479	127	352	26.
Handlers, equipment cleaners, etc.	935	326	609	34.
Service workers				
Private household	1,358	182	1,172	13.
Other	10,020	3,161	6,859	31.
Farming, forestry, and fishing	654	172	482	26.
Total	56,296	27,383	28,913	48.

Women who work full-time are disproportionately concentrated, compared with men, in low-paying industries and occupations. Firms with a high proportion of low-wage workers are less apt to provide much by way of health benefits (Rossiter and Taylor, 1982). In the poorer plans, a larger share of the premium comes from the employee, and the employer contributes little or nothing to the coverage of dependents of the employee. Premium outlays and employer contributions are less for firms with a large proportion of part-time workers and for firms in service and trade. These are "markers" for a female presence.

The tax law passed by Congress in 1986 made continuation of the tax privileges of health plan benefits for higher-paid employees of a firm dependent on the firm's offering nondiscriminatory coverage to lower-paid and part-time employees. But the implementation of the plan for nationwide employers with a mix of ages, retirees, and active workers, and

TABLE 4.2 (continued)

Occupation Group	All Workers	Year-Round Full-Time	Part-Time or Part-Year or Both	Percentage Year-Round Full-Time
B. MEN				
Executive, administrative, and managerial	8,300	7,110	1,190	85.7
Professional specialty	7,225	5,652	1,573	78.2
Technical and related support	1,894	1,455	439	76.8
Sales	7,236	5,243	1,993	72.5
Administrative support including clerical	3,858	2,719	1,139	70.5
Precision production, craft, and repair	13,567	9,214	4,353	67.9
Machine operators, assemblers, and inspectors	5,267	3,577	1,690	67.9
Transportation and material moving	4,617	2,883	1,734	62.4
Handlers, equipment cleaners, etc.	4,807	1,901	2,906	39.5
Service workers				
Private household	64	3	61	4.7
Other	7,060	3,458	3,602	49.0
Farming, forestry, and fishing	3,776	1,649	2,127	43.7
Total	67,809	44,943	22,866	66.3

Source: U.S. Department of Commerce, Bureau of the Census, *Statistical Abstract of the United States, 1987.* (107th ed.) (Washington, DC, 1986), table 681.

facing local diversity of HMOs and Preferred Provider Organizations, remained problematic (Freudenheim, 1986). Some employers are expected to substitute salary increases for upper-level employees for benefits, rather than to expand benefits to lower-level staff.

I noted earlier that an employed woman who is married may have better benefits through her spouse's plan than through her own. Whether or not this is so, the benefit package she gets through her own employer may duplicate benefits to which she is entitled through her husband. But she is not necessarily able to redirect the employer contribution, or her own, to such services as prevention and day care that would be more useful to her. Some employers have addressed this problem by adopting flexible benefits, or "cafeteria" plans, which permit employees to choose among health care, child care, pensions, and so forth. Employers may restrict such options to certain categories of workers, and, in selecting the level of benefit, salary class is the leading criterion used (Mercer-Meidinger, 1986). While these rules limit the value obtained by lower-income workers, the general idea is a good one.

Current concern with costs of health care may have special implications for working women. The Consolidated Omnibus Budget Reconciliation Act of 1985 held down government liabilities by making Medicare the second payer for all employed eligible persons. This is one of several sources of recent financial pressure on employers (Equitable HCA Corporation, May 1986). In response, they have sometimes ceased their previous contributions to dependents' coverage and have introduced many other changes (short of simple cancellation) in benefit plans to control their financial outlays. Such changes often involve new or increased cost sharing by employees, in the form of payment toward premiums, deductibles that must be satisfied annually before the insurance is applicable, and copayment for services received. A 1986 survey showed that 91 percent of employer health plans had deductibles, 40 percent of which were $150 or more; 63 percent required coinsurance for inpatient hospital care, and 72 percent required it for surgery; 41 percent required an employee contribution toward premiums; and only 30 percent paid the full cost of family coverage. Nine-tenths of the plans had raised deductibles in the previous four years. Employers whose work force was largely female required higher contributions for dependent coverage (47 percent of the premium for those with 60 percent or more female, as compared with 31 percent of the premium for firms with less than 60 percent female) (Johnson and Higgins, 1986).

In relation to the total burden of health care costs on individuals, employer contributions to premiums are less significant than they used to be because copayments imposed by employers reduce the share of total benefit costs met through premiums. A more sensitive measure of third party support is the percentage of the health care bill met by insurance. The low proportion of private consumer expenditures on health care met by insurance—only 53 percent in 1984 (U.S. Department of Commerce, 1986, p. 98)—comes from the growth of employer cost controls, as well as the uninsured. It represents the weakened efficacy of insurance as a device for financing health care, as cost controls shift part of the burden to consumers. The health care bill that employers attempted to keep down arose from several causes whose relative importance continues to be debated: heavy administrative costs of claim-based financing in fee-for-service medicine; overperformance by physicians seeking to maximize revenue; utilization necessitated by deficient quality of care; and unneeded service patterns entrenched by provider habit, such as the routine battery of admission tests. The incidence of illness triggering utilization and expense is also affected by past and present failure to cover preventive services. Lack of restraint on the part of covered consumers has often been blamed as well, reasoning from the public's enhanced expectations about medicine's potential and increased use by those with low out-of-pocket cost because of insurance. But time constraints and the unpleasantness of certain processes act as deterrents to discretionary utilization, suggesting that, when financial deterrents are imposed, they may cut into needed, nondiscretionary care, as, indeed, research has shown to be the case.

Although deductibles and other cost-sharing provisions tend to be uniform across classes of employees within a firm, the burden of out-of-pocket payments is greater for low-income workers. A $200 deductible means more sacrifice of other consumer needs for a worker earning under $20,000 than for one earning $50,000. When a sex wage gap exists, women are more burdened by health care expenses than men, particularly since they tend to use more care. Women's use of hospital care, measured in days per 1,000 population in 1986 for persons age 15 and over, was 44 percent greater than men's (National Center for Health Statistics, 1987), and their use of physician services in 1980, measured in visits per person per year, was higher than men's in all age groups over 15 (McLemore and Koch, 1982). There is a similar regressive effect for stop-loss provisions: 94 percent of plans with an employee stop-loss (out-of-pocket) maximum have the same maximum for all employees (Johnson and Higgins, 1986). The low-income workers must spend a higher proportion of their income in order to benefit if the cap is uniform.

FERTILITY-RELATED CARE

Maternity

Women make far greater use than men of reproductive, or fertility-related, services, and such care is increasingly a concern for employed women. Even in the early 1970s, work during pregnancy was widespread. Over two-fifths of the 3 million women who had a live birth in a 12-month period, 1972–1973, worked at some time during pregnancy. Over half of these women were under 25, and the likelihood of working while pregnant was higher for nonwhites (National Center for Health Statistics, 1977). Many of these women left the labor force for extended periods as the time of delivery approached, but they do so less frequently today. In the June 1987 survey by the Census Bureau, among women with a live birth in the preceding year, 51 percent were in the labor force, compared with 31 percent in June 1976 (*New York Times,* 19 June 1988).

Pregnancy care frequently involves expensive, high-technology services (see chapter 7, on reproductive care). These are often complements of, rather than substitutes for, regular prenatal care, since procedures such as ultrasound, amniocentesis, and, more recently, chorionic villus sampling are done to identify problems that would affect clinical decisions (including pregnancy termination).[2] As more women are now having first births in their thirties and even after age thirty-five, the prevalence of chronic conditions that could affect a pregnancy is increasing. There is more risk of miscarriage and stillbirth, and older women have an increased interest in skilled management of their pregnancy through a physician and hospital model, rather than through midwives as attendants and birthing centers or homes as the delivery sites. They may also be rejected by alternative birthing centers if they apply (Fay and Smith, 1985).

While older women may be seeking motherhood, the orderly development of careers (and family formation) of younger women is obstructed by unplanned adolescent pregnancy. A variety of interventions have been used to help adolescents avoid untimely pregnancy and to improve pregnancy outcomes and parenting skills if they do become pregnant. These programs are usually not financed through the workplace, either because the younger women involved are not yet in the labor force or because, lacking skills, they hold the least advantaged jobs. (Some, however, may be served under employed parents' policies.) Generally, low-income adolescents need a spectrum of social and medical services to deal with the problems generated by ill-timed and unwanted fertility.

Federal legislation of 1978 obliged employers to discontinue provisions for pregnancy-related health services that were more restrictive than those applicable to other health care in a group plan, and this was an important step toward equality of the sexes in the workplace.

Before that time, the history of maternity benefits in group insurance reveals sustained differential treatment of reproductive services. I have studied board minutes and other archival materials of the New York City "Blue" plans spanning a fifty-year period to see what happened to maternity benefits and why (Muller, 1989). In New York City's major nonprofit health insurance plan, maternity was less adequately covered than other conditions, including those that occur in men only, for many

---

[2]The enhanced protocol may be cost-effective if high-risk deliveries and poor fetal outcomes are averted.

years. Family policies were required for maternity coverage, a special waiting period was imposed, and payment was on an indemnity basis (partial reimbursement) instead of meeting the full cost of service. This last restriction was especially important for in-hospital care. Benefits were later modified so that coverage for complications of pregnancy was similar to that for nonmaternity illness. However, this applied only after the termination of the pregnancy. In addition, "false labor" days were deducted from the total days allowed for maternity. These restrictions further contributed to the discriminatory and inferior position of maternity benefits until laws of the 1970s mandated equality with other conditions.[3]

A blend of factors sustained the special provisions for maternity. The Blue plans adhered to the casualty insurance philosophy, rather than to a goal of covering noncatastrophic health needs and prevention in particular. This stance was in accord with the separation of prevention (public health agencies) from treatment (private practice sector), a split that was preferred by fee-for-service practitioners and the voluntary hospitals, which by and large accommodated the interests of the physicians affiliated with them. The connection between prevention and reduction of eventual social costs, both direct and indirect, was largely lost from view outside the realm of communicable disease. Nonprofit insurance operated as part of a system in which it advanced the objectives of the nonprofit hospitals used by private physicians as their workshops, and this limited funds available for benefit expansion.

But the limitation of maternity benefits requires further explanation. The governance of nonprofit insurance firms was not broadly representative of the community but favored providers, and women had little voice. As the specialty of obstetrics grew and controlled a market whose size was sustained by a high birthrate, providers improved their earnings. They did not challenge the restricted maternity coverage. This implied that outside economic and political influences (employed groups and regulation) would have to be the bearers of change. But labor's economic and bargaining difficulties in the New York market restricted its choices of alternatives (such as organizing its own delivery system), and employed groups that were predominantly male did not, for the most part, make equal maternity coverage a key issue in their negotiations for health benefits. The state regulatory body, the Insurance Department, often resisted the pass-through of predicted costs of benefit expansion into premiums, although it did not attempt to regulate the pass-through

---

[3]A New York State law of 1976, the Donovan Act, required insurers to provide maternity benefits equal to benefits for other conditions.

of hospital costs in the retrospective reimbursement system. In the circumstances, it was possible for the plan leadership to avoid responding to expressions of subscriber preference for improved maternity benefits.

A full benefit, which was of interest to women for health and economic reasons and as a symbol of equality, was not attained by voluntary adaptation. Blue plan leaders did not defend the differential treatment with an overt philosophy regarding women, but the issue was repeatedly given low priority in the context of the objectives and constraints that determined the actions of decision makers. Women's general position in society strongly influenced the results.

Most workers in the United States have long had some maternity benefits through employment. In 1977, 87.4 percent of the privately insured under 65 and 89.2 percent of women age 15–44 had some maternity benefit. But only 79.6 percent of these women had any coverage for normal pregnancy; for cesareans, 74.3 percent had hospital coverage and 61.9 percent had physician coverage (Farley, 1986b). Combining these data with 1978–1979 data showing some health coverage for 88 percent of the 97 million employees in the United States (Rossiter and Taylor, 1982), we find that about 70 percent of women in the nation had any coverage for normal pregnancy (88 percent × 79.6 percent).

Protection for normal delivery was less than for other disabilities. For hospital stays, either the covered period was shorter or the benefit was limited to a lump sum, and higher deductibles were imposed. (The Blue plans usually gave shorter regular benefits, and commercial carriers often gave a lump sum.) Only half of women of childbearing age (15–44) who had benefits for normal delivery were fully covered for a semiprivate room without a limit on the days of care. About three-fifths of those with benefits for the physician's delivery fee were insured for the full usual/customary/reasonable charge, 12 percent had partial coverage, and most of the rest were reimbursed according to a fee schedule allowing less than $500. Either a waiting period for maternity or enrollment at the time of conception was required by plans covering four-fifths of insured women of childbearing age. Some women employees had to buy dependent coverage to be insured for maternity (Farley, 1986b).

Maternity benefits were more often found in collectively bargained plans than in employer-created plans, and in Blue plans, rather than in commercial plans (Kittner, 1978). For many women, however, absence of any health insurance, not specific discrimination against maternity, was the access-limiting problem. But it could not be linked to unequal treatment in comparison with male employees within a given health plan of a given firm and, therefore, was not affected by civil rights laws.

Even after the Pregnancy Discrimination Act of 1978, conceptions prior to the date of entitlement to group health benefits were still excluded from coverage in plans that denied benefits to preexisting conditions. Restrictions on preexisting conditions are facially sex-neutral, but they were expected by insurers to have the same effect on maternity claims as the previous waiting period specifically for pregnancy.

According to Bundy (1985), the percentage of insured employees with maternity protection for themselves or their spouses rose to 89 percent after the Pregnancy Discrimination Act. However, there are some gaps. The act is restricted to employers who have 15 or more full-time employees and already offer insurance to their workers. Furthermore, compliance is reported to decrease as firm size goes down, to a low of 55 percent in firms of 15 to 100 employees. Some states have passed similar laws covering employers with under 15 employees (U.S. Department of Labor, 1987).

Bergstahler (1984) studied the effects of the act on employer health insurance benefit levels in Iowa firms that offered a full range of health benefits. Before the 1978 law, Iowa, like eleven other states, merely required that benefits for pregnancy complications, for female employees and wives and daughters of male employees, be on a par with those for other illnesses. Plans from Missouri and Indiana, states that had no insurance requirements for pregnancy before 1978, were compared with the Iowa plans.

Before the act, none of the plans had treated pregnancy equally with other conditions in either basic or major medical benefits, but all the Iowa plans went beyond their state law by covering normal pregnancy at all.

After the act, there were no changes in general benefit levels, and no firms shifted costs to employees either by converting employer-financed plans into contributory ones or by changing the copayments under major medical insurance. Changes were, however, made that limited care for conceptions prior to entitlement and jeopardized delivery coverage in high-risk cases where the women had to leave work before the third trimester (Bergstahler, 1984). Concurrent changes in the health care market in the late 1970s may have diverted the attention of carriers from making other changes to reduce their maternity costs.

The federal law of 1978 does not require employers to provide benefits for abortion, except for complications or where the mother's life would be endangered. But employers are not precluded from providing abortion benefits, and they may not fire or refuse to hire a woman because she has "exercised her right to have an abortion" (U.S. Department of Labor, 1980).

Whether a woman's reproductive system care is covered depends on the type of service she uses and the carrier's policies. As an example, in the government-wide indemnity plan for federal workers, administered by the Aetna Life Insurance Company, maternity coverage includes certified midwives and birthing centers, as well as sonograms, amniocentesis, and related tests. Waiting periods are prohibited by the federal program, and all eligible family members can get maternity benefits. Voluntary sterilization is covered, but artificial insemination, in vitro fertilization, and reversals of sterilization are not covered. Since conservative opposition to abortion and to use of federal funds for abortion resulted in eliminating abortion coverage from the Federal Employees Health Benefits Program, abortion is excluded from the Aetna plan unless the mother's life is in danger (Aetna Life and Casualty, 1987). Aetna policies for other employee groups do not have to exclude abortion and may differ in other respects from the federal employees' plan.

Abortion Coverage and Privacy

Abortion coverage expanded after several states legalized elective abortion in the late 1960s and the Supreme Court handed down its decision of 1973 protecting the right to abortion under the doctrine of privacy. Unmarried employees and unmarried minor dependents became eligible for maternity benefits (including abortion) under Blue plans. Following the federal lead, bills have been introduced in state legislatures that would exclude abortion from coverage in state and local employee plans supported by public funds (*Insight and Instatus*, 1986). A Rhode Island law to this effect was declared unconstitutional in 1985 by a U.S. district court (Charles D. Spencer and Associates, 1985, pp. 108–109).

Use of insurance to pay for abortions has been constrained, because privacy is impaired in the claim-filing process when it is administered wholly or in part by the firm or because employees are uncertain as to just how much disclosure filing a claim would entail, and they do not wish to ask. Even if the employer is informed by the carrier only of dollar amounts paid out for specific claimants in a given month, and not of the specific service, that may be more information than the claimant would wish the employer to have. "Unbundling" of insurance services by employers who now buy selected services from carriers makes internal administration more likely and increases the privacy problem for abortion.

Privacy was acknowledged as essential to individual autonomy in the 1973 Supreme Court decision on abortion and is recognized as an ethical element in the doctor–patient relationship; yet it has not been fully implemented in the financial administration of health benefits. This is important for women because of economic discrimination and the attitudes that support it. Since judgments about women's sexual, reproductive, and contraceptive behavior still influence the treatment they receive in the workplace, women may sacrifice financial benefits to protect their privacy and implicitly to safeguard their future on the job.

Insurance is rarely used as a payment source at clinics, where most abortions are performed. The clinics insist on cash at the time of service (Henshaw and Wallach, 1984). Yet most abortions are received by single women over twenty (Powell-Griner, 1987), most of whom are in the labor force and many of whom are covered by group insurance.

A special benefit for abortion was devised by the Social Service Employees Union Welfare Fund in New York City, one of the early funds to honor abortion claims after New York legalized abortion in 1970. The Health Insurance Plan of Greater New York (HIP), in which many of the union's members were enrolled, covered abortion only in hospitals at that time. The Welfare Fund set up a special benefit fund through which members and dependents could use a private practitioner for abortions and be reimbursed up to $200. Claims that identify the service received must be filed, but these are handled by the employee's union fund and do not involve the employer (the City of New York) (Social Service Employees Union Local 371, 1986). Women workers may perceive this as partial privacy; in any case the fund was continued, even though out-of-hospital abortions are now common in HIP (Pilson and Brown, 1987).

Stigmas, stereotypes, and privacy issues are not confined to women or abortion. The patient may be reluctant to file claims for mental and emotional disorders, alcoholism, and, more recently, AIDS and HIV infection. Despite legal protection of employment as handicapped workers, men who have AIDS or are HIV positive may be reluctant to use workplace benefits because of others' prejudice against a homosexual lifestyle, fear, and misinformation about AIDS.

The carrier (or employer) may be influenced by prevailing stereotypes in deciding what health conditions to cover (Johnson, 1987), especially if the problem is attributed to character and behavior. To illustrate from health insurance history, a 1938 report on group purchase of medical care by employers describes the limitations of benefits in the Allis-Chalmers Manufacturing Company as follows: "No cash benefits or medical service of any kind are given for disability resulting from venereal disease, disorderly conduct, excessive use of alcohol or narcotics, professional sports, or maternity cases" (Brown, 1938, p. 30). The public eventually accepted the insurability of services for mental illness and alcoholism; indeed, so many persons were willing to use insurance to pay for treatment that carriers typically limited the benefits to control claims cost. Yet mental health diagnoses remain underreported on insurance claims "due to fear of confidentiality" (Tsai, Reedy, and Bernacki, 1987). For alcoholism, women may be especially reluctant to use their benefits. The administrator of a professional workers' union benefit fund, which honors a number of claims for alcoholism treatment annually in a state where coverage is mandated (New York), reports that no claims are received from women (Frey and Giammusso, 1987). This could reflect denial by the person with the problem, lack of recognition of the problem by providers, gender-related shortcomings of treatment programs (see chapter 2), or avoidance of the insurance system when treatment is sought. It has been reported that alcoholism among women is undertreated, and privacy in use of insurance is a factor (National Institute on Alcohol Abuse and Alcoholism, 1986).

For reproductive health care, as in treatment for alcoholism and the like, women may feel a special concern for privacy because the work environment in which they decide whether to use their coverage for "sensitive" services may be perceived by them as discriminatory and is not free of stereotypes.

Privacy problems in connection with using group health insurance for abortion (and insurance coverage itself) may seem secondary in view of the onslaught on the constitutional right to have an abortion backed by the administration. However, it is not trivial, and it is connected to the current legal struggle. Public controversy will make many individuals hesitate to risk disclosure, even if the procedure is legal in their states. And opponents of abortion have targeted restrictions on insurance and financing as a method of eliminating elective abortion.

EMPLOYERS AND FAMILY NEEDS

An important question for society is whether employers can successfully reconcile the adaptation of workplace policies to the emerging needs of women and men in their family roles and the changes in the family with their own interest in controlling costs of health care and other benefits and protecting managerial prerogatives. Absent a legal requirement, both basic protection and the degree of innovation incorporated into benefit packages depend on where one works. Whether this is ultimately equitable depends on the degree of equality in choice of jobs.

So far as their core workers are concerned, employers' capacity for adaptation is shown by the evolution of specific programs and a mood of flexibility. Yet programs tailored to certain family or health situations may not be supported by workers with different needs unless there is a quid pro quo (New York Business Group on Health, 1987). Both employers acting unilaterally and unions planning their bargaining demands try to develop packages that will balance diverse interests, within the limits set by funds available and health care costs. But a costly, high-technology benefit that applies to a limited number, such as infertility treatment services, may be disputed, especially if an expanded concept of medical need or illness is involved.

The recent changes in the family and in work patterns have obliged employers to consider pregnancy-related and child-rearing issues. Working mothers are now over 60 percent of all wage-earning women, and, as noted earlier, women commonly work until shortly before delivery and return to work after a leave of limited duration. Single-parent households, whose heads have financial responsibility for children, have increased in number, and two-earner households have tied their living standards to continued work by wives. Teenagers who become pregnant are usually daughters of members of the labor force and may be covered for maternity under employee plans; hence, the prevention of unwanted teenage pregnancies may become a concern of plan managers. The productivity of women who delay childbearing while developing their careers through formal training and accumulation of experience is an asset to their employers. The era of dismissing women during their pregnancy seems to be closing, and there is a trend toward requiring employers to allow at least unpaid maternity leave with job security. It is argued that this will end patients' pressure on medical practitioners to supply evidence of disability to employers when the real reason for taking leave is psychosocial and is related to bonding, adjustment, and deferment of the double load borne by many working mothers.

Health care is involved in the reshaping of employer policies in several ways. Pregnancy is the most common reason for employee hospitalization, and even a normal delivery with a normal infant generates an average cost for hospital care alone of $2,378 (New York Business Group on Health, 1987). Reduction of risk through prenatal education covering nutrition, exercise, cessation of smoking, use of medication, and avoidance of stress has the potential to be cost-effective. On-site prenatal care, which can be offered in lunch hours or at the end of the day, and the alternative of sanctioning absences in working hours for prenatal care protect the pregnant woman against having to choose between medical care and job security. Family planning services fit into a family-oriented cluster of services.

If the employer adequately informs the health care provider of the health hazards of the job of an individual pregnant employee, the practitioner can make intelligent recommendations for continued work, job modification, or avoidance of a hazardous environment. (Whether these can be carried out depends on the woman's economic circumstances and bargaining strength—and informing the practitioner in the first place assumes an enlightened employer.) Cases wherein employers removed pregnant women and women of childbearing age from an environment that was hazardous to reproductive outcome became controversial because of the conflict with equal job opportunities for women. It was argued that blocking women from certain jobs within a firm based on assumptions concerning their family plans was paternalistic and that women should decide for themselves if they wished to take the risks of a given job. In addition, as awareness of work-related risks to men's reproductive health increased, policies addressed to women alone became viewed as one-sided, and removal of male or female workers from an area does not change the hazardous environment. After it was determined that there were risks of miscarriage in the manufacture of semiconductors, certain employers offered paid medical leave or a transfer but were reluctant to order a transfer (*Wall Street Journal*, 13 January 1987; 14 January 1987). But women in similar situations are trying to establish the right to a transfer. At least two courts have ruled that forcing pregnant X-ray technicians to leave their jobs is sex discrimination under Title VII of the Civil Rights Act (U.S. Department of Labor, 1987). The issue is difficult to resolve because employees even of the same sex may be dissimilar as to personal goals (including the value they place on their fertility and reproductive outcomes) and awareness of risks, and employers' goal of protecting employees and preventing liability suits may conflict with assuring production and avoiding major costs of changing the work environment.

The employer's role as a third-party payer of employee health care costs has stimulated employer-sponsored pregnancy-related programs that are beneficial to physical and psychological health and are expected to constrain the costs of high-risk births. These programs safeguard the health and morale of members of the permanent work force of a given employer. Unfortunately, they do nothing for the women who are less securely connected with a given employer.

Employer maternity leave policies affect health care. Disability leave provisions for maternity were protected against unequal treatment by the Pregnancy Discrimination Act of 1978. A woman receiving paid leave usually retains the right to group health insurance. If no paid leave is granted, the employee may lose her coverage while absent. Larger employers are reported to be more likely than smaller employers to grant a protected leave of eight or more weeks, but even among the larger firms the terms vary (New York Business Group on Health, 1987).

TABLE 4.3
Prevalence of Selected Reported Chronic Conditions, by Sex,
for Working-age Population, 1986

	Number of Conditions per 1,000 Persons			
	Male		Female	
	Under 45	*45–64*	*Under 45*	*45–64*
Arthritis	24.7	218.7	35.7	344.7
Orthopedic impairments				
Back	44.9	101.6	69.2	83.2
Lower extremities	45.8	83.1	28.9	57.7
Hearing impairments	45.0	180.0	34.3	96.4
Visual impairments	31.2	55.8	13.6	37.7
Dermatitis	36.1	26.1	50.7	43.9
Frequent indigestion	16.8	33.5	17.4	29.2
Ulcer	13.0	27.5	13.6	28.8
Migraine	18.1	25.0	53.7	64.2
Heart disease	26.3	140.4	38.7	107.6
High blood pressure	45.6	237.0	38.6	263.0
Hemorrhoids	25.0	78.6	33.1	68.2
Chronic sinusitus	115.0	164.8	145.1	207.3
Chronic bronchitis	41.4	38.8	52.1	52.3
Diabetes	4.4	68.5	8.1	59.4
Total	533.3	1479.4	668.5	1543.6

Source: Deborah A. Dawson and Patricia F. Adams, *Current Estimates from the National Health Interview Survey: United States, 1986.* (Hyattsville, MD: National Center for Health Statistics, October 1987), table 58.

Even if a delivery-related leave with benefits is available, women who take a child care leave for the early months of the baby's life may have no group health insurance or may have to pay for it themselves. For example, in a health services agency now employing about 450 workers, 85 percent of them women, unpaid maternity leave up to one year is available with a guarantee of a similar job upon return. Group health insurance is provided for the first three months of the leave, which would carry a woman with a normal pregnancy through her delivery. For the remaining nine months, she has the option to continue in the group but must pay the premium herself (Batkin, 1987).

Group insurance so far has not covered the services of a caregiver who may be needed for a woman with a high-risk pregnancy, because of both her medical condition and the fact that the infant may need extra attention (Pego, 1987).

The Supreme Court has upheld a California law requiring employers to give unpaid pregnancy leave and to guarantee reinstatement, stating that there was no congressional intent to prohibit preferential treatment

TABLE 4.4
Measures of Illness, by Sex, for Working-age Adults, 1986

	Age in Years	
	18–44	45+
A. ACUTE CONDITIONS		
1. Acute conditions per 100 persons/year		
Male	144.3	98.6
Female	205.6	143.0
2. Percentage medically attended		
Male	51.3	63.1
Female	56.2	67.2
3. Restricted activity days per 100 persons/year—acute conditions		
Male	607.0	594.0
Female	787.8	1010.9
4. Bed days per 100 persons/year—acute conditions		
Male	253.1	210.6
Female	359.4	490.7
5. Work-loss days per 100 currently employed persons/year—acute conditions		
Male	310.1	256.7
Female	371.6	385.5
6. Injury episodes per 100 persons/year		
Male	33.2	18.6
Female	23.0	21.6
7. Restricted activity days from injury per 100 persons/year		
Male	298.4	377.6
Female	172.5	407.9
8. Bed days for injury per 100 persons/year		
Male	80.0	108.6
Female	55.7	178.6

for pregnancy (*Monthly Labor Review*, 1987). Federal legislative proposals would grant extended unpaid leave up to twenty-six weeks, with the right to medical benefits protected but without requiring the employer to pay for them. (The Secretary of Labor has said that she will advise President Bush to veto a current bill mandating the offer of unpaid leave (*The Nation's Health*, 1990).) According to several studies, few women take any unpaid leave to care for new children, preferring to use available paid leave. A General Accounting Office (GAO) survey of firms shows that 40 percent of women in firms with disability leave had six weeks of such leave, and other women had paid sick and vacation leave that they could use after childbirth, with an average of three and a half weeks' entitle-

TABLE 4.4 (continued)

B. ACTIVITY LIMITATION AND HEALTH STATUS

1. Percentage of persons with activity limitation due to chronic conditions, for working-age population

Activity Limitation Status	Percentage with Limitation, by Age			
	Male		Female	
	Under 45	45–64	Under 45	45–64
With limitation	9.2	24.2	8.1	24.2
Limited in major activity	6.5	17.3	5.0	17.3
Limited, but not in major activity	2.7	6.9	3.1	6.9
No limitation	90.8	75.8	91.9	75.8

2. Activity restriction due to acute and chronic conditions, for working-age population, days per person per year.

Type of Restriction	Days, by Sex and Age Group					
	Male			Female		
	18–24	25–44	45–64	18–24	25–44	45–64
Bed disability	3.0	4.4	6.9	5.2	5.4	9.6
Work loss	3.5	4.6	6.0	6.6	5.5	7.2
All types	7.8	10.9	18.1	12.4	13.3	22.9

3. Respondent-assessed health status for working-age population

Health Status	Percentage, by Sex and Age Group					
	Male			Female		
	18–24	25–44	45–64	18–24	25–44	45–64
Excellent	49.1	46.3	29.4	40.4	38.5	24.0
Very good	28.1	29.1	25.7	32.0	30.6	26.5
Good	19.8	18.7	27.5	23.2	23.9	30.7
Fair	2.5	4.5	11.4	3.8	5.8	13.0
Poor	0.5[a]	1.4	6.0	0.5[a]	1.2	5.9

Source: Deborah A. Dawson and Patricia F. Adams, *Current Estimates from the National Health Interview Survey: United States, 1986.* (Hyattsville, MD: National Center for Health Statistics, October 1987), tables 2, 12, 17, 27, 37, 42, 53, 67, 69, 70.
[a]Relative standard error exceeds 30%.

ment (General Accounting Office, 1988). In one survey, "over 84 percent of women taking leave returned to work within 10 weeks" (p. 13). The GAO believes that leave to care for new children will be used predominantly by women. Health care continuance during unpaid leave will cost about ninety million dollars annually. Proposals for family or medical leave have emerged in many states (*Wall Street Journal,* 12 October 1987), but employer opposition to making this a paid leave is expected, as voiced in California, where the legislation that was passed provided for unpaid leave. These bills at least express recognition of the problem. Neither employer-initiated leave policies nor proposed laws resolve the problem of women who are reluctant to stay away from the job because they expect that they will jeopardize their future status in the firm by doing so. Unfortunately, there is no simple remedy for this.

Employers may oppose mandating certain health benefits, despite their concern with workers' family needs. Some employers with generous plans would like to see their competitors obliged to provide similar coverage. But less successful and smaller firms may find the premium cost burdensome, and even large employers may wish to keep benefits at the bargaining table and out of the legislature, in order to retain control. Carriers, too, may resist mandated benefits because they prefer to divide the market according to employers' ability to pay and the preferences and demographic makeup of employed groups. They may wish to offer various packages at different price levels to make their marketing effective. In the past, Blue plans have expressed fear of public resentment if premium costs go up to cover mandated benefits.

CONCLUSION: SEX SIMILARITIES AND DIFFERENCES

In many respects the positive and negative aspects of the method of financing health care through the workplace are similar for the two sexes once they are part of the system. Employers do not provide different benefit packages by sex. Unlike pensions and other fringes, health benefits are generally similar across classes of employees (professional and administrative, technical and clerical, and production) (Charles D. Spencer and Associates, 1985), although some firms provide supplemental medical coverage to executives (Johnson and Higgins, 1986). Therefore, if there is sex-based occupational segregation within the firm or lower pay for women in a given occupation, this does not usually imply lower benefits. Claims are processed according to contract: if a service specified in the master policy is rendered by a legitimate provider to a covered person, male or female, the reimbursement proceeds in a routine fashion. Maternity is now protected against inequality of benefit levels. The language of cost control, including preservice review and certification, is neutral as to gender. The procedures commonly singled out for mandatory second surgical opinions are a mixture of those confined to or concentrated in men, such as prostatectomy and hernia repair; those that are exclusive to women, such as hysterectomy; and those that are not confined to one sex, such as gallbladder surgery.

Nevertheless, the foregoing review suggests that employed women's health care needs differ from those of men in certain respects. The differences listed next are based on the economic status and reproductive needs of women and on problems rooted in sexual stereotypes and women's reactions to them.

1. Workplace coverage is an imperfect social instrument to assure coverage for those whose employment is interrupted. Other tools must be added to conventional employee group-negotiated benefits to serve those who have gaps of varying duration in their work history. Waiting periods at the start of employment may be substantial in otherwise attractive plans. These problems are worse for contingent workers and women with absences from employment for child care.

2. Cancer screening for two sites specific to women is potentially cost-effective, but insurance benefits for these, and all preventive services, are often limited. The cost of the Pap smear test is not high, but screening of asymptomatic women is not a standard benefit. (Doctors sometimes write plausible diagnoses to justify reimbursement.) Breast cancer screening is well established scientifically but is often costly, and in many policies it is not a covered service, although this situation is changing.[4]

3. For various reasons, certain cost controls that employers hoped would be very useful have had weak effects or one-time effects (Latham, 1983). In the 1986 survey cited earlier, few employers (about 10 percent) reported any savings from second-opinion programs, and most could not judge if savings were realized (Johnson and Higgins, 1986). Only 42 percent of those offering HMOs believed them to be effective in controlling costs. It has been speculated that some devices to limit utilization could even expose employers to lawsuits if health outcomes are poor (Forbes, 1986). Therefore, more pressure to reduce health benefit levels is likely. If the patient's share of costs is increased, the outlay is a larger percentage of income for low-income workers, who may find higher out-of-pocket costs a barrier to care. Thus, sex-neutral cost-sharing (actually cost-shifting) policies may have "side effects" for women.

---

[4]Required coverage for mammography and cervical cytology screening has been legislated in Minnesota and Massachusetts, and for mammography only in Oklahoma. California now requires group plans that already cover mastectomy (which is generally covered) and prosthetic devices and reconstructive surgery after mastectomy (usually covered) to cover mammography as well (*Commentary Report on State Legislation,* 1988).

4. Early discharge from hospitals after surgical or medical treatment shifts the completion of recovery to the home setting. To a greater extent than formerly, the convalescent patient must rely on family members to supply personal care, meals, and health-related services, tasks often performed by women as family caregivers. These situations apparently have become more common with the adoption of Diagnosis-Related Groups as a hospital reimbursement method by Medicare (and other payers). Use of outpatient surgical settings, now widely encouraged by employer benefit plans, similarly relies on supportive services in the home. A working woman with a family member (child, husband, or functionally disabled parent) who undergoes outpatient surgery or is discharged from the hospital is thus subject to more demands on her time and the stress of intensified responsibilities. Working women may have to pay for help if they are unable to meet both family and work demands. At the same time, if the patient is a woman without sources of assistance in her family household, such as a single parent, she may have to purchase help for herself or risk a slower or less satisfactory recovery.

5. Employers' discontinuance of contributions for dependents' coverage is harmful for single-parent households, although it may be quite acceptable to some two-earner households (Reimers, 1987). Interests of different subclasses of women must be reconciled.

6. Threats to privacy may be generated by utilization review and other devices used by employers for cost control. (A sociopolitical atmosphere that is hostile to abortion heats up the atmosphere around women's decision making and intensifies the importance of privacy to the individual.) Quality of care may be reduced because of cost cutting by employers (for example, requiring or promoting use of low-cost alternative providers) (Egdahl, 1987; Forbes, 1986). Employees who feel insecure in their jobs may be reluctant to complain.

7. Absence from work for maternity, especially if a period of absence for child care follows the postpartum disability period, may interrupt coverage if there are no formal leave provisions, which is the situation for the majority of employed women in the United States, unlike in European industrialized countries ("When the Stork Brings the Sack," Economist, 1986).

8. Women may have preferences for women-centered providers who combine reproductive and other health services in one setting and who differ from conventional providers in offering a more communicative style, more health reference materials, and

adaptation to employed women's time constraints. Among firms with plans surveyed in 1986, 56 percent covered birthing centers and 25 percent covered midwives (Johnson and Higgins, 1986). These figures show growth over past years but also indicate that a gap in access remains. In contrast, coverage for physician and hospital services for maternity is typical in employer plans.

9. Sex stereotypes that result in overtreatment, undertreatment, or misdirected treatment for women waste resources of the system or compromise the patient's health. The payment system has no internal checks against prescribing of psychotropic drugs (more common for women patients and believed to be a gray area of quality of care). The treatment of alcoholism in women has been inhibited by the established focus, now being challenged, on disease models derived from and tested on men (National Institute on Alcohol Abuse and Alcoholism, 1986). The debate as to whether premenstrual symptoms constitute a syndrome and whether needs for care are widespread is sociopolitical: On one side a fear that acceptance of premenstrual distress as a disease reinforces traditional social attitudes about women's fragility, and on the other, a fear that real health needs have been neglected (Watkins, 1986; see also chapter 2, on treatment issues).

The earlier years of adult life offer a window of opportunity for health care and related programs that will maximize wellness in the later years of life and will improve ability to pay or prepay for needed care in old age. Thus, the equity and sensitivity of services associated with the workplace have vital connections with the situation of the elderly, the subject of the next chapter.

References

Aetna Life and Casualty. Indemnity Benefit Plan: A Governmentwide Plan Administered by the Aetna Life Insurance Company. Washington, DC, 1987.

American Public Health Association. *The Nation's Health.* Washington, DC, August 1987.

Batkin, Miriam. Interview, October 23, 1987.

Bergstahler, Janet Witte. "The Impact of the Pregnancy Discrimination Act of 1978 on Employee Health Insurance Benefit Levels." Ann Arbor, MI: University Microfilms, 1984.

Berk, Marc L., and Amy K. Taylor. *Women and Divorce: Health Insurance Coverage, Utilization and Health Care Expenditures.* Rockville, MD: National Center for Health Services Research, October 11, 1983.

Brown, Leahmae. *Group Purchase of Medical Care by Industrial Employees.* Princeton, NJ: Princeton University, Industrial Relations Section, 1938.

Bundy, Darcie. *The Affordable Baby.* New York: Harper & Row, 1985.

Charles D. Spencer and Associates. *Employee Benefit Plan Review.* Chicago: March 1985, 198–199.

Christensen, Kathleen. Testimony before Employment and Housing Subcommittee, Committee on Government Operations, U.S. House of Representatives, February 26, 1986.

Commentary Report on State Legislation, vol. 3, no. 1, June 1988.

Cooney, Joan P. "What Determines the Start of Prenatal Care? Prenatal Care, Insurance, and Education." *Medical Care,* vol. 23, no. 8 (August 1985): 986–997.

Dawson, Deborah A., and Patricia F. Adams. *Current Estimates from the National Health Interview Survey: United States, 1986.* Series 10, No. 164. DHHS Pub. No. (PHS) 87-1592. Hyattsville, MD: National Center for Health Statistics, October 1987.

Economist, "When the Stork Brings the Sack," vol. 301, no. 7467 (October 11, 1986): 34.

Egdahl, Richard. "Maintain Quality When Cutting Health Costs." *Wall Street Journal,* 5 January 1987, 16:3.

Equitable HCA Corporation. *Commentary from Equicor,* vol. I, no. 8 (April, 1986); vol. I, no. 9 (May 1986); vol. II, no. 2 (June 1987); vol. III, no. 2 (November 1987); vol. III, no. 4 (February 1988).

Farley, Pamela, J. "Hospital and Ambulatory Services for Selected Illnesses." *Health Services Research,* 21:5 (December 1986a): 587–616.

———. *Private Health Insurance in the United States.* Data Preview 23. DHHS Pub. No. (PHS) 86-3406. Rockville, MD: National Center for Health Services Research, September, 1986b.

Fay, Francesca C., and Kathy S. Smith. *Childbearing after 35: The Risks and the Rewards.* New York: Balsam Press, 1985.

Forbes, Daniel. "Cut Health Care Costs, Get Sued?" *DUN's Business Month* (July 1986): 38–40.

Freudenheim, Milt. "Business and Health-Discrimination in Benefit Plans." *New York Times,* 11 November 1986.

———. "Insurers Seek Help for Uninsured." *New York Times,* 4 January 1990, pp. IV, 1, 7.

Frey, Norma, and Estelle Giammusso. Interview, October 7, 1987.

General Accounting Office. *Parental Leave, Estimated Costs of H.R. 925, the Family and Medical Leave Act of 1987, November 1987.* GAO/HRD-88-34. Washington, DC, 1988.

Henshaw, Stanley K., and Lynn S. Wallach. "The Medicaid Cutoff and Abortion Services for the Poor." *Family Planning Perspectives,* vol. 16, no. 4 (July/August 1984): 170–172, 177–180.

Insight and Instatus. Chatsworth, CA: NILS Publishing Co., January–December 1986.

Johnson, Dirk. "High Court Faces Alcoholism Issue." *New York Times,* 25 October 1987.

Johnson and Higgins. *Corporate Health Care Benefits Survey, 1986.* Princeton, NJ, 1986.

Kittner, Dorothy. "Maternity Benefits Available to Most Health Plan Participants." *Monthly Labor Review* (May 1978): 53–55.

Latham, W. Bryan. *Health Care Costs—There Are Solutions.* AMA Management Briefings. New York: American Management Association, 1983.

McLemore, Thomas, and Hugo Koch. *1980 Summary: National Ambulatory Medical Care Survey.* Advance Data No. 77. Hyattsville, MD: National Center for Health Statistics, February 22, 1982.

Mercer-Meidinger, Inc. *Survey, Multi-Opinion Flexible Benefit Plans.* New York, 1986.

Monheit, Alan C., Michael M. Hagan, Marc L. Berk, and Pamela J. Farley. "The Employed Uninsured and the Role of Public Policy." *Inquiry,* vol. 22 (Winter 1985): 348–364.

Monthly Labor Review, vol. 110, no. 3 (March 1987): 43–44.

Muller, Charlotte. "Change and Resistance to Change: Maternity Provisions in New York City Blue Plans." Chapter in History Project (book) of Empire Blue Cross and Blue Shield, edited by Daniel M. Fox. New York: Health Services Improvement Fund, 1990 (in press).

———. "Health and Health Care of Employed Women and Homemakers: Family Factors." *Women & Health,* vol. 11, no. 1 (Spring 1986a): 7–26.

———. "Review of Twenty Years of Research on Medical Care Utilization." *Health Services Research,* 21:2 (June 1986b): 129–144.

National Center for Health Statistics. *Pregnant Workers in the United States.* Advance Data No. 11. Hyattsville, MD, September 15, 1977.

———. *1986 Summary: National Hospital Discharge Survey.* Advance Data No. 145. Hyattsville, MD: Hospital Care Statistics Branch, September 30, 1987.

National Institute on Alcohol Abuse and Alcoholism. "Women and Alcohol: Health-Related Issues." Research Monograph No. 16, DHHS Pub. No. (ADM) 86-1139. Rockville, MD, 1986.

The Nation's Health, vol. xx, no. 2 (February 1990): 6.

NBER Digest. National Bureau of Economic Research, March 1985.

New York Business Group on Health, Inc. *Pregnancy and the Workplace.* Discussion Paper. vol. 7, supp. no. 5 (November 1987).

New York Times, "Working Mothers." 19 June 1988, IV, 28:5.

Pego, Maria. Interview. November 20, 1987.

Perman, Laurie, and Beth Stevens. "Industrial Segregation and the Gender Distribution of Fringe Benefits." *Gender and Society,* vol. 3, no. 3 (September 3, 1989): 388–404.

Pilson, Judith, and John Brown. Interview. October 27, 1987.

Powell-Griner, Eve. "Induced Terminations of Pregnancy: Reporting States, 1984." *NCHS Monthly Vital Statistics Report,* vol. 36, no. 5, supp. 2 (September 8, 1987): 1–36.

Reimers, Cordelia D. Interview. September 1987.

Rossiter, Louis F., and Amy K. Taylor. "Union Effects on the Provision of Health Insurance." *Industrial Relations,* vol. 21, no. 2 (Spring 1982): 167–177.

Social Security Administration, Office of Research and Statistics, Research Report No. 56, *Disability Survey 72, Disabled and Nondisabled Adults,* compiled by Donald T. Ferron. SSA Publication No. 13-11812. Washington, DC, 1981.

Social Service Employees Union Local 371. *Benefit Funds: Your Membership Benefits.* New York, 1986.

Tsai, Shan P., Susan Miller Reedy, and Edward J. Bernacki. "The Effect of Redesigning Mental Health Benefits." *Business and Health* (April 1987): 26–29.

U.S. Department of Commerce, Bureau of the Census. *Characteristics of Households and Persons Receiving Selected Noncash Benefits: 1983.* Current Population Reports, Series P-60, No. 148. Washington, DC, 1985.

U.S. Department of Commerce. *Statistical Abstract of the United States.* 1987 (106th ed.) Washington, DC, 1986.

U.S. Department of Labor. *Program Highlights, Maternity Leave.* September 1980.

———. Bureau of Labor Statistics. *Handbook of Labor Statistics.* Bulletin 2217. June 1985.

———. Women's Bureau. *Pregnancy and Employment: Federal and State Legal Requirements, Facts on U.S. Working Women.* Fact Sheet No. 87-1. 1987.

Wall Street Journal, 12 August 1986, 2:3.

Wall Street Journal, 13 January 1987.

Wall Street Journal, 14 January 1987.

Wall Street Journal, 12 October 1987.

Warshaw, Leon M. Interview. September 19, 1987.

Watkins, Linda M. "Premenstrual Distress Gains Notice As a Chronic Issue in the Workplace." *Wall Street Journal,* 22 January 1986, 31:4.

CHAPTER FIVE

The Elderly

IN THIS CHAPTER SEVERAL themes recur as to the ways in which gender influences the "careers" of the elderly as users of the health care system. Lifelong adherence to gender-based social roles greatly affects the income, assets, and insurance of older persons and, thus, their ability to gain access to the system. The current economic status of the elderly is affected by their past; for women this includes sex-typed jobs and discontinuous careers, the persistence of wage discrimination in the U.S. economy, and marriages in which the bride was typically younger than the bridegroom (and therefore survived him). Moreover, the informal resources available to help an elderly person with mobility and self-care limitations are affected by whether one has a living spouse or is dependent on adult children, who tend to be less available than a spouse. Thus, much of the extra burden falling on women because of functional limitations (including, in many cases, inability to get needed help) is connected with their greater life expectancy.

Health financing programs and reimbursement approaches that do not make any distinctions whatsoever between the two sexes nevertheless may have a special impact on women because of their vulnerability to poverty and their problems obtaining regular help from caregivers. Finally, age biases may interfere with rational care and equal opportunity to achieve the highest attainable functional level and, even, protect life. Such biases, although embracing all elderly, are especially hurtful for women, because the oldest age groups are largely female.

Gender differences are only part of the health care scene of the elderly. There is heterogeneity within each sex as to health levels, prevalence of poverty, and use of care. Gender is, in many respects, a proxy for ability to pay, living arrangements, and so forth, but it is not an exact indicator:

the poor (or functionally impaired) male and the poor (or functionally impaired) female may be far more alike as clients, buyers, or program targets than the poor and the well-to-do, the vigorous and the frail, within each sex. Furthermore, the progress that has been achieved in improving health levels and increasing equity of access for the elderly should be acknowledged. It gives us examples to build on and a reminder of what we lose by insufficient or ill-conceived resource allocation such as ignoring opportunities for prevention, paying providers without guarding quality levels, and reerecting financial barriers to needed care.

THE ELDERLY: A FEMALE MAJORITY

Elderly persons of both sexes, but especially women, have increased their life expectancy by the continuous drop in mortality since the late 1960s and the overall drop in mortality from 1940 to 1980. In these four decades, the drop for women 65+ was 47.3 percent; for men, 30.7 percent (Verbrugge, 1984). The sex difference in life expectancy reflects sex-linked genetic factors, but there are other causes as well: life-long exposure to environmental pollutants, the physical demands of specific occupations, and health habits. Another factor is variations in the pace of discovery and general adoption of methods able to resolve, contain, or prevent health problems affecting each sex, such as cancer of different sites. Almost two-fifths of today's elderly of both sexes have some degree of chronic limitation (U.S. Congress, 1984). Such impairment, and, indeed, all the health problems and needs of the elderly, concern a larger proportion of the population than in previous eras. In 1984, 28 million persons, or 11.8 percent of the population, were 65 and older, and the projected figure for 2010 is 13.9 percent (United Hospital Fund of New York, 1986b). Elderly women make up 13.8 percent of the entire female population; the comparable figure for men is 9.8 percent: there are 16,741,000 women 65+ and 11,299,000 men (U.S. Department of Commerce, 1985, p. 24).

Since the longevity advantage of women gives them 18 more years of life at age 65, compared with 14 for men, the population becomes increasingly female in each succeeding age group after 65, and after 85 there are only 45 men per 100 women. As a result, such gender-related problems as may exist in our health care system (e.g., obstacles to access related to living arrangements and income status of elderly women and the residue of sex bias that may remain in medical treatment situations) are translated into deficits in the care of the elderly. Conversely, generic deficits in the health care of the elderly have an adverse effect on large numbers of women.

The pattern of sex differences in the situation of today's elderly, as shown by statistics on life expectancy, health needs, health care, and ability to pay, is based on the experience of specific birth cohorts. Projections into the future must be guarded, for some trends may be augmented, others reversed. Today's elderly women include those who reached adulthood during World War II and had fewer children than later cohorts. This reduced the number of adult children who could serve as caregivers to the functionally limited. For future elderly women, family size, age of mother at time of birth, births to nonmarried women, and other demographic characteristics will affect the probability of having effective personal networks in old age. The higher educational level achieved by today's younger women (U.S. Department of Commerce, 1986, table 191) predisposes to occupational attainment, and occupational distribution and industry of employment in turn affect whether group health insurance is available and will be extended into retirement. Health habits too are affected by educational level.

In recent years (1975–1985), for both blacks and whites, the percentage of young wives expecting to have only one or two children in their completed families increased (U.S. Department of Commerce, 1986, table 97), and the proportion of married women who were childless rose (table 93). First births after age thirty also increased from 1980 through 1985 (table 90), which may mean smaller families but more career development, and the number of births to unmarried women grew dramatically from 1960 through 1984 (table 86). Labor market statistics show a rise in the number of women employed full-time from 1976 through 1985 (table 644), and a further increase is projected. The proportion of women with four or more years of college who enter managerial or professional jobs is now slightly higher than for men: 69.3 percent versus 65.0 percent (table 658). The numbers involved are substantial, as there were 9.7 million women at that educational level in 1986.

Cohort differences in health levels and ability to pay for health care in old age reflect environmental changes and public policies, as well as personal health habits, reproductive history (for women), and private human-capital investment. A variety of public policies not limited to the last phases of the life cycle can ultimately affect the elderly. The status of programs for equalizing educational opportunity, strategies for promoting equity in hiring and promotion, and integrity of income maintenance, public maternity care, and other current programs all figure in the set of policies that will influence the needs and resources of future elderly. Meanwhile, Haug and Folmar (1986) have found that elderly women have a lower quality of life than elderly men, as measured by physical health, functional ability, income adequacy, social contact, lack of distress, and cognitive ability.

POVERTY, CHRONIC ILLNESS, AND MEDICAL EXPENDITURES IN OLD AGE

Poverty, chronic illness, and medical expenditures among the elderly are interactive, with special impact on women because of their higher rates of poverty and chronic limitations.

Many elderly women are poor because, having worked only in second-class industries and occupations, they earned little and acquired few pension rights, and because their domestic roles conflicted with continuous work careers (Minkler and Stone, 1985). Services that women supply as homemakers and caregivers for minor children, working or retired husbands, and disabled parents or husbands do not result in rights to retirement income and old-age health benefits. Women's pension benefits have not kept pace with those of men in the manufacturing labor force of the United States and four other industrial countries over the period 1960–1980 (Tracy and Ward, 1986). Women past sixty-five are less likely than men of that age to have group insurance through their employers because of the occupations and industries in which they were employed and the likelihood of a part-time and/or discontinuous work history. Many women acquire retirement income and medical benefits as wives of employed men, but various contingencies can strip away their protections and cause impoverishment and hardship in meeting health needs. If the husband becomes disabled and enters a nursing home, the state can claim his social security and pension income when he becomes eligible for Medicaid (American Association of Retired Persons, 1987), although recent changes in federal law have modified this (see page 123). If the husband dies, pension payments may cease, while most of the cost of maintaining the household continues. As the widow grows older, assets may be depleted, and informal networks are disrupted by moving, disability, or death of kin and friends. Use of hospitals and purchase of home-based services by those lacking sources of informal assistance further diminish asset accounts.

The association between illness and poverty is generally strong among the elderly. Among elderly women, the poor have disproportionate health problems, compared with those above the poverty line: more of them have major limitations on usual activities, fewer report no limitations, and they have poorer self-assessed health. Many of the elderly have intense fears of the future, revolving around health, money, and dependency (Louis Harris and Associates, 1986).

Reform of the social security system significantly reduced the prevalence of poverty in the elderly after 1970. The proportion of poor persons among elderly men dropped from 19.2 percent in 1970 to 8.7 percent in 1984, and from 28.6 percent of women to 15 percent (Stone, 1986a). Because women's poverty rate is higher (as shown by these figures) and they constitute the majority of the population over sixty-five, women make up 71.2 percent of the elderly poor. The poverty rate is three times as high for unrelated individuals (living alone or with nonrelatives) as it is for those living in families, and, in the former group, which is heavily dominated by women (Louis Harris and Associates, 1986), the proportion who are poor is higher for women (27.7 percent versus 22.1 percent for men). The poverty rate among ELAs (elderly living alone) is especially high for black and Hispanic women: 63.4 percent and 45.7 percent, respectively, versus 24.5 percent for whites (Stone, 1986b). Female disabled ELAs are more often poor than disabled men living alone.

Poverty among the elderly affects use of health care. It can hinder receipt of health care, especially when no third party will pay and when care is not urgent; consequently, preventive care may be reduced. For illness-related care, the elderly poor are high utilizers. This is due to the access they have obtained through the social programs set up in 1965 (Medicare and Medicaid) and to their long-standing health problems that, in their earlier years, either caused low income or resulted from and were worsened by low incomes. Of course, they have newer problems as well, and these may be traced in part to a shortfall in preventive care.

A study of the "crossover population," aged persons entitled to both Medicare and Medicaid, provides information on use of health care by the elderly poor in 1978. (Sex differences in enrollment and utilization for all Medicare enrollees are discussed on pages 127–128.) Dual coverage was held by 14 percent of the elderly who were on Medicare (U.S. Department of Health and Human Services, 1986b, p. 5). The dually entitled, or crossover group, were older than those with Medicare only[1] (mean age 76.6, versus 73.6, years), and 71 percent were women (versus 59 percent for the Medicare-only group). Their health difficulties were not, however, merely the result of age, for the crossovers had a death rate 50 percent higher than the others after standardization for age, and for specific age groups under 80 the difference was substantial. Dual enrollees had a higher proportion who received Medicare-covered services, and reimbursement per enrollee was 1.6 times as high for the crossovers un-

---

[1]In this context, "Medicare only" means without Medicaid. See pages 108–109 for comparisons including those with "Medigap" private insurance.

der both hospital insurance and supplementary medical insurance (covering physicians' and other medical services). Even after standardization for age, the crossovers had 2.6 times as many hospital discharges per 1,000 enrollees as the others. Much of their high utilization was due to their increased mortality, because persons in their last year of life incur 6 times as much expense for medical care as patients who survive (McMillan and Gornick, 1983).

A further study based on the National Medical Care Utilization and Expenditure Survey, with data from 1980, separates out the noninstitutionalized crossovers, to clarify whether the utilization and health experience of all crossover elderly was dominated by those living in long-term care facilities (McMillan and Gornick, 1984). This analysis confirmed that the community-dwelling crossovers, like the larger group of which they are a part, were older, were more often female, and contained more minority members. They were in poorer health than Medicare-only enrollees. For males, the proportion with moderate to severe functional limitations was 1.7 times as high as for noncrossovers; for women, 2.0 times. The percentage with limitations of that level of severity was 56.8 percent among the women crossovers, compared with 44.3 percent among the men. The dually entitled living in the community had much higher per capita health care expenses than the singly entitled. Medicaid coverage is more comprehensive than Medicare, and this contributed to the expenditure difference. (As an exception, crossovers used only half as many dental services as the others, due to loss of teeth as well as socioeconomic status.) The crossovers had lower income and education levels than the elderly with Medicare only.

Medicare's limitations are themselves a source of financial hardship if much care is used. Medicare was expected to pay only 44 percent of health care expenditures of a couple and 33 percent of those of female ELAs in 1986 (Stone, 1986b). Because cost-sharing provisions are linked to service use, the elderly who are in poor health have the highest beneficiary liability under Medicare (Gornick et al., 1985). The burden of medical costs as a percentage of income is inversely related to income and is "still quite high for the lowest income group," among whom 18 percent have out-of-pocket expenses of 10 percent or more of their income (Gornick et al., 1985, p. 53). This makes it harder to meet nutritional and housing needs.

Despite the health difficulties of the dually entitled, compared with all other elderly, the poor and near-poor who have Medicaid (29 percent and 8 percent, respectively, in 1984) are in a better position to get medical care than other low-income elderly. Near-poor elderly in fair or poor health with neither Medicaid nor "Medigap" insurance to supplement

Medicare use fewer physician services in a year (6.5 visits) than those with private insurance (8.7 visits) and those with Medicaid (13.1 visits). Poor elderly in fair or poor health obtain fewer physician services if they have either private insurance or no supplemental coverage than if they have Medicaid. The Commonwealth Fund Commission on Elderly People Living Alone has concluded that there are many elderly who forgo needed care (Rowland and Lyons, 1987).

If low-income elderly without Medicaid wish to buy private insurance, they must pay a premium, averaging $500 a year, that represents over 10 percent of the income of a poor elderly person. About one-third of the elderly poor are exposed to substantial out-of-pocket expenses for deductibles, copayments, and uncovered services. Medical expense drives about 8 percent of near-poor elderly living alone into poverty.

The Medicare Catastrophic Coverage Act of 1988 assists states to buy Medicaid coverage for Medicare Part A beneficiaries with incomes up to 100 percent of the federal poverty level. The covered benefits are limited to Medicare cost sharing and, if the state chooses, premiums for enrolling a beneficiary in a risk-sharing HMO (Health Care Financing Administration, 1988). The near-poor are not affected.

The 1988 law introduced a number of Medicare benefit expansions including

1. unlimited hospitalization after a single annual deductible
2. improved skilled nursing facility and hospice benefits
3. unlimited duration of home health care
4. a stop-loss on outpatient services under Part B
5. home respite care (an aide to replace a family caregiver)
6. mammography screening
7. outpatient prescription drugs, plus insulin

The act, however, was criticized because it duplicated existing benefits held by many elderly, taxed retirees for the additional hospital benefits (those with income tax obligations, or about 40 percent of retirees), and imposed a new premium under Part B for the catastrophic (stop-loss) feature, while both custodial nursing home care for chronic conditions and assistance with activities of daily living at home remained uncovered (Health Care Financing Administration, 1989b). Congress repealed the Medicare benefit additions in November 1989. Clearly, if contributions based on ability to pay are to be used, there is no reason to tax only the elderly. Alternatively, using a payroll tax on the economically active and their employers to support these expansions would conform to social security principles.

GENDER DIFFERENCES IN HEALTH

Health Status

For the elderly, gender differences in health vary according to the measure used. Self-reported health status shows no difference: according to National Center for Health Statistics (NCHS) data published in 1978, the same proportions of elderly men and women reported poor or fair health, rather than excellent or good health (Verbrugge, 1984). Findings in National Medical Care Utilization and Expenditure Survey (NMCUES) data for 1980 are similar (Schlenger, Wadman, and Corder, 1983).

Acute Disability

A measure of health used for the general population is acute disability, which refers to conditions causing restricted activity or need for medical attention and lasting less than three months. Acute disability is distinguished from long-lasting activity limitations due to chronic disease. Figures on acute disability among the elderly from NMCUES indicate that the average number of restricted activity days in 1980 was similar, both for all men and women (30 and 33, respectively) and for those with one or more restricted activity days (49, 51). But women had more illness conditions (4.8 versus 3.9 for men) in the year, and among those with any conditions, women again had more (Schlenger, Wadman, and Corder, 1983).

The NCHS now considers restricted activity days a "less than ideal indicator" of the health status of older people and prefers bed-disability days (1986, p. 12). The reasons are not presented, but they may be related to the increase with advancing age in the proportion of both sexes reporting that they do not do shopping, housework, and other activities that are considered instrumental to self-maintenance in a household. Just how usual activities are interpreted by a respondent also may depend on whether the person has a history of paid employment or full-time homemaking, whether there is household help, and, especially for women who have worked, the specific daily activities that constitute the frame of reference. Hence, questions on restriction are interpreted by respondents against a varied and ever-changing background, and the answers are difficult to interpret. When bed-disability days are used as the measure, women 65+ have both higher rates than their male peers and longer duration per condition (Verbrugge, 1984). But this may be due to women's higher age levels, rather than to a gender difference.

Injuries are considered acute conditions. Older women have a much higher rate of injuries than older men and frequently acquire permanent disabilities from them (Kovar, 1977). Women 65+ are more likely to use emergency rooms and less likely to use doctors' offices (than men) for care of their injuries, a difference that may be due to having more severe injuries (Collins, 1985).

Limitations in Usual Activity

Among those in the 65+ age group, a larger percentage of men report that they are limited in their major activities because of a chronic condition: 43 percent versus 35 percent for women (Verbrugge, 1984). However, among the elderly poor, women have more activity limitations caused by chronic conditions than men. As with interference with usual activity in acute illness, gender roles may bias the information available through self-report on activity limitation due to chronic conditions. Men interpret the questions asked in national surveys in relation to ability to perform paid work, but women who have been primarily homemakers interpret them in relation to housework. They may say they are not disabled if they can adapt household routines to their limitations. Men whose past occupations were sedentary may report limitations less often than men with similar impairments but different job histories. In future surveys, older women will have spent more time in paid work, possibly in occupations with heavy physical demands, before reaching 65 than in previous survey years. If so, they may perceive themselves as more limited for a given amount of physical impairment.

Work-related Activities

To avoid these problems of interpretation, special criteria of sample selection were used in a recent study based on the Supplement on Aging (SoA) to the National Health Interview Survey of 1984 (Kovar and LaCroix, 1987). In this study, the subjects were men and women age 55–74 who were in the labor force after age 45 (they either continued to work or returned to work). Women, it was found, had less ability to perform work-related activities. The difference was greatest for the proportion who had trouble lifting or carrying 25 pounds (women 31 percent, men 16 percent), and was less for walking up 10 steps; stooping, crouching, or kneeling; and lifting or carrying 10 pounds. For all four of these activities, the sex differences were sharpest in the oldest age category, 70–74 years (Kovar and LaCroix, 1987). At that age, more women than men had difficulty standing on their feet for 2 hours, sitting for 2 hours, reaching up over their heads, and grasping with their fingers, as well as with the four functions previously mentioned. Fewer of the women than the men in the study were currently employed, and women were more likely to have left the work force earlier than men. Persons who had retired, especially those who had retired for health reasons, had less capacity to perform the work-related activities than those who were still working.

Ability to perform these activities evidently affects ability to remain in the labor force and probably is related to ability to maintain personal independence after retirement. In previous studies of activity limitation, sex differences, related to labor force participation, in the way questions were understood by respondents are believed to have affected findings. In this study, however, only men and women with work experience in the recent past were compared, and, therefore, the revelation of greater disability among women is more reliable. The study was also distinctive in that respondents were asked whether they had difficulty in doing the activity, not whether they received help; this overcomes the possible sex bias due to women's being offered help when they do not actually need it and accepting help merely because it is expected female behavior to do so when help is offered.

It has been suggested that higher rates of disability in women may be due in part to failure to develop appropriate exercise programs for women's health needs. According to this view, load-bearing exercises that are responsive to musculoskeletal problems displayed by older women should be emphasized, rather than the aerobic exercises that are useful for cardiovascular problems (chiefly male) and have been widely promoted. (See page 120 for a discussion of medications as a factor in falls.)

Daily Living

In addition to work-related disability, the NCHS has studied functional limitations in self-maintenance among the elderly, using the 1984 Supplement on Aging to the National Health Interview Survey. The study covers seven personal care items (activities of daily living, or ADLs) and seven home management items (instrumental activities of daily living, or IADLs). The personal care items were bathing, dressing, eating, transfer (from bed to chair, etc.), toileting, walking, and getting outside. The home items were preparing meals, shopping, telephoning, handling money, light and heavy housework, and transportation. More women than men were found to have trouble in all ADLs except dressing and eating, but this is due to women's higher average age (the percentage with trouble rises with age), and there are no significant sex differences within five-year age groups after sixty-five. The percentage with difficulties in home management also increases with age. Here women reported difficulty more often than men within each age group after sixty-five, except for handling money and telephoning, but the results are questionable because elderly men who had not customarily taken responsibility for meals and housework would not have been likely to report difficulty. Men are more apt to report that they do not prepare meals, shop for personal items, or do heavy or light housework (National Center for Health Statistics, 1986b), but the proportion reporting that they "don't do" various IADL items rises with age for both sexes. Thus, both respondents' reappraisals of usual tasks following onset of disability and gender-based household roles enter into these replies.

The study examined whether help was received, and it is possible to compute what percentage of those needing help got it. In personal care, there was no sex difference in the proportion of the sample getting help with dressing, eating, or toileting, but women got more help with walking after age 75 and with going outside after age 70. Of those needing help, women were less likely to get help than men with bathing, dressing, eating, transfer, and toileting, and they were more likely than men to receive help only for walking outside. In home management tasks, women got more help with meals and light housework. Although this is explainable by age, within 5-year age groups, women did get more help with heavy housework and, at age 70+, with shopping. Of those needing help, women were less likely than men to get help with meals and both light and heavy housework (Dawson, Hendershot, and Fulton, 1987). Thus, there is a sex difference in the proportion of those with needs who actually receive help. Women's lower probability of receiving help with personal care, meals, and housework is very likely related to their dependence on adult children, rather than on spouses, and their deficit arises well before extreme old age. However, the sex differences in the proportion of those needing help who received it are not very large, with the highest difference being 12 percentage points for meal preparation (81.6 percent of women with difficulty receive help, versus 93.6 percent of men). For both sexes, the greatest unmet needs exist in walking and transfer, but there are substantial numbers who need help with bathing, dressing, and eating and do not receive it. To sum up, functional limitations tend to be more burdensome to women to the extent that there are sex differences in need and in help received at a given age. But many of both sexes who report having difficulty with basic self-care do not receive help.

Sensory Impairments and Mobility

Data from the 1984 Supplement on Aging show that "the presence of visual impairments in persons is associated with a higher frequency of limitations" (Havlik, 1986, p. 5). The same is true of hearing impairments. Elderly women are slightly more likely than men to use eyeglasses and have a higher prevalence of cataracts up to age eighty-four, but men have higher rates of hearing impairments than women at all age levels past sixty-five (although the rise in prevalence with advancing age is greater for women).

For both sexes, these sensory impairments may not be an independent cause of mobility problems. The SoA data show that arthritis, cardiovascular disease, and hypertension are more often present in those with vision or hearing defects. The medical condition could cause the sensory problem, or a single etiological factor could cause both.

Impaired functional ability for daily living is one of the most significant measures of health status among the elderly, because it strongly affects the possibility of remaining in the community. Because of women's financial problems and their reduced access to caregivers within the household, those with functional limitations would benefit from programs that facilitate obtaining help in activities of daily living, such as subsidized personal care and congregate housing opportunities, and, of course, from efforts to prevent disability.

USE OF HEALTH SERVICES

Office Visits

The proportion of women 65+ with one or more physician contacts in 12 months slightly exceeded that for men in all age subgroups after 65 in 1975–1976: 81.7 percent versus 76.1 percent (Kovar and Drury, 1978, table 5).

Among older persons receiving ambulatory care from physicians, the proportion who used private health insurance to pay for it was slightly higher for men, but the proportion using any public payment sources was about equal for the two sexes (Kovar and Drury, 1978, table 9). Men have more veterans' entitlements, and women are more apt to be on Medicaid (U.S. Department of Health and Human Services, 1986a).

Data on use of physician office services in the 1985 National Ambulatory Medical Care Survey,[2] based on physician records of encounters, show that elderly women had slightly more visits per person per year than elderly men: 5.0 versus 4.6 (McLemore, 1987). (At 45–64, women had 38.5 percent more visits than men, but men's visit rate rose with age, narrowing the gap.) A higher proportion of women had five or more visits.

---

[2]The period actually studied was March 1985 through February 1986.

For both men and women, visit rates after sixty-five were higher than for the population as a whole. Older men were slightly more likely than women to visit a hospital outpatient department or a freestanding clinic; women were more apt to go to private offices (Kovar and Drury, 1978, table 7) and to use them as the sole source of ambulatory care (table 8).

A number of studies have reported that widowed persons are more likely to use physician services than married persons, but most of the studies have considered women only. Homan et al. have studied both sexes and have included labor force participation and living arrangements in their model. They used 1978 National Health Interview Survey data on persons aged fifty-five and over: 56 percent female, 23 percent widowed, and 34 percent gainfully employed. They report that widows made more use of physician services than widowers, both as to probability of use and as to number of visits. The difference is, however, traceable to the higher probability of living alone after loss of a spouse and to a lower probability of being gainfully employed (Homan et al., 1986). Widowhood per se does not appear to have an independent effect.

Elderly women had more visits per 1,000 persons in 1979 than men, even after visits for sex-specific diagnoses were excluded (Hing, Kovar, and Rice, 1983). For both sexes, circulatory, nervous system and sense organ, respiratory, and musculoskeletal disorders were the leading causes of visits. For 8 top categories, each of which had 200 or more visits per 1,000, the sex difference was greatest in musculoskeletal conditions, notably various forms of arthritis (men's visit rate being .68 that of women, which closely approximates the sex difference in prevalence), and circulatory disease, for which men had .80 of the women's visit rate. Within circulatory conditions, however, many of women's visits were for hypertension, rather than for coronary artery disease, which was much more prevalent among men and is more serious (Cypress, 1979).[3] Although sex differences in visits were in the same direction as sex differences in prevalence, this does not show (as has been inferred on occasion) that enough care was received by either sex. For example, there may be persons with uncomfortable symptoms and limitations due to arthritis who do not obtain care because of access problems. Additional indicators are needed to reveal whether such a gap exists.

It has been claimed that the office visits of the elderly are not long enough for adequate care, that doctors do not spend enough time with

---

[3]Within a visit for coronary disease, men and women did not differ significantly in the frequency of examinations, laboratory tests, X rays, and ECGs. Given a symptomatic serious disease and access to care, intensity of services seems to have been in keeping with clinical needs and not affected by sex of patient.

them. The elderly do not have a higher percentage of visits lasting ten minutes or less than do younger persons (National Center for Health Statistics, 1987, table 60), but visits may still be too short to disclose all the treatable conditions that a patient has. In the mistaken belief that there is nothing to be done, the patient may not mention chronic complaints, and the physician may not inquire deeply into chronic conditions (Meier, 1987). Furthermore, the elderly need more time for undressing, dressing, and carrying out procedures. It has been argued that physician behavior may be due to the focus of medical education on acute illness and a payment structure that, by rewarding cognitive services less than surgical procedures, discourages making a complete problem assessment in primary geriatric care. A reimbursement method effective January 1, 1992, will increase Medicare allowed fees for evaluation and management of patients and reduce those for "invasive and imaging procedures" (Altman and Rosenthal, 1990). However, few of the case vignettes used to develop a proposed standard for payment involve the elderly (Physician Payment Review Commission, 1989).

Preventive Care

Visits for preventive services at the doctor's office were studied using NAMCS data for 1977–1978. These visits were usually made by asymptomatic patients and were likely to be "patient motivated rather than physician initiated"; they accounted for 17 percent of all visits for the population (Cypress, 1981). Preventive services that are not sex specific (all the sex-specific ones listed are female) include general medical examinations, blood pressure tests, prophylactic immunizations, and eye examinations. For all of these, the average annual visit rate per 1,000 at age 65+ was higher for women than for men, according to NAMCS, but the difference was substantial only for blood pressure tests, 37.0 percent higher for women:

Preventive Services, by Sex

	Female/Male
General medical examination	224.4 vs. 211.3
Blood pressure test	238.2 vs. 173.9
Immunization	22.2 vs. 21.4
Eye examination	56.5 vs. 51.3

These numbers do not reveal preventive services included in a visit for treatment purposes.[4] This is a significant omission, since doctors often disguise preventive services to get around Medicare restrictions when they fill out the forms.

Information on receipt of sex-specific preventive care by women is provided by the survey. For older women, gynecological examinations were far less common than for women under 65 (21.6 visits per 1,000 persons per year). (Breast examinations and Pap smear tests were also less frequent for older women, but the numbers were too small to be reliable.)

According to a national survey of health habits, women 65+ are less likely to know how to do breast self-examination than younger women (Thornberry, Wilson, and Golden, 1986), and they are less likely to have had a Pap smear or a breast examination within the past year. Of the older women, 39 percent said they had had a breast examination during the year, versus 50 percent for all ages,[5] and 25 percent had had a Pap smear test during the year, versus 46 percent for all ages. Since the efficacy of breast self-examination has not been definitely established, the lower rate for older women is perhaps not an important problem. However, self-examination for all older women is considered a definite part of a cancer prevention strategy. Data from other surveys in the 1980s indicate that over half of older women, perhaps up to 60–63 percent, had had a Pap smear within three years (Muller et al., 1990). But 11 percent of women aged 65+ reported that they had never had the test (Hayward et al., 1988).

Medicare has just begun to cover the Pap test for cancer screening, and, until fairly recently, elderly women were omitted from screening guidelines of national organizations. Yet, when elderly women who had previously been infrequently screened received the Pap test, a high percentage of abnormal smears was observed, and such screening has been shown to be cost-effective, entailing a modest cost per life year saved by early treatment (Mandelblatt and Fahs, 1988).

Mammography among the elderly has been underutilized. A survey by the National Cancer Institute (NCI) showed that 62 percent of women 40+ had never had a breast X ray, and only 6.5 percent had had a mammogram in the last year. The recommended frequency for women over

---

[4]In addition, a substantial number of visits were made with preventive care as the second reason for the visit, but these were not analyzed by age and sex. These visits equaled in number 10 percent of the visits with prevention as the principal reason.

[5]1973 data show that, for women 65+, as for younger women, the proportion who never had a breast examination declines as income goes up: 40.3 percent at under $5,000, 29.9 percent at $5,000–$9,999, and 24.6 percent at $10,000 and over (National Center for Health Statistics, 1975).

50 is annually (*New York Times,* 30 June 1988). As a partial step, Congress included mammography every two years at a fee of up to $50 for women 65+ in the Medicare Catastrophic Coverage Act of 1988 (Advocates Senior Alert Process, 1988), but when this law was repealed in 1989, the mammography provision was canceled.

Prescribing

In 1980 males 65+ had over 60 million drug "mentions," or 1.52 per visit, according to NAMCS data; women 65+ had 105 million drug mentions, or 1.72 per visit (Koch, 1982). Men had 2.19 drugs per "drug visit" (a visit at which prescribing occurred), versus 2.37 for women. The rate of drug mentions per visit is significantly higher for women. Since older women also have more visits per person per year than men, their per capita drug use is also higher. These differences could be due in part to the higher average age of women over 65, but information on minor tranquilizers suggests that this is not the whole story (see more on this later).

Total drug mentions for women 65+ were 15.4 percent of those for the whole population, and those for men 65+ were 8.9 percent. Women 65+ had 158 mentions of analgesic drugs per 1,000 visits in 1980–1981, whereas men had 126; women 65+ had 126,383,000 visits, versus 81,532,000 for men. Thus, older women's total use was about 20,000,000 analgesic prescriptions; men's, 10,000,000 (Koch and Knapp, 1984). Use of analgesics by women 45+ has been attributed to their proneness to musculoskeletal disease after menopause (Koch, 1986).

Use of psychotropic drugs has been compared for elderly men and women. In the National Medical Care Expenditure Survey of 1977 "utilization" of psychotropic drugs refers to households' reports that the doctor prescribed them and that the drug was bought or otherwise obtained. The NMCES data show 23.3 percent of women 65+, but only 14.3 percent of men, as having at least one psychotropic drug prescription in 1977. However, the number of prescriptions per person with at least one was equal for women and men (p. 2). Widowed persons had a higher proportion of users, and more drugs per user, than other marital status groups, which may have reflected in part their age and the observed association of drug use with activity limitation. For older women, 9.5 percent of all prescribed medicines were psychotropic, compared with 7.9 percent for men (Cafferata and Kasper, 1983).

Additional information is provided by NAMCS. The term "utilization of psychotropic drugs" here is applied to ordering or prescribing of such drugs by an office-based physician; it does not include compliance by the patient in purchasing the ordered drug. (Neither NMCES nor NAMCS shows how many persons actually took the drug.) In NAMCS the number of psychotropic drug mentions per 1,000 visits peaks at ages 45–54 and begins a "gradual if fluctuating descent" thereafter for both sexes. Prescribing for males and females is equal up to age 45, but thereafter the rates "diverge dramatically," with women having a rate one-third higher than men from 45 to 64 and 60 percent higher at 65+. This is said to "correlate positively" with diagnostic evidence, since older women have more mental disorders and essential hypertension than older men (Koch and Campbell, 1983). This is a weak argument. First, the relation of the drugs to essential hypertension is questionable.

Second, prescribing for mental disorders of women has come under critical scrutiny. More than three-fifths of the mentions of anti-anxiety agents, sedatives, and hypnotics in 1980–1981 were at visits to general and family practitioners and internists, as were a similar fraction of anti-depressants and close to half of antipsychotic and antimanic drug mentions. In all, over half of the prescribing of psychotropic drugs was done by primary care physicians. There were 25 million drug mentions for mental disorders in all specialties but only 14 million in psychiatry (Koch and Campbell, 1983, tables 2, 5, pp. 4, 7). Whether there is excessive use of psychiatric diagnoses by primary care physicians cannot be settled from currently published data. It is interesting, however, that the use of minor tranquilizers goes up far more for women than for men after age 75.

Use of Minor Tranquilizers, by Sex
(Rate per 100)

	Under 75	75+
Men	35	38
Women	44	66

Source: Hugo Koch and Mickey C. Smith, *Office-based Ambulatory Care for Patients 75 Years Old and Over: National Ambulatory Medical Care Survey, 1980 and 1981.* (Hyattsville, MD: National Center for Health Statistics, 1985), table 10, p. 8.

It has been argued that physicians use psychotropic drugs inappropriately as a way of dealing with the expressive aspects of patients' behavior (especially of women) that do not fit into their clinical treatment models. This reasoning about physician behavior is supported by the observation that women's cultural role leads to a life-long record of ability to form relationships and engage in mutual dependence. Therefore, it is argued, they should not be at high risk of depression. Nevertheless, loss of family roles without other gratifying roles to replace them can create depression in old age or intensify character traits that have a depressive aspect. Financial problems, physical illness, and side effects of medications used for physical illness can create depression. (Absence of effective caregiver sources could also be depressing.) It has also been suggested that hormonal deficiency after menopause provides an explanation for depression and that estrogen replacement therapy, rather than psychotropic drugs, may be appropriate. McKinlay, McKinlay, and Brambilla (1987), however, find that depression is apt to be found with a surgical menopause but not a natural one and is associated with multiple roles and causes of worry among married women. (They do caution, however, that psychic morbidity might lead to a hysterectomy, rather than the other way around.)

Physicians may miss a diagnosis of depression because mental illness appears less socially acceptable to patients than physical illness, and older patients, therefore, present somatic complaints when depressed; or the physician may mistake depression for senile dementia. These diverse possibilities can be handled best by a thorough evaluation by the physician (Lobel and Hirschfeld, 1984). Many elderly women have dependence problems that would respond to economic and social improvement and medical problems for which diverse therapies other than psychotropic drugs would be the treatment of choice. Prescribing of such drugs should be studied to see if it is supported by confirmed clinical diagnoses for which tranquilizers and the like are considered appropriate therapy.

It has been reported that the risk of falling, which is higher for women, is greater among users of hypnotics, tranquilizers, and diuretics, suggesting additional reasons for monitoring of drug use (Mossey, 1985). Ray et al. (1987) have shown by a case-control study of elderly persons on Medicaid that the use of psychotropic drugs that have long elimination half-lives (over twenty-four hours) was associated with an increased risk of hip fracture. The effect was dose-related and was not explainable by the presence of dementia. Short-acting hypnotic-anxiolytic drugs did not increase the risk of falling. (In this study, 77 percent of the cases of hip fracture and 78 percent of the controls were women.)

Hospital Use

Hospital discharge rates increase with age, and, in 1981, those 65+, representing 11 percent of the population, used 39.3 percent of all short-stay hospital days (U.S. Congress, 1984, p. 70). Older males have higher discharge rates at each age level after 65 than older females; the difference increases after age 85 (Graves, 1986).[6] Discharges per 1,000 enroll-ees under Medicare in 1982 were 405 for men and 363 for women (U.S. Department of Health and Human Services, 1987, p. 43), and reimburse-ments per enrollee for 1982 were $1,179 for men and $1,078 for women (p. 37). The 1985 data from the National Hospital Discharge Survey show a hospital discharge rate for men 65+ of 395.6 per 1,000; for wom-en, 348.1. But women's length of stay was slightly longer: 8.7 days ver-sus 8.2 (National Center for Health Statistics, 1987). Reported sex differences in discharge rates vary, depending on the year and the source (hospital records versus household interviews), but the higher rates for men persist. (However, because so many of the elderly are women, ad-missions of women 65+ numbered 6 million, or 29.1 percent more than those of men, and total days for elderly women were 37.0 percent more than for men, making up one-fourth of all days for the population.) For both sexes, the rate of procedures performed in hospitals also increases after age 65, and again the rate is higher for males (U.S. Congress, 1984, p. 71).

The most common cause of hospitalization after age 40 is coronary atherosclerosis. For males, narrowing of blood vessels develops rapidly in middle age, but for women it starts after menopause. This is reflected in gender differences in hospitalizations for the condition. At ages 40–64, over 70 percent of admissions are male, but at age 65 the percentage with this condition who are women increases, rising to 60.0 percent at 80+. Severity increases with age. Length of stay and number of procedures are similar for both sexes in each age subgroup (Garnick and Short, 1985). Another leading cause of admission is hip fractures. Women account for 72 percent of all elderly patients admitted for hip fractures and, at age 80+, 83 percent. Over 87 percent have surgery. Length of stay averages over 20 days, and this is often the result of waiting for nursing home placement.

Hospitals can respond to prospective payment incentives by reducing services per case, shifting more patients to nursing homes, or restricting admissions to less severe cases entailing less resource use. If hospitals take such steps, patients who are vulnerable for medical or social reasons (such as lack of caregivers at home) may have worse outcomes or trouble getting needs met, even though hospital policies are apparently objective and based on clinical criteria or financial problems of the institution. A

---

[6]This is based on 1975–1976 data from the National Hospital Discharge Survey (NHDS) (National Center for Health Statistics, 1987). The National Health Interview Sur-vey for the same period shows a higher female rate for 85+, but the NHDS, based on hospital records, does not depend on recall, as the interview survey does.

study done for the Health Care Financing Administration (HCFA) by Forgy and Williams found that severity of illness at the time of discharge increased from 1982 to 1985, implying greater need for posthospital services (Gornick and Hall, 1988). The Medicare Catastrophic Coverage Act of 1988 made more skilled nursing facility days (SNF) and home health visits available, but these provisions were repealed in the following year.

Nursing Homes

"Elderly females are twice as likely as elderly males to be residents of nursing homes" (Hing, 1987, p. 2), according to the 1985 National Nursing Home Survey. Sixty out of every 1,000 elderly women and 29 out of every 1,000 elderly men lived in nursing homes. For each age group past 65, women used nursing homes at significantly higher rates, and, at 85+, one in 4 women, versus one in 7 men, lived in nursing homes. Females made up three-quarters of the nursing home population. The figures are a reflection of higher use by persons without spouses and in poor health. The women residents were older than the men (average age of 84, versus 81, years).[7] Because functional dependence increases with age, women require more help with activities of daily living and have an average of 4.0 ADL disabilities, whereas men have 3.6. These limitations are, as expected, even more frequent than in the part of the community-dwelling elderly population most at risk for nursing home admission. Women's length of stay is 41 percent greater than men's, and the difference is substantial even for women and men over 84 (Sekscenski, 1987, tables 2, 4).

The female residents were much more likely to be widowed than the male (74 percent versus 37 percent), whereas 33 percent of the men were married, compared with 11 percent of the women. Being married is conducive to a shorter stay (Sekscenski, 1987, p. 3). More of the women had living children, but it is not known whether the children lived close enough and were able to provide informal care at home.[8]

The women residents were more likely to have lived alone before admission and to have been admitted from a short-stay hospital rather than

---

[7]New York City data for 1983 show, not only that female residents in skilled nursing facilities and health-related facilities (HRFs) are older than male residents, but also that a substantial number are old-old: 47.2 percent of female SNF residents and 38.4 percent of female HRF residents were 85+. The end-of-the-year patient census for New York City SNFs and HRFs for 1983 shows 90 percent of patients in both types of facilities to be on Medicaid (United Hospital Fund of New York, 1986a).

[8]Elderly black residents were less likely than whites to have children, and other evidence shows that the black impaired elderly are more likely than whites to live with children, rather than to enter a nursing home.

a private residence. The latter is taken as evidence of their being in poorer health. Women were also more likely to have Medicaid as their primary payment source. This may be a reflection of their lower incomes: in 1982 46 percent of elderly women living in the community had family incomes of under $7,000, a level reported by only 31 percent of their male counterparts (Hing, 1987). However, assets are often transferred to family members, to qualify under current eligibility rules for Medicaid that preclude partial contributions from families, with the result of fostering excessive dependence and institutionalization (United Hospital Fund of New York, 1986b).

Reasons for sex differences in long-term care are best identified by prospective multivariate studies, but good studies of this kind are unfortunately few (Wingard, 1987). Some factors, though, are known. It appears that women's high use rate is due to their high disability levels, in part a correlate of age and their low incomes, which limit receipt of paid help. Together these factors affect the ability of elderly women living alone to continue in the community. Fortunately, information from recent national surveys of nursing homes and long-term care clients will permit fresh analyses that may add to our understanding of the factors resulting in institutionalization and prolonged stays, and of sex differences. Meanwhile, the public share of nursing home expenditures has declined and self-pay sources have become more prominent, thus making income levels more important in determining access to nursing homes (Gornick et al., 1985).

The Medicare Catastrophic Coverage Act of 1988 amends Medicaid provisions in order to help prevent impoverishment of spouses whose partners enter long-term care facilities. For instance, in any month in which a husband is institutionalized, no income of the wife is considered to be available to the husband in determining eligibility for Medicaid. Once eligibility has been established for the husband, income paid in the name of both spouses is deemed to be divided equally. A resource allowance is protected for the community spouse, equal to the greater of $12,000 annually or the spouse's share (half) of the couple's total resources. A state can set a figure higher than $12,000, and a community spouse can show in a fair hearing that more is needed to achieve the minimum protected amount of monthly income. This amount is specified, unless an exception is made, to equal one-twelfth of 150 percent of the federal poverty level for a two-person household by 1992, with additional allowances for family dependents. The protected income is deductible from the institutionalized spouse's income in calculating how much of the latter amount is available for monthly costs of care. The new provisions help resolve the problem created by previous linkage of

Medicaid eligibility to actual or potential receipt of Supplemental Security Income (SSI) cash assistance, and they set a federal standard for the
protected income of the community spouse (U.S. Department of Health
and Human Services, 1988). These improvements survived the repeal of
most MCCA provisions in 1989.

Community-based Care

Relatively few of the elderly use formal home health services, but such
use is more common among women, according to the 1977 National
Medical Care Expenditure Survey (5.2 percent versus 3.2 percent). Use
was more common for those who lived alone, rather than with a spouse,
children, or other relatives; who were limited in ability to perform usual
activity or outside activity; and who were in fair or poor health. Neither
these associations nor the correlation of use of home health services with
source of payment and hospitalization were analyzed by sex. The bulk of
these services came from publicly financed sources. For all elderly, only 5
percent of home health visits were paid by a private insurance source,
and a substantial proportion (29 percent) of visits to elderly users involved some out-of-pocket expenses. Nonmarket services rendered by
family members can replace market services to which poverty would be a
barrier, but this substitution depends on having available children or a
living spouse (Berk and Bernstein, 1985) and on the types of services that
sons and daughters typically supply (see page 126).

Women are generally thought to have strong affiliative capacity and
interest in affiliation (West and Simons, 1983), based on their family
roles, and to have the ability to make and keep friends. Yet their network
for health maintenance purposes and for dealing with health problems is
often frayed by widowhood and raided by age. Living past eighty-five
reduces the number of surviving peers with whom new friendship ties do
not have to be created. For those elderly who do not have serious impairments, friends and neighbors are useful for exchange of information on
health practices and the health care market, expression of positive concern and encouragement to seek medical advice, and general protection
of morale. The more seriously impaired need a regular flow of services
that cannot usually be supplied by friends and neighbors when the
spouse has died and adult children are living elsewhere.

Fifteen percent of men 65+ and 41 percent of women of that age were
living alone in 1984; the women made up 80 percent of the elderly living
alone and were equally divided between those under and those over age
75. The male ELAs were slightly more likely to be under 75 (Kovar,
1986).

The position of ELAs is not necessarily problematic. Most ELAs lived close to their families and had frequent contacts with them: about 90 percent had gotten together with either family or friends in the two weeks before the interview, and a similar proportion had talked to them on the telephone. Those living alone did not use less health care than other elderly or spend fewer days in bed, but they reported themselves as being in better health than those living with others (70 percent said health was excellent, very good, or good), possibly because many elderly stop living alone when health declines. Only 22 percent said they were limited in their usual activity or unable to perform it. Four-fifths said they were in control of their future health. While some ELAs may need to see their situation in a positive light, or may be naturally optimistic, many are evidently well able to manage—unless there is a change in health. Most ELAs felt they would have someone to take care of them for a few days, but 24 percent said they would have no one to take care of them for a few weeks if needed. About three-fourths of persons aged 70 and older who live alone "with some type of limitation receive no help and manage on their own" (Kasper, 1988, p. 54).

Social contacts are part of the coping pattern of these elderly and provide, to some extent, a substitute for living with others. There is evidence that having many friends and relatives and seeing a great deal of them fends off mortality. The effect seems to be stronger for men (*New York Times*, 4 August 1988). It would be interesting to know whether or not male and female ELAs differ in the amount of support received when ill, of encouragement to participate in activities, and of reminders to visit doctors and follow their diets. Men are more likely than women to fall into a small subgroup of ELAs who do not have social contacts, recent medical care, or good self-reported health. Clearly, the ELAs are heterogeneous in their health level and resources, and some are quite vulnerable to a change in health.

A Virginia study of disabled elderly with one or more ADL limitations shows that, after control for other factors, gender was important in use of services. Women used more "social," or supportive, services such as home health care, homemaker services, personal care, community health services, and physical therapy than did men.

Disabled women did not use more physician and hospital services per person than did disabled men. However, more of the women were disabled: 43 percent versus 38 percent (Wan and Arling, 1983). The disabled elderly were older than the nondisabled, more likely to have incomes below $5,000, more likely to be on Medicaid, and slightly more likely to lack a regular source of care.

Among the community-dwelling elderly, women are more likely than men to use senior centers and to eat meals at the centers. Persons living alone are more likely to use the centers and eat center meals, and they also receive more homemaker services and home-delivered meals. Elderly persons with activity limitations also use more in-home services; and so, women, who are more likely to live alone and have a higher rate of limitations, are more frequent users of in-home services. The use of centers by women does not increase after age 75, implying that, as limitations increase, they can't get to the centers even though they could benefit from the social support and the meals (Stone, 1986a).

CAREGIVING

Compared with men, women are more commonly faced with role demands as caregivers as they enter old age. The receivers may be husbands (usually older than their wives in the cohorts in or near old age) or elderly parents: a woman of 65 may have a parent of 85 or 90 who needs services. Even if the parent is cared for in a nursing home, energy is expended in traveling to the facility, providing emotional support through regular visits, and interacting with nursing home management and staff to protect the patient's rights and welfare. Parents-in-law also receive care and attention from aging women who are married or widowed.

One-third of those giving informal care to the disabled elderly, according to the National Long-Term Care Survey (Stone, Cafferata, and Sangl, 1986) were over sixty-five, and over 70 percent were female. When the caregiver was a wife, in three-fifths of the cases she did the job alone. This happened almost as often for husbands giving care to wives. But where the child was the source of aid, daughters were twice as likely as sons to do the tasks alone and were less likely to serve as secondary caregivers. One-third of all caregivers reported their own health to be fair or poor.

A New York study by Horowitz (1985) found that adult sons are less likely than daughters to render "hands-on" assistance to their elderly parents in personal care, household chores, meal preparation, and transportation or to step into the role of primary caregiver. For financial tasks and negotiations with bureaucracies, however, sons and daughters did not differ in involvement. There was no significant sex difference in frequency of telephone contact or visiting, but three-fifths of children in a caregiving role came only once a week or less, too rarely for basic personal care and household maintenance. Eighty-five percent of the parents in need of care were mothers. Sons had less perceived stress because of caregiving, even if they provided the same level of care as daughters; it is believed that the latter had more conflicting demands (62 percent were working) and also more emotional connection with their impaired mothers. Of the children identified as caregivers by older subjects, 70 percent were daughters. A study by Brody and colleagues (Brody et al., 1987) notes that women are more vulnerable to possible conflict between work and elder care. Even though work provides some respite from caregiving, pressures may increase as the capacities of the parent decline over time.

The relation of informal caregiving to purchased care in the last twelve months of life figured in a study in a West Coast group practice. Women had higher out-of-pocket expenses than men, both in dollars ($6,610 versus $2,963) and as a percentage of total health care expenditure (27.4 percent versus 14.7 percent). They had higher expenditures on nursing home and home health care but were less likely to have insurance coverage for these services (Scitovsky, 1986). Scitovsky thinks women might be using more nursing home and home health services because they have fewer sources of social support than men. However, differences in the percentage with daily contact (which was used in this study as a measure of social support) did not help explain the sex differences in expenses. (A study that would take account of sex of adult children might have a different result.)

THIRD-PARTY PAYERS

Medicare

Medicare enrollment and utilization data by sex reflect the various factors of demography, needs, and resources mentioned in the previous sections. Between 1966 and 1984 the number of aged women enrolled under Medicare grew at an annual compound rate of 2.2 percent; the number of aged men enrollees, at 1.7 percent. In 1984 three-fifths of the Medicare elderly population was female. At the same time, the ratio of those 75+ to those 65–74 in Medicare increased. Thus, the survival of women to older ages explains the high proportion of women among enrollees (U.S. Department of Health and Human Services, 1989a, table 2.2). The amount reimbursed per person served was 23 percent higher for men ($3,116 versus $2,536 in 1984), and the amount reimbursed per enrollee was 10.6 percent higher for men. This occurred mainly because, for every 1,000 enrollees, women are more likely than men to be served under supplementary medical insurance (SMI), or Part B, which covers ambulatory services (in addition to physician services in hospitals and nursing homes), with relatively small average expense, and less likely to be served as inpatients. For both sexes, 70 percent of total expenditures was under hospital insurance (Medicare, Part A). Per enrollee, expense for men was $1,435 under Part A (hospital) and $952 under Part B (medical); comparable figures for women were $1,261 and $799. The user rate (proportion of enrollees receiving service) for SMI services went up with age (U.S. Department of Health and Human Services, 1989a, table 3.3).

Although men used more hospital care, women were more likely than men to use skilled nursing facilities or home health services under Medicare (see table). For other categories of service, the sex difference was small.

Persons Served per 1,000 Aged Medicare Enrollees, 1984

Service Type	M	F	M/F (%)
Hospital insurance (HI)			
Inpatient hospital	238.1	222.0	107.3
Skilled nursing facility	8.3	12.3	67.5
Supplementary medical insurance (SMI)			
Physician & other medical	643.7	699.5	92.0
Outpatient	314.0	335.1	93.7
HI and/or SMI			
Home health agency	45.0	56.0	80.4

Source: U.S. Department of Health and Human Services, *Medicare and Medicaid Data Book, 1988.* (Baltimore, MD, 1989a), table 3.

Private Insurance

Medicare's limitations, even for acute illness, have resulted in wide marketing of supplementary coverage. Several central findings on health insurance coverage of elderly men and women from the National Health Care Expenditures Survey of 1977 (Cafferata, 1984b) are explained by women's inferior position in the labor market during their earlier years. Women are only slightly less likely than men to have private coverage in old age. But women who are covered are much less likely to have group plans or an employer contribution, and they have considerably lower annual premiums.[9] The premium difference seems to have little effect on benefit scope, but for some benefits the dollar amounts or units of service allowed may be restricted.

A major problem for aging women is the gap between widowhood and eligibility for Medicare. In 1980, at age 55–59, 14.2 percent of women

---

[9] Percentages for women and men are 64.0 percent versus 66.9 percent (private coverage); 29.7 percent versus 45.4 percent (group plans); 19.0 percent versus 41.3 percent (employer contribution); and annual premiums are $232 versus $391.

were widowed and at 60–64, 22.6 percent. Black women were widowed at younger ages (Bianchi and Spain, 1986). If coverage was obtained through the husband and is not continued for the widow, and if it is not replaced by benefits through women's own employment, widows are not likely to have good quality insurance for their health care needs.

Elderly persons have flawed knowledge of their actual coverage, according to data from the National Medical Care Expenditure Survey (Cafferata, 1984a). Their best showing was 80 percent correct as to hospital and surgical coverage; and their worst, 12.6 percent as to outpatient mental health coverage. These percentages are based on the response of the most knowledgeable person in the household. Elderly respondents tend to think they are not covered when they really are, rather than the reverse. Thus, one-fourth of the sample wrongly believed they were not covered for physician office visits. (To a lesser extent, this was also a problem in younger age groups.) Among the elderly, knowledge of coverage went down with age, but this was not so for those with private insurance. It was inferred from this that, having shopped for insurance, they had learned the details. Nevertheless, because of ignorance and confusion, as shown by the many "don't know" responses, the elderly may underuse covered services, fail to obtain reimbursement, or buy duplicative policies.

Long-term Care

Among the elderly, chronic illness is a more important problem than acute illness. This is especially true for women, who have higher rates than men of arthritis and functional limitations. Yet the financing and delivery of health care have focused on acute illness. Public programs for long-term care are subject to many restrictions. Improvements legislated by Congress in 1988 obliging Medicare to pay for one hundred and fifty skilled nursing home days per year and dropping the requirement of a prior stay in the hospital were reversed in the following year. Copayments are collected for the first eight days. Home health services are still limited to acute and postacute situations; 1988 provisions increasing services per week and the duration were also repealed. Medicaid, the main public payer for nursing home care, requires spending down of savings for eligibility. Administration on Aging agencies must offer home care and congregate and home-delivered meals, but funds are severely limited. Two-thirds of all long-term care spending goes to nursing homes; community-based care is underdeveloped (Ruchlin and Braham, 1986).

Private insurance for long-term care is believed to be in its infancy, although the market is changing rapidly. Potential beneficiaries are apparently reluctant to plan on needing the care and do not realize the limitations of the coverage they now have (they may be aware, too, that Medicaid serves as an insurer of last resort). State insurance regulations were said to have inhibited introduction of new products, but several states passed laws providing incentives for long-term care insurance. A few years later, allegedly "outrageous practices" in the sale of such coverage were charged (Tolchin, 1990).

The insurance companies reportedly fear that beneficiaries interacting with fee-for-service providers will inflate demand and push costs up. Some observers believe that case management to avert demand escalation and make the insurance workable can be attained through HMOs. Stop-loss insurance, in which payment by the carrier starts only after a certain amount of outlay by the patient, has been proposed to protect insurers against adverse selection. This would keep premiums more affordable, but the protection provided would be too meager for some elderly (Knickman and McCall, 1986). The need for government programs to supplement private group and individual policies has been noted (New York Business Group on Health, 1988).

VULNERABILITY TO REIMBURSEMENT ISSUES

Women may be particularly affected by certain features of the health care reimbursement system for the elderly because they frequently lack family caregivers, have income constraints, and less often receive supplementary insurance through an employer. One such feature is the prospective payment system for hospitals, which motivates them to discharge patients sooner, with the risk that they will need substantial care from others (U.S. Congress, 1986a). Another is payment schedules that penalize doing certain procedures on an inpatient basis. These may relocate recovery to the home, often making satisfactory recovery depend on caregiver availability (U.S. Congress, 1986b). Such effects need to be measured through well-designed research that could include determining if the effects vary by gender.

Both sexes share the need for a geriatric care system that encompasses nonphysician services for health maintenance and rehabilitation and supportive services such as special transport and home-based or community-based meals. Multidimensional functional assessment should be incorporated in geriatric primary care. Whether it will be encouraged by a reimbursement system that honors cognitive services equally with surgical procedures is something we will be able to determine when the new Medicare physician payment method incorporating this intent has been implemented. Physician training that helps practitioners recognize age differences in the presentation of illness would raise the detection power of the medical encounter and clarify the interpretation of tests. This would improve cognitive services.

Both sexes are affected by deficiencies in financing arrangements. Long-term care coverage is too expensive for most elderly. Balance billing (charging more than the Medicare-allowed charge) results in substantial out-of-pocket expenses. Elderly enrollees in HMOs may find them predisposed toward rapid processing of the patient caseload for financial reasons.

Both sexes are injured by termination of retirees' health benefits when employers file for bankruptcy or face financial difficulties. Congressman Edward R. Roybal of California has stated that an important factor in current threats to retirees' health benefits is the changes in Medicare mandated by Congress that have shifted costs of protection for older workers to employers. Other changes have been proposed that would further shift to private employers' plans the costs of their retirees' care. The Medicare Part A deductible increased from $40 in 1966 to $520 in 1987; the daily copayment, from $10 in 1965 to $130 in 1987 (U.S. Congress, 1984; U.S. Department of Health and Human Services, 1987, p. 41). Changes in either Part A or Part B deductibles or copayments could drive up the cost of supplementary coverage to employers.

In a survey reported by Anthony J. Gajda, testifying before the House of Representatives Select Committee on Aging, 57 percent of the firms surveyed provide health benefits to retirees, and, of these, 89 percent also cover the spouse. Two-thirds of the firms with retiree benefits require retirees to pay something, and 31 percent require them to pay 50 percent or more of the cost. The General Accounting Office estimates the total accrued retiree health benefits liabilities of employers for 1988 at one-fourteenth the value of stocks of publicly held U.S. corporations, or $227 billion (General Accounting Office, 1989).

The legal status of firms' obligations to continue retiree benefits is muddy. Courts have ruled that employers who have not clearly reserved the "right to terminate or award retiree benefits in their written contract communications" or in their conduct are not free to do so. But, in another case, absent a specific agreement not to change or drop benefits, the court said the employer could cease to cover retirees (Equitable HCA Corporation, Dec. 1988–Jan. 1989).

As the probability of having employer-sponsored benefits is greater for men, the loss of benefits is more of an issue today for male employees than for female employees. However, as women enter the primary labor market in greater numbers, they acquire more benefit rights and are thus placed at similar financial risk. Women may be vulnerable if they retire early before they are eligible for Medicare, to join (typically) older spouses in retirement, and if they are spouses of retired men, with supplementary entitlements based on their husbands' employment. Both sexes are vulnerable if they retire early for health reasons without qualifying for Social Security disability benefits that would entitle them to Medicare before age 65.[10] Both sexes are at financial risk, too, if employer benefits stop years after the retirement of the employed persons in the household and they cannot afford Medigap (supplementary coverage) or are rejected because of adverse health histories, as happened to a retiree whose plight was described to the House Select Committee on Aging.

Health maintenance organizations, once a dream in the minds of health care reformers, became attractive across a broad political spectrum as a way of attaining a cost-effective delivery system. General application of HMOs to Medicare has been the subject of several bills that encourage choice among alternative delivery systems through vouchers. Schlesinger (1986) expresses strong doubt that elderly persons with chronic illness will be well served through the HMO model. A key reason is that costs can be shifted out of the acute care system by placing the responsibility with family members or by nursing home placement followed, in due course, by Medicaid eligibility. This weakens the HMO's incentive to deal effectively with chronic problems. Similarly, prevention is not provided unless clearly cost-effective to the HMO, which is more difficult to show for the elderly than for younger clients, unless different outcome targets are chosen. Professional norms for care of the elderly are not well established and have not penetrated noticeably into HMOs, which were created to serve young employed populations in good health. Extended care benefits are rarely offered and, when they are, it is only for a few months. The HMOs refer enrollees to other providers for long-term care. (Of course, private practice outside HMOs is also deficient in its adaptation to total needs of the elderly.)

Doctor–patient communication is reported to be less than satisfactory in HMOs, which interferes with the case management approach often necessary for care of the elderly. But Hibbard and Pope (1986) report that elderly patients in an HMO are more likely than younger ones to form an attachment to one doctor, and, when they do, they make more office visits. Gender, however, did not affect total visits, initial (i.e., patient-initiated) visits, or preventive visits by those 65+ in study models that considered need, education, and other factors. The HMOs use wait-

---

[10]Medicare eligibility starts 24 months after a Social Security Disability Insurance (SSDI) award and 29 months after onset of the disability. Retiring after age 62 years and 7 months on SSDI would not create any Medicare eligibility before age 65.

ing time as a means of nonfinancial rationing of care; while this may not be onerous to older patients in general, who are reported to be less bothered than the young by waiting, the disabled elderly may have a problem when waiting is prolonged. Centralized locations of HMO facilities are a handicap to older people, who tend to need more time to travel a given distance for care, possibly because they rely more on public transportation (which, in turn, is traceable to poverty, disability, and lack of special transport arrangements).

Elderly persons are said to be ill-equipped to assess alternative insurance policies and providers (see page 129). Schlesinger argues that informed choice among HMOs is even more difficult for the elderly, because they underestimate the importance of long-term care benefits. Meanwhile, cost incentives motivate HMOs to screen out Medicare beneficiaries whose care will be expensive because of chronic illness or to disenroll them. This behavior is difficult to control through regulation.

These potential HMO problems are not gender-specific. However, women tend to have inferior resources, compared with men, for the purchase of outside services if their needs are not met fully within an HMO or if they are rejected by HMOs. Moreover, women who have chronic conditions and are members of an HMO that is not prepared to provide all the services they need may lack access to unpaid supportive services to fill the gap. Modification of HMO practices to meet needs of the elderly presents a challenge to policymakers who are attracted by potential efficiencies of HMOs.

GENDER WITHIN THE TREATMENT PROCESS

Does gender affect what happens to elderly patients once they enter the health care system? Evidence suggests that many important influences on medical care adequacy and quality at all ages are not gender-linked. Studies have analyzed medical misadventures due to errors of physicians' judgment and have described the damage done (or opportunities for improvement lost) by translation of findings from poor research into treatment protocols, circumstances that are not confined to either sex. Many aspects of patient processing are dictated by physiological, anatomical, and humanistic considerations—all universalistic. In the sphere of health policy, the debate over ways of financing the health care system, including long-term care, is conducted without mention of gender, as seen by titles of articles in leading health care journals.

Yet it seems likely that, for the elderly, economic and cultural differences related to gender are more clearly relevant in dictating whether the system works well for the patient than they are for younger groups. This is because of the strong relation of social factors to preservation of functional level and quality of life in old age. Not only must the total patient be understood, but also the patient in his or her total setting, in which the continuation of the desired medical regimen, nutritional support, and so forth occur. This means that the correlates of gender among the elderly cannot be omitted from consideration. In addition, cultural stereotypes regarding women's response to pain (that they overstate it and that they perceive it when an organic basis is absent) may distort physicians' cognitive processes of arriving at correct diagnoses and appropriate treatment plans.

Drug prescribing appears to be affected by the patient's sex. Psychotropic drugs are more frequently prescribed for women, and the prolonged use of these drugs without medical indications has often been criticized. Moreover, drugs (and other treatments) may be prescribed for older women on the basis of research done on younger, male subjects; the appropriateness of the dosage and of the drug itself may be unsupported. Use of only male subjects for clinical testing of new treatments is being discouraged by federal granting agencies following criticism by two women scientists from the National Institute of Mental Health (Hamilton and Parry, 1983) and recommendations from a Public Health Service Task Force on Women's Health (U.S. Department of Health and Human Services, 1986c). Investigators using only male subjects are now asked to state this explicitly in their reports.

Do Elderly Women Receive Enough Care?

According to Verbrugge (1984), the specific conditions bothering elderly women in daily life, such as their sensory or musculoskeletal problems, are not life-threatening. The diseases to which women eventually succumb, heart disease, cancer, and stroke, are similar to the causes of mortality for men. But older men, in contrast with women, die of the same diseases that cause them difficulty in daily life. The proportion of cases receiving medical attention is less for women's disabling or limiting conditions than for other conditions such as heart disease. Verbrugge considers this difference to be rational, because cures are not known for arthritis and similar conditions. But it is also possible that care is not received that could relieve symptoms and preserve functional level (e.g., prevent joint deterioration in arthritis). Patients may be unaware that relief is possible or hampered by poor mobility. Their finances may preclude use of less urgent care. Similarly, assistive devices and palliative and corrective surgery that can help sensory impairments exist, but NCHS notes that "such therapy has an impact on out-of-pocket expenses" (Havlik,

1986, p. 6). Evidence from cataract care in relation to condition prevalence also suggests undertreatment for women, for there is no sex difference in surgery rates, despite a higher prevalence of cataracts in women. Furthermore, grading of lens opacification in a population-based sample in Framingham indicated that women's cataracts were no less severe than men's, so that the difference in probability of treatment cannot be explained by less frequency of disabling eye disease among women (Havlik, 1986). There is currently concern about overuse, namely, that cataract surgery is done excessively because it is now feasible on an outpatient basis and reimbursable in that setting. But it is possible for overtreatment and undertreatment to coexist.

According to data from three sites used for epidemiological study of the elderly, women have more prevalence than men of past fractures of the hip and other sites (Cornoni-Huntley et al., 1986). Postmenopausal osteoporosis, as a contributing factor, appears to be influenced by activity level, calcium intake, and estrogen therapy, although its dynamics are still being studied (Butler, 1985). If the relationships are valid, the medical care system can help reduce future risk of fractures by appropriate prescriptions and diet advice and by encouraging women to participate in sports and maintain a high general activity level. However, this is only one factor in preventing falls among the elderly, since sensory, neurological, and other system problems, including feet, and environmental hazards, including lighting and clothing, have been identified as risk factors (Tinetti and Speechley, 1989). Fall prevention is thus a challenge to be met by a comprehensive approach.

AGEISM

If the potential of medical care to improve the health and functioning of the elderly of both sexes is not fully used, one reason for this is ageism.

Ageism is a generalized attitude in society as to the decline in personal capacities with age and the consequent illegitimacy of great expectations as to the yield from social investment in the elderly. If this stereotype is shared as a self-perception by the elderly, it acts as a constraint on their goals and assertiveness. Ageism limits what health care can do for both men and women past sixty-five by infiltrating the management of encounters and the underlying premises of the reimbursement system. Providers who are influenced by age stereotypes overlook reversible elements in the patient's presenting condition, and their attitudes are colored by frustration with the slower or different response of an elderly patient to treatment. The right of each person to the maximum attainable functional level may not be accepted or really understood. An illustration is what happened to a patient, then in her early sixties, who was examined several years ago by an otologist of around forty years of age with excellent credentials and a very delicate touch with instruments that minimized the discomfort of the procedures that were performed. When told that her sinus blockage was probably related to an anatomical problem, a deviated septum, the patient asked whether a surgical correction was available. She received the reply: "Oh, you've lived your life— we do it on younger people." Reason suggests, of course, that the desirability of surgery would have to be carefully weighed, but the ready categorization was indicative of an ingrained attitude.

Greenfield et al. (1987) have found that older women with breast cancer often get less treatment than they should because of their age. Only 83 percent of those 70+ got appropriate care, whereas 96 percent of those 50–69 did so. It was suggested by the chief medical officer of the American Cancer Society that physicians may have withheld treatment (presumably radiation) because they feared that patients would not tolerate serious side effects (New York Times, 22 May 1987). However, the women selected for this study did not have medical problems except for their cancer and were likely to have lived a long time if the cancer had been successfully treated. Whether similar differences would be found in treatment of a serious condition specific to, or most common among, men would be worth looking into.

Low rates of use of mental health services by the elderly are deemed underuse because the stresses of retirement, widowhood, and inability to care for oneself frequently occur and imply a need for help. The elderly of today may be influenced by a lingering social stigma attached to emotional illness (Kovar, 1977). It has been suggested, based on a study of around three hundred persons, that women are more vulnerable than men to life changes in old age (West and Simons, 1983) (they rate standard events as more disruptive) and also that income serves as a buffer against adverse life events. But for both sexes, self-efficacy, a coping element in younger groups, is less useful in dealing with those life changes that occur in old age.

The element of gender in physician attitudes toward the elderly has not been empirically studied, but such research would add to our understanding of health care issues. Physicians are thought to be considerate and compassionate toward the frail, suffering, or anxious older person: perhaps they are even particularly so toward a woman who resembles in some way a loved mother or grandmother. But the male physician may not be oriented to autonomy needs of older women and to their full participation in decision making. Doctors' social class fosters professional dominance (Haug and Ory, 1987), and this may be encouraged by a sex difference between doctor and patient, especially with older doctors, who are more likely to be male. Male doctors' judgment and goals may be more similar to those of their male patients than to those of women. Their interpretations of symptoms may depend on patients' communication style, and they may ascribe to emotional causes the symptoms reported by patients who have an expressive style (Bernstein and Kane, 1981). Whether different cohorts of women have different expressive styles could be examined, along with their interaction with younger cohorts of doctors who have grown up in a more sex-equal society.

CONCLUSION

The interpretation of gender's influence on the appropriateness of health care received by the elderly is a task calling for subtlety. One problem concerns the type of statistics to use. Women dominate many statistics about the elderly's health and their use of the health care system because of their greater life expectancy, and, therefore, a proper perspective is supplied by considering rates per 1,000 population, rather than absolute numbers, and by examining 5-year age groups rather than all over 65. Additional insight is gained by ascertaining the proportion of a specific market, such as the market for psychotropic drugs, accounted for by the demand of each sex, so that the parties at interest can be identified when change is contemplated. Another problem is the selection of findings for review and discussion. Statements regarding sex differences in various rates can be misleading if the differences are small, which they sometimes are, or if only those dimensions and conditions are brought into view for which women have demonstrated excess of undertreatment, overtreatment, or unmet need for care. Both a focus on substantial differences and a sense of the whole are necessary.

The gender issue in old age manifests itself, with regard to health care, as an accumulation of special risks and needs based on the previous position of women in the economy and the family structure. As wives of somewhat older men and as caregivers, they become, partly as a result of men's higher mortality, survivors with a mismatch of needs to informal caregiving sources. As individuals who have spent their adult years in less advantaged, sex-typed jobs and whose work careers have often been interrupted, they enter old age with fewer financial resources than their male counterparts that can be used to translate their health needs into effective demand. They are currently bumping up against cost-containment approaches that emphasize self and family care—admirable if feasible and voluntary, difficult if Procrustean in application. Facial neutrality to gender is typical of policy proposals and analyses in health care financing for the elderly, and it is often difficult to ascertain whether there will be a differential effect on one sex. Cohort changes in work opportunities, spousal sharing, health practices, and environmental exposures make it necessary to continue assessing gender issues among the elderly and noting those that are waning—and new ones that may arise. The ebb and flow of financial protection against the health needs of the elderly and of trends toward equality in the workplace prevent any assumption that the problems of the elderly female are merely transitional. Medicare, in place since 1965, has been retreating from being the first payer for group insurance policyholders at the same time that employers are reviewing their commitments to both retired and economically active elderly workers. Medicare dropped its commitment to a mammography benefit before implementing it, but did add Pap smear coverage. We shall need to study how this addition affects utilization of preventive services and cancer rates.

A somewhat hidden aspect of the various statistics and analyses of gender aspects of health and health care in old age is the emphasis on women as disabled and dependent, perhaps victimized by poorly regulated nursing homes, sometimes literally out of sight, and sometimes with their positive qualities rendered psychologically invisible because of how they are categorized. Almost one out of seven females is sixty-five or over. Part of gender equality must surely involve distribution of preventive services and development of effective treatments that will reduce the amount of disability now accompanying old age.

References

Advocates Senior Alert Process. *A.S.A.P.*, vol. 4, no. 2 (June 1988).

Altman, Lawrence K., and Elaine Rosenthal. "Changes in Medicine Bring Pain to Healing Profession." *New York Times*, 18 February 1990, I: 1, 35.

American Association of Retired Persons. *AARP News Bulletin*, vol. 28, no. 5 (May 1987).

Berk, Marc L., and Amy Bernstein. "Use of Home Health Services: Some Findings from the National Medical Care Expenditure Survey." *Home Health Care Services Quarterly*, vol. 6, no. 1 (Spring 1985): 13–23.

Bernstein, Barbara, and Robert Kane. "Physicians' Attitudes toward Female Patients." *Medical Care*, vol. XIX, no. 6 (June 1981): 600–608.

Bianchi, Suzanne M., and Daphne Spain. *American Women in Transition*. New York: Russell Sage Foundation, 1986.

Brody, Elaine M., Morton H. Kleban, Pauline T. Johnsen, et al. "Work Status and Parent Care: A Comparison of Four Groups of Women." *Gerontologist,* vol. 27, no. 2 (1987): 201–208.

Butler, Robert N. Reply to Questions to Witnesses from Senator John Glenn. In *Women in Our Aging Society.* Hearing before the Special Senate Committee on Aging. 98th Cong., 2nd sess., October 8, 1984. Washington, DC: Government Printing Office, 1985, 91.

Cafferata, Gail Lee. "Knowledge of Their Health Insurance Coverage by the Elderly." *Medical Care,* vol. 22, no. 9 (September 1984a): 835–847.

———. *Private Health Insurance Coverage of the Medicare Population.* National Health Care Expenditures Study, Data Preview 18. Rockville, MD: National Center for Health Services Research, September 1984b.

Cafferata, Gail Lee, and Judith A. Kasper. *Psychotropic Drugs: Use, Expenditures, and Sources of Payment.* NCHSR National Health Care Expenditures Study, Data Preview 14. DHHS Pub. No. (PHS) 83-3335. Rockville, MD: National Center for Health Services Research, January 1983.

Collins, John Gary. *Persons Injured and Disability Days Due to Injuries, 1980–81.* Data from the National Health Survey. Series 10, No. 149. DHHS Pub. No. (PHS) 85-1577. Hyattsville, MD: National Center for Health Statistics, March 1985.

Cornoni-Huntley, Joan, et al., eds. *Established Populations for Epidemiologic Studies of the Elderly—Resource Data Book.* NIH Pub. No. 86-2443. Bethesda, MD: National Institute of Aging, 1986.

Cypress, Beulah K. *Office Visits for Diseases of the Circulatory System: The National Ambulatory Medical Care Survey: United States 1975–6.* Series 13, No. 40. DHEW Pub. No. (PHS) 79-1971. Hyattsville, MD: National Center for Health Statistics, January 1979.

———. *Office Visits for Preventive Care: The National Ambulatory Medical Care Survey: United States, 1977–8.* Advance Data No. 69. Hyattsville, MD: National Center for Health Statistics, April 1, 1981.

Dawson, Deborah, Gerry Hendershot, and John Fulton. *Aging in the Eighties: Functional Limitations of Individuals Age 65 Years and Over.* Advance Data No. 133. Hyattsville, MD: National Center for Health Statistics, June 10, 1987.

Equitable HCA Corporation. "Can Employers Reduce or Terminate Retiree Health Plans?" *Commentary from Equicor,* vol. 4, no. 4 (December 1988–January 1989).

Garnick, Deborah W., and Tobin Short. *Utilization of Hospital Inpatient Services by Elderly Americans.* HCUP Research Note 6. DHHS Pub. No. (PHS) 85-3351. Rockville, MD: National Center for Health Services Research and Health Care Technology Assessment, 1985.

General Accounting Office. *Employee Benefits: Companies' Retiree Health Liabilities Large, Advance Funding Costly.* Washington, DC, June 1989.

Gornick, Marian, Jay N. Greenberg, Paul W. Eggers, and Allen Dobson. "Twenty Years of Medicare and Medicaid: Covered Populations, Use of Benefits, and Program Expenditure." *Health Care Financing Review*, 1985 Annual Supp., 13–59.

Gornick, Marian, and Margaret Jean Hall. "Trends in Medicare Use of Post-hospital Care." *Health Care Financing Review*, 1988 Annual Supp., 27–38.

Graves, Edmund J. *Utilization of Short-Stay Hospitals, United States, 1984, Annual Summary*. Series 13, No. 84. DHHS Pub. No. (PHS) 86-1745. Hyattsville, MD: National Center for Health Statistics, March 1986.

Greenfield, S., D. M. Blanco, R. M. Elashoff, and P. A. Ganz. "Patterns of Care Related to Age of Breast Cancer Patients." *Journal of the American Medical Association*, vol. 257, no. 20 (May 22-25, 1987): 2766–2770.

Hamilton, Jean, and Barbara Parry. "Sex-Related Differences in Clinical Drug Response: Implications for Women's Health." *Journal of the American Women's Medical Association*, vol. 38, no. 5 (September/October 1983): 126–132.

Haug, Marie R., and Steven J. Folmar. "Longevity, Gender, and Life Quality." *Journal of Health and Social Behavior*, vol. 27 (December 1986): 332–345.

Haug, Marie R., and Marcia G. Ory. "Issues in Elderly Patient-Provider Interactions." *Research on Aging*, vol. 9, no. 1 (March 1987): 344.

Havlik, Richard J. *Aging in the Eighties: Impaired Senses for Sound and Light in Persons Age 65 Years and Over*. Advance Data No. 125. Hyattsville, MD: National Center for Health Statistics, September 19, 1986.

Hayward, R. A., M. Shapiro, H. F. Freeman, et al. "Who Gets Screened for Cervical and Breast Cancer?" *Archives of Internal Medicine*, 148 (1988):1177–1181.

Hibbard, Judith, and Clyde R. Pope. "Age Differences in the Use of Medical Care in an HMO." *Medical Care*, vol. 24, no. 1 (January 1986): 52–66.

Hing, Esther. *Use of Nursing Homes by the Elderly: Preliminary Data from the 1985 National Nursing Home Survey*. Advance Data No. 135. Hyattsville, MD: National Center for Health Statistics, May 14, 1987.

Hing, Esther, Mary Grace Kovar, and Dorothy P. Rice. *Sex Differences in Health and Use of Medical Care: United States, 1979*. Analytical and Epidemiological Studies, Series 3, No. 24. Hyattsville, MD: National Center for Health Statistics, September 1983.

Homan, Sharon M., Cynthia Carter Haddock, et al. "Widowhood, Sex, Labor Force Participation, and the Use of Physician Services by Elderly Adults." *Journal of Gerontology*, vol. 41, no. 6 (1986): 793–796.

Horowitz, Amy. "Sons and Daughters as Caregivers to Older Parents: Differences in Role Performance and Consequences." *Gerontologist*, vol. 25, no 6 (1985): 612–617.

Kasper, Judith A. *Prescribed Medicines: Use, Expenditures and Sources of Payment*. NCHSR National Health Care Expenditures Study, Data Preview 9.

DHHS Pub. No. (PHS) 82-3320. Hyattsville, MD: National Center for Health Services Research, April 1982.

———. *Aging Alone, Profiles and Projections.* Baltimore, MD: Commonwealth Fund Commission on Elderly People Living Alone, 1988.

Knickman, James R., and Nelda McCall. "A Prepaid Managed Approach to Long-Term Care." *Health Affairs* (Spring 1986): 90–104.

Koch, Hugo. *Drug Utilization in Office Practice by Age and Sex of the Patient: National Ambulatory Medical Care Survey, 1980.* Advance Data No. 81. Hyattsville, MD: National Center for Health Statistics, July 26, 1982.

———. *The Management of Chronic Pain in Office-based Ambulatory Care: National Ambulatory Medical Care Survey.* Advance Data No. 123. Hyattsville, MD: National Center for Health Statistics, August 29, 1986.

Koch, Hugo, and William H. Campbell. *Utilization of Psychotropic Drugs in Office-based Ambulatory Care: National Ambulatory Medical Care Survey, 1980 and 1981.* Advance Data No. 90. Hyattsville, MD: National Center for Health Statistics, June 15, 1983.

Koch, Hugo, and Deanne E. Knapp. *Utilization of Analgesic Drugs in Office-based Ambulatory Care: National Ambulatory Medical Care Survey, 1980–81.* Advance Data No. 96. Hyattsville, MD: National Center for Health Statistics, March 14, 1984.

Koch, Hugo, and Mickey C. Smith. *Office-based Ambulatory Care for Patients 75 Years Old and Over: National Ambulatory Medical Care Survey, 1980 and 1981.* Advance Data No. 110. Hyattsville, MD: National Center for Health Statistics, August 21, 1985.

Kovar, Mary Grace. "Elderly People: The Population 65 Years and Over." In *Health—United States—1976–1977.* USDHEW Pub. No. (HRA) 77-1232. Washington, DC: Government Printing Office, 1977, 3–26.

———. *Aging in the Eighties, Age 65 and Over and Living Alone, Contacts with Family, Friends, and Neighbors.* Advance Data No. 116. Hyattsville, MD: U.S. Department of Health and Human Services, Public Health Service, May 9, 1986.

Kovar, Mary Grace, and Thomas F. Drury. *Sex Differences in Health and Illness Behavior of the Elderly.* Prepared by the National Center for Health Statistics for distribution at the meeting of the Gerontological Society, Dallas, Texas, November 19, 1978.

Kovar, Mary Grace, and Andrea Z. LaCroix. *Aging in the Eighties: Ability to Perform Work-Related Activities.* Advance Data No. 136. Hyattsville, MD: National Center for Health Statistics, May 8, 1987.

Lobel, Brana, and Robert M. A. Hirschfeld. *Depression—What We Know.* Rockville, MD: National Institutes for Mental Health, 1984.

Louis Harris and Associates, Inc. *Problems Facing Elderly Americans Living Alone.* Report of the Commonwealth Fund Commission on Elderly People Living Alone. New York, 1986.

Mandelblatt, Jeanne S., and Marianne C. Fahs. "The Cost-Effectiveness of Screening for Cervical Cancer in Elderly Indigent Women." *Journal of the American Medical Association*, vol. 259 (April 22–29, 1988): 2409–2413.

McKinlay, John G., Sonja M. McKinlay, and Donald Brambilla. "The Relative Contributions of Endocrine Changes and Social Circumstances to Depression in Mid-Aged Women." *Journal of Health and Social Behavior*, vol. 28 (December 1987): 345–363.

McLemore, Thomas, and James DeLozier. *1985 Summary: National Ambulatory Medical Care Survey.* Advance Data No. 128. Hyattsville, MD: National Center for Health Statistics, January 23, 1987.

McMillan, Alma, and Marian Gornick. "The Dually Entitled Elderly Medicare and Medicaid Population Living in the Community." *Health Care Financing Review*, vol. 6, no. 2 (Winter 1984): 73–85.

———. "A Study of the 'Crossover Population': Aged Persons Entitled to Both Medicare and Medicaid." *Health Care Financing Review*, vol 4, no. 4 (Summer 1983): 19–46.

Meier, Diane. Personal communication, June 1987.

Minkler, Meredith, and Robyn Stone. "The Feminization of Poverty and Older Women." *Gerontologist*, vol. 25, no. 4 (1985): 351–357.

Mossey, J. M. "Social and Psychologic Factors Related to Falls among the Elderly." *Clinic-Geriatric Medicine*, vol. 1, no. 3 (August 1985): 541–553.

Mount Sinai School of Medicine. Tables on Coronary Bypass Operations for 1984 (unpublished).

Muller, Charlotte, Jeanne Mandelblatt, Clyde Schechter, et al. *Costs and Effectiveness of Cervical Cancer Screening in Elderly Women.* Washington, DC: U.S. Congress, Office of Technology Assessment, 1990.

National Center for Health Statistics. "Health Interview Survey, NCHS, Characteristics of Females Ever Having a Breast Examination and Interval since Last Examination, United States, 1973." *Monthly Vital Statistics Report*, vol. 24, no. 6, supp. Rockville, MD, September 12, 1975.

———. *Health United States 1985.* DHHS Pub. No. (PHS) 86-1232. Hyattsville, MD, December 1985.

———. *Health United States, 1986 and Prevention Profile.* DHHS Pub. No. (PHS) 87-1232. Hyattsville, MD, December 1986a.

———. *Supplement on Aging to the National Health Interview Survey of 1984.* Unpublished tables. Hyattsville, MD, 1986b.

———. Hospital Care Statistics Branch, Division of Health Care Statistics. *1985 Summary: National Hospital Discharge Survey.* Advance Data No. 127. Hyattsville, MD, September 25, 1986c.

———. *1986 Summary: National Hospital Discharge Survey.* Advance Data No. 145. DHHS Pub. No. (PHS) 87-1250. Hyattsville, MD, September 30, 1987.

———. *Health, United States, 1987.* DHHS Pub. No. (PHS) 88-1232. Washington, DC: Government Printing Office, March 1988.

New York Business Group on Health, Inc. *Long-Term Care.* Discussion Paper, vol. 8, supp. no. 1 (July 1988).

New York Times, "Age Bias Found in Cancer Treatment," 22 May 1987.

New York Times, "Laxity on Breast X-Rays," 30 June 1988.

New York Times, 4 August 1988.

Physician Payment Review Commission. *Annual Report to Congress, 1989.* Washington, DC, 1989.

Ray, W. A., M. R. Griffin, W. Schaffner, et al. "Psychotropic Drug Use and the Risk of Hip Fracture." *New England Journal of Medicine*, vol. 316, no. 7 (February 12, 1987): 363–369.

Rowland, Diane, and Barbara Lyons. *Medicare's Poor.* Baltimore, MD: Commonwealth Fund Commission on Elderly People Living Alone, 1987.

Ruchlin, Hirsch S., and Robert L. Braham. *Long-Term Care of the Elderly: The Growth and Problem Area of the Future.* New York: Cornell University Medical College, 1986. Xerox.

Schlenger, William E., William M. Wadman, and Larry S. Corder. *Health Status of Aged Medicare Beneficiaries.* Series B, Descriptive Report No. 2, NMCUES. Baltimore, MD: Health Care Financing Administration and National Center for Health Statistics, September 1983.

Schlesinger, Mark. "On the Limits of Expanding Health Care Reform: Chronic Care in Prepaid Settings." *Milbank Quarterly*, vol. 64, no. 2 (1986): 189–215.

Scitovsky, Anne A. *Medical Care Expenditures in the Last Twelve Months of Life.* Final Report to the John A. Hartford Foundation. Palo Alto, CA, March 1986.

Sekscenski, Edward S. *Discharges from Nursing Homes: Preliminary Data from the 1985 National Nursing Home Survey.* Advance Data No. 142. Hyattsville, MD: National Center for Health Statistics, September 30, 1987.

Stone, Robyn. *Aging in the Eighties, Age 65 Years and Older Women: Use of Community Services.* Advance Data No. 124, Hyattsville, MD: National Center for Health Statistics, September 30, 1986a.

———. *The Feminization of Poverty and Older Women: An Update.* Rockville, MD: National Center for Health Services Research, February 1986b.

Stone, Robyn, Gail Lee Cafferata, and Judith Sangl. *Caregivers of the Frail Elderly: A National Profile.* Rockville, MD: National Center for Health Services Research, 1986.

Thornberry, Owen T., Ronald W. Wilson, and Patricia M. Golden. *Health Promotion Data for the 1990 Objectives.* Advance Data No. 126. Hyattsville, MD: National Center for Health Statistics, September 19, 1986.

Tinetti, Mary E., and Mark Speechley. "Current Concepts: Geriatrics: Prevention of Falls among the Elderly." *New England Journal of Medicine*, vol. 320, no. 16 (April 20, 1989): 1055–1059.

Tolchin, Martin. "States Are Criticized Over Insurance for the Elderly." *New York Times*, 3 May 1990, I: 23.

Tracy, Martin B., and Roxanne L. Ward. "Trends in Old-Age Pensions for Women: Benefit Levels in Ten Nations, 1960–1980." *Gerontologist*, vol. 26, no. 3 (1986): 286–291.

United Hospital Fund of New York. *Health and Health Care in New York City, 1986*. New York, 1986a.

———. *New Directions in Health Care: Consequences for the Elderly*. New York, 1986b.

U.S. Congress. Senate. *Aging America, Trends and Projections*. Prepared by the Special Committee on Aging in conjunction with the American Association of Retired Persons. PL3377(584). Washington, DC, 1984.

U.S. Congress. House. Select Committee on Aging. *Hearing on Corporate Retiree Health Benefits: Here Today, Gone Tomorrow?* 98th Cong., 2nd sess., 1984. Washington, DC: Government Printing Office, 1985.

U.S. Congress. Senate. Committee on Finance. *Hearing on Examination of Quality of Care under Medicare's Prospective Payment System*. 99th Cong., 2nd sess. Washington, DC: Government Printing Office, 1986a.

U.S. Congress. Senate. Committee on Finance, Subcommittee on Health. *Hearing on Proposals to Modify Medicare's Physician Payment System*. 99th Cong., 2nd sess. Washington, DC: Government Printing Office, 1986b.

U.S. Department of Commerce, Bureau of the Census. *Statistical Abstract of the United States*. 1986 (106th ed.). Washington, DC, 1985.

———. *Statistical Abstract of the United States*. 1987 (107th ed.). Washington, DC, 1986.

U.S. Department of Health and Human Services, Health Care Financing Administration. *Health Services Utilization in the U.S. Population by Health Insurance Coverage*. NMCUES, Series B, Descriptive Report No. 13. DHHS Pub. No. 20213. Washington, DC, December 1986a.

———. *Medicare and Medicaid Data Book, 1984*. Health Care Financing Program Statistics. HCFA Pub. No. 03210. Baltimore, MD, 1986b.

———. Public Health Service. *Women's Health*. Report of the Public Health Service Task Force on Women's Health Issues, vol. II. Washington, DC, 1986c, IV-59.

———. *Medicare and Medicaid Data Book, 1986*. Health Care Financing Program Statistics. HCFA Pub. No. 03247. Baltimore, MD, 1987.

———. *The Medicare Catastrophic Coverage Act of 1988*. Legislative Summary. Baltimore, MD, November 7, 1988.

———. *Medicare and Medicaid Data Book, 1988.* Health Care Financing Program Statistics. HCFA Pub. No. 03270. Baltimore, MD, 1989a.

———. *The Medicare Handbook 1989.* HCFA Pub. No. 10050. Baltimore, MD, 1989b.

Verbrugge, Lois M. "A Health Profile of Older Women with Comparisons to Older Men." *Research on Aging,* vol. 6, no. 3 (September 1984): 291–322.

Wan, Thomas T., and Greg Arling. "Differential Use of Health Services among Disabled Elderly." *Research on Aging,* vol. 5, no. 3 (September 1983): 411–431.

West, Gale E., and Ronald L. Simons. "Sex Differences in Stress, Coping Resources, and Illness among the Elderly." *Research on Aging,* vol. 5, no. 2 (June 1983): 235–268.

Wingard, Deborah L., Denise Williams Jones, and Robert M. Kaplan. "Institutional Care Utilization by the Elderly: A Critical Review." *Gerontologist,* vol. 27, no. 2 (April 1987): 156–163.

CHAPTER SIX

Medicaid: The Lower Tier of Health Care for Women

B EING POOR, LIKE BEING old, is a socially defining characteristic that affects one's potential relationship to the health care system in the United States. If one is poor, Medicaid eligibility and service coverage become crucial for determining whether health care needs will be met. Since women's social problems place many of them at risk for poverty, the burdens created by certain features of the Medicaid system have become a gender issue. This chapter draws on information contained in various statistical reports and research documents to review Medicaid program elements that affect both younger and older women. Younger women's access to health care is affected by features of Aid to Families with Dependent Children and federal and state policies regarding pregnancy care. Older women are affected by regulations regarding eligibility for long-term care.

The Medicaid program is described as the "primary source of health care coverage for the poor in America" (National Pharmaceutical Council, 1986). Characteristics of the Medicaid program are determined by both the legislative guidelines of the federal statute and federal regulations and the power given to each state to determine its own eligibility and benefit pattern and to control costs through measures affecting the volume and mode of delivery of service. Besides being influenced by state discretionary powers within federal guidelines, the types of health needs that will be met, the personal circumstances that qualify, and the sources of care that will be reimbursed are also influenced by specific program elements determined by federal law and the states' responses thereto. These characteristics affect the well-being of the poor who depend on the Medicaid system for care.

Also affected are those poor who are kept outside the system by income ceilings and other rules and, hence, receive less service. Among adults, there are more poor without Medicaid coverage than with it (Kasper, 1986). Although some of the non-Medicaid poor have private insurance, insurance coverage tends to be associated with income level and a favorable type of employment. This means that many poor are dependent on the variable kindness, interest, and financial strength of sources of low-cost care. Unfortunately, the ever-increasing financial pressure on both public and voluntary hospitals, which now compete for paying patients, makes them reluctant to charge paying patients prices that are high enough to cover deficits from uncompensated care or care for which charges are set below costs (Texas Task Force, 1984).

When a medically needy program was curtailed for financial reasons in 1982 in California, 270,000 recipients were turned back to the counties for care. This led to a measurable drop in health status, access, and satisfaction with care. The drop was not confined to a brief adjustment period, for the various indices used failed to regain, during the subsequent six months, most of the loss incurred in the first six months. In this research, reported by Lurie et al. (1986) from the UCLA Group Practice in Los Angeles, the population studied was 69 percent female. Similar findings of deterioration in health status, decline in physician visits, and less access were reported from a San Francisco population (Pittman-Lindeman et al., 1985). Although the latter group was equally divided between males and females, women reported worse health status than men throughout the study. Although hospital days at first dropped after the curtailment of the program, they later increased, implying that reduced access may have produced severe illness and some erosion of cost savings to the program.

Historically, private practitioners have been disinclined to accept Medicaid clients, an attitude perhaps created, and certainly reinforced, by program payment levels and payment procedures. Because of these features, doctors perceive involvement with Medicaid as both time-consuming and less remunerative. Over 25 percent of the nation's privately practicing physicians refuse to treat Medicaid patients, and participation by obstetrician-gynecologists and other key specialists is even lower (National Pharmaceutical Council, 1986). Only 56 percent of the general and family practitioners and gynecologists who provide contraceptive care accept Medicaid patients (Blank, 1985). Additionally, hospital admissions under the care of a personal physician, the norm for insured and self-pay patients, are precluded when Medicaid clients are not accepted by practitioners. Low participation rates of private physicians have driven urban Medicaid patients, who are the majority, to more costly, often less effective, hospital settings for routine primary care (or to those practitioners who specialize in Medicaid practices for economic reasons and may exploit their clientele). Clinic environments, resources, and rules that form the context within which many of the poor receive care have often been described as impeding timely, appropriate, and good-quality care (Pittman-Lindeman, Berkowitz, and Rundall, 1985; Children's Defense Fund, 1976). In fortunate areas, hospital arrangements have been made more humane and medically more effective through efforts of community organizations, public hospitals, voluntary hospitals, and other groups.

Sources of Variability

Within Medicaid there is a core of uniformity surrounded by many sources of variability. Access to covered care in each state depends on the basis of eligibility, the type of service, and the place of service. States must cover certain *groups* of categorically needy, such as dependent children and their caretakers, and aged, blind, and disabled adults, who meet income tests and other criteria, and they may cover other groups. If a state covers an optional group, it must provide Medicaid to all eligible individuals in that group. For the mandatory categorically needy, states must cover certain mandatory *services*, five of which were specified in the 1965 law enacting Medicaid and six of which, including family planning, were added later. States are now permitted to offer certain services to some groups without offering them to all covered groups.

States may provide clinic services in a nonhospital setting and (under waiver) home and community-based services needed to avoid institutionalization. They may cover emergency hospital services, even though the hospital does not fulfill the conditions for participation. They may also provide limited dental, podiatric, and certain other services. States may cover the medically needy (those who do not meet income tests for cash assistance payments). If a state does this, it must provide prenatal care and delivery services, plus, for those qualifying for institutional care, certain other services.

In their efforts to control costs, states impose many limitations on health care services received under Medicaid. The limitations include a maximum number of hospital days or visits per year; required prior authorization or reauthorization for care (as in skilled nursing facilities) and special numerical limits for psychiatric and allergy visits; maximum quantities per drug prescription and numbers of prescriptions and refills. Certain services are sometimes simply excluded from coverage (U.S. Department of Health and Human Services, 1989, table 4.8). Each state determines its own limits and exclusions within federal regulations.

States have been permitted since 1972 to require cost sharing by clients, limited to a nominal sum, for *optional* health services to recipients of income assistance; and for *any* services to the medically needy. As of 1982, both the categorically and the medically needy may be required to make a contribution in the form of a deductible or copayment for any service offered; however, this state option does not apply to services to persons under 18, pregnancy-related care, family planning services and supplies, and services to categorically needy HMO enrollees. (States may also exempt from cost sharing persons between 18 and 21 and medically needy enrollees in HMOs.) Since 1985 emergency care and certain institutionalized persons have also been exempted from cost sharing.

Those who depend on Medicaid for their health needs are not assured of a uniform standard of eligibility. The variation in the percentage of the poverty level represented by the income cutoff for Medicaid eligibility is a major factor in this lack of uniform protection. Although each state's Medicaid program must cover all those receiving cash payments under AFDC, each state defines its own income level of eligibility. The need standard used for this purpose, for a two-person family, varied in 1983 from $1,704 in Tennessee to $5,292 in Vermont (U.S. Department of Health and Human Services, 1986, table 4.2). The actual payment level, however, does not correspond to the need standard; for example, the payment was only $1,212 in Tennessee and $3,444 in Vermont, and, therefore, the income level for eligibility overstates the maximum income that might be available to each applicant for private medical care, copayments, services not covered by Medicaid, or general living needs.

Women, Poverty, and Medicaid

The burdens imposed on individuals through various restrictions in Medicaid have become a gender question, as well as a class question, because of the increased predominance of females among the poor. The risk of poverty arises from, or is intensified by, problems commonly encountered by women in society. Both younger and older women are at risk for poverty and, thus, for Medicaid. Single parenthood without good earning ability and inadequate child care are problems for younger women. Widowhood is also more likely for women and is often accompanied by depletion of economic assets. Women generally have lower retirement income because of lower earnings records. Female householders with no husband numbered 10,100,000 in 1984 and had a median family income of $12,003, versus $29,612 for married-couple families. Of these female householders, 1.9 million had incomes below $5,000, and 2.2 million had between $5,000 and $9,999; one-third of the female householders were in poverty in 1985, and 41 percent were below 125 percent of the poverty level. This compares with 14 percent of all persons in 1985 being under the poverty level and 17 percent being under 125 percent of it. The poverty level is defined on the basis of the Department of Agriculture's 1961 economy food plan and reflects the consumption requirements of families of different size and composition. Only money income is counted. The cutoff point for poverty for a family of four in 1986 was $11,203, with $14,003 equaling 125 percent (U.S. Department of Commerce, 1986, p. 415, tables 746, 439, 745; 1987, p. 406).

These facts influence the sex and age composition of Medicaid (see table 6.1.). Females account for between 59.9 percent and 70.0 percent (72 percent in the Virgin Islands) of Medicaid recipients in the 52 jurisdictions and 64.1 percent overall (U.S. Department of Health and Human Services, 1989, table 4.6).

Recipients of Aid to Families with Dependent Children are the largest component of Medicaid-eligibles. In fiscal year 1984, 78 percent of all Medicaid-eligibles were in AFDC, in which 9.8 million children and 5.6 million adults are enrolled. It is largely because of this program that there are two females age 18+ on Medicaid for every male (Kasper, 1986). Table 6.2 shows the income distribution of the 2.3 million female-headed family households receiving Medicaid in 1984; two-thirds are below the poverty level.

Aid to Families with Dependent Children is largely a program for unmarried parents and their children: 46.5 percent of the children in the program arrive there because of unmarried parents (Gornick et al., 1985). Over half of out-of-wedlock births in 1980 appeared in the AFDC caseload the following year. Another 39.6 percent of AFDC children are eligible because of divorces or separations. Among adult women aged 35–64, according to 1977 data, those who were divorced or widowed were much more likely than married women to be on Medicaid; the percentages were higher if they were not in the labor force. There were, additionally, substantial numbers not currently married who had neither Medicaid nor private insurance (Berk and Taylor, 1983). Thus, membership in the poverty clientele for health care is generated by problems related to marriage, childbirth, and the absence of economic support from fathers. The proportion of adults on AFDC rolls has increased, owing to the decline of family size of recipient families. This decline will perhaps ease the transition of AFDC mothers to work status, but the issue of Medicaid coverage for the working poor and their families remains.

TABLE 6.1
Medicaid and Non-Medicaid Population, by Age and Sex, 1980

Group	All Ages	Age in Years				
		18–34	35–44	45–64 (in thousands)	65–74	75+
Both sexes						
Without Medicaid						
Poor	28,777	7,489	2,425	4,447	2,685	2,196
Nonpoor	169,013	51,044	21,887	36,590	10,223	4,393
With Medicaid	25,087	5,720	972	2,508	2,327	1,079
Men						
Without Medicaid						
Poor	12,642	3,439	1,150	1,833	910	582
Nonpoor	84,769	26,024	10,935	18,056	4,747	2,034
With Medicaid	10,128	1,651	[a]	922	861	436
Women						
Without Medicaid						
Poor	16,135	4,050	1,275	2,614	1,775	1,614
Nonpoor	84,244	25,020	10,952	18,534	5,476	2,359
With Medicaid	14,959	4,069	972	1,586	1,466	643
Percentage female						
Without Medicaid						
Poor	56.1	54.1	52.6	58.8	66.1	73.5
Nonpoor	49.8	49.0	50.0	50.7	56.2	53.7
With Medicaid	59.6	71.1	100.0	63.2	63.0	60.0

Source: Based on Judith A. Kasper, "Health Status and Utilization: Differences by Medicaid Coverage and Income." (*Health Care Financing Review*, vol. 7, no. 4, summer 1986).

[a]Excluded because of small cell size or large standard error.

TABLE 6.2
Female-headed Family Households Receiving Medicaid,
by Income Level, 1984

	Number (000)	%
Total	3,232	100.0
Under $5,000	1,254	38.8
$5,000–$9,999	1,131	35.0
$10,000–$14,999	374	11.6
$15,000 and over	473	14.6
Below poverty level	2,201	67.2

Source: U.S. Department of Commerce. *Statistical Abstract of the United States, 1987,* (107th ed.). (Washington, DC, 1986), table 609.

Among those age 65+ years on Medicaid, women are again the majority, making up 61.9 percent of Medicaid-eligibles. The aged with dual enrollment in Medicare and Medicaid are older, and more often female, than the aged with Medicare only (Rymer, 1984). At all adult ages, women are a higher percentage of the poor with Medicaid (and of the poor without Medicaid) than they are of the nonpoor (those with incomes above the poverty level).

Fully 60 percent of the males on Medicaid are under 18, and only 25 percent are 18–64. In contrast, only 13 percent of the females on Medicaid are under 18, and 44 percent are 18–64. Table 6.3 shows that 10 percent of expenses for all personal health services for females (all ages) and 6 percent of those for males were met by Medicaid in 1977. Medicaid was most important as a payment source for inpatient hospital services (14 percent of expenses for females and 8 percent for males). For families with a female head, 21 percent of expenses for all personal health services was covered by Medicaid, but only 5 percent was covered for families with a male head.

Utilization of physician services under Medicaid has been analyzed by Buczko (1986), based on data from a four-state survey of full-year Medicaid-eligibles that was part of the National Medical Care Utilization and Expenditure Survey of 1980. In the sample, 62 percent were female, and only 13 percent were married; 88 percent had a regular source of health care. After controlling for demographic, enabling, and health status factors that could affect use of services, sex was shown to be an important predictor of the probability of a visit, the number of visits, and the expenditure on care (being female had a positive effect). Two other influential factors for probability of a visit were having a regular source of care and small family size, the latter of which could reflect widow-

TABLE 6.3
Medicaid as a Source of Payment, by Type of Service and Sex, 1977

	Total Population with Expense (in thousands)	Mean Expense per Person with Expense (in dollars)	Percentage of Expense Paid by Medicaid
1. Inpatient hospital services			
Male	9,116	2,322	7.9
Female	14,049	1,742	13.7
2. Ambulatory physician services			
Male	67,221	132	5.8
Female	82,374	148	9.1
3. Nonphysician health care providers			
Male	17,122	97	6.1
Female	23,976	92	6.9
4. Personal health services			
a. Individual			
Male	82,656	567	6.0
Female	95,561	618	10.0
b. Family			
Male head	55,852	1,453	5.0
Female head	19,625	1,271	21.0

Sources: National Center for Health Services Research, *Inpatient Hospital Services: Use, Expenditures and Sources of Payment.* (Rockville, MD, 1983), table 4; Amy K. Taylor, *Contacts with Physicians in Ambulatory Settings: Rates of Use, Expenditures, and Source of Payment.* (Rockville, MD: National Center for Health Services Research, 1983), table 5; Mark L. Berk and Claudia L. Schur, *Nonphysician Health Care Providers: Use of Ambulatory Services, Expenditures and Sources of Payment.* (Rockville, MD: National Center for Health Services Research, 1985), table 6; Judith A. Kasper, Louis F. Rossiter, and Renate Wilson, *A Summary of Expenditures and Sources of Payment for Personal Health Services from the National Medical Care Expenditures Survey.* (Rockville, MD: Center for Health Services Research, 1987), table 9.

hood or divorce, as well as fewer children and fewer time constraints on seeking care. Health variables (number of bed days and dying within the year) were also predictors of having one or more visits. For number of visits and expenditures, health status and all the other named variables were influential. Use varied among the states, probably reflecting the effect of program reimbursement levels and limits on number of services, as well as doctor supply and costs of care.

SPECIAL GROUPS

The Working Poor

The impact of eligibility changes affecting the working poor has fallen primarily on women AFDC clients striving to become earners. In 1980 Medicaid covered 49 percent of the poor and 23 percent of the near-poor, those between 100 percent and 150 percent of the poverty level (Kasper, 1986). One of the changes in federal law regarding public assistance after 1981 was a requirement in the Omnibus Budget Reconciliation Act (OBRA-1981) that affected the interpretation of earned income.

In determining eligibility for AFDC, only a limited amount of income could be disregarded because of expenses of working and child care, a rule that restricted eligibility to those whose incomes were not greater than 150 percent of the state's need standard. This rule severely affected the working poor. Sixteen states raised their need standard to avoid dropping people from the rolls; nevertheless, the proportion of AFDC families with earned incomes fell from 11.8 percent to 5.7 percent in one year (Gornick et al., 1985). This played a large part in the drop from 51 percent to 45 percent in the ratio of Medicaid enrollees to the poverty population between 1982 and 1983 (Feder and Holahan, 1986). As an offset, a 1984 federal law, the Deficit Reduction Act (DEFRA) required states to grant eligibility for nine months after transition to work and allowed a further such extension of six more months. This option was adopted, however, by only thirteen states (Hill, 1987). Thus, coverage of the working poor is both uneven and limited; in its absence Medicaid tends to become a program for only the chronically and severely poor, which may affect attitudes of both providers and clients.

Data from 1981–1982, a recession period, indicate that 35 percent of those who lost Medicaid coverage obtained private insurance, but this coverage was less adequate than the Medicaid they had lost. Those deprived of Medicaid paid over half their bills out of pocket and reported significantly more delays in seeing doctors and dentists then those remaining on AFDC (Feder and Holahan, 1986). The 45 percent who obtained no private insurance at all sustained a substantial drop in receipt of professional services and prescription drugs.

Pregnancy Coverage   Medicaid coverage for pregnancy reaches only a minority of the poor. Recently, changes have been made to make it easier for pregnant women to obtain Medicaid, but problems remain. Nationally, among women of reproductive age, in the early 1980s, 43 percent of those with incomes under $5,000 and 31 percent of those with incomes of $5,000–$9,999 had Medicaid coverage; only 20 percent of women in these brackets had group health insurance (Blank, 1985).

Despite a general trend to restrict social programs, coverage of pregnancy was targeted as a special need after a worsening of indicators of maternal and child health in certain states. This was believed, based on the research literature, to be due to lack of access to prenatal care. Averting delay in starting prenatal care may help prevent low birthweight and other adverse outcomes of pregnancy and may result in savings in health care costs for a state program (Texas Task Force, 1984).

Federal law (DEFRA-1984) required states to cover first-time pregnant women who would qualify for AFDC after the birth and pregnant women in two-parent families whose principal earner was unemployed. Ten states changed their Medicaid programs to meet the first condition, and twenty-five did so to meet the second condition. A federal law in the following year (OBRA-1985) required states to provide pregnancy care for all women meeting the state's financial tests, a change that affected twenty states (Hill, 1987). The proportion of births covered by Medicaid in 1985 ranged from 3 percent in Alaska to 25 percent in Michigan; the national average was 17 percent (Alan Guttmacher Institute, 1987). Coverage of pregnant women was further encouraged by a provision of another federal law (OBRA-1986) allowing states to cover those with incomes between current eligibility standards and the federal poverty level. Hill called this the most potentially profound reform of Medicaid in many years. However, a survey of state Medicaid directors indicates that only one-third felt their states would cover pregnant women up to the federal poverty level, although most felt that day would eventually come. This coverage was made mandatory by the Medicare Catastrophic Coverage Act of 1988.

The federal legislation of 1985 authorized state plans to offer to pregnant women an expanded service package that might include social work assessment, nutritional evaluation, health education, and transportation, without having to offer the same services under Medicaid to other categorically eligible groups. Three states responded by adopting this option, and a few had previously provided such services, but most states' Medicaid programs offer a narrower band of services for pregnant women. States that do not offer these optional services for pregnant women exclusively may reach at least some through the WIC (Women-Infants-Children) nutrition and health education program.

The 1985 federal law also stated that presumptive eligibility could be granted to pregnant women by providers while their Medicaid application was being processed (and errors would be disregarded in computing the state's error rate). But few administrators (under 10 percent) thought adoption of such presumptive eligibility was probable in their states. States are currently allowed forty-five days from the date of application to determine Medicaid eligibility, which is a potential source of delay in receiving care. Only nine of forty-eight reporting states take any steps to expedite processing of Medicaid applications for pregnant women. Moreover, only four states "make aggressive efforts" to inform pregnant women of their eligibility (Alan Guttmacher Institute, 1987).

Granting more liberal eligibility during pregnancy involves disregarding state spend-down provisions. In a state with a medically needy program, any categorically related person (aged, blind, disabled, a dependent child, or the child's caretaker) may qualify for Medicaid if medical bills are large enough to bring income down to the medically needy income standard, that is, to 133 percent of the AFDC payment level. But for a pregnant woman with income above the medically needy level, spending down would take time, causing a loss of access to early prenatal care under Medicaid. A woman above the state's usual income standard for eligibility who already had children would not be eligible under the federal option (along with her family) unless she spent down. Eligibility for low-income pregnant women without spending down would assure prompt medical care when it counts.

Another problem in regard to income standards is the status of pregnant teenagers. In all but two states, it is the parents' income that is considered in determining eligibility for pregnant teenagers who live at home. If the parents are not already Medicaid-eligible, the adolescent is not eligible either, unless she leaves their home. This may be a factor in delaying prenatal care (Alan Guttmacher Institute, 1987) and could discourage staying at home in some cases.

The newly mandated coverage applies only to pregnancy-related care, including complications, with the state defining "pregnancy-related." A gray area is left in reimbursement criteria: when are the health problems of a pregnant woman pregnancy-related? The Tax Equity and Fiscal Responsibility Act of 1982 had exempted pregnancy-related care from cost sharing by recipients; the difficulty of interpretation prompted states to adopt the permitted approach of exempting all medical care from cost sharing during pregnancy. This might suggest that, in the same spirit, states would cover all care during pregnancy. Under the new law, however, this is not a valid assumption because of the potential costs involved with a larger clientele. Whether provision of fairly comprehensive services during pregnancy is actually allowed by states should be ascertained.

Absence of abortion coverage, a significant limitation for those with unwanted pregnancies, is very likely to affect use of other services, including care of high-risk pregnancies and, ultimately, care of infants with severe problems. States are prohibited from treating abortion as a federally assisted family planning service, but they may provide abortion using state funds, as New York State does. The federal government has promulgated rules to force family planning clinics to give up abortion counseling, but the rules are being challenged in the courts of several states (*New York Times*, 30 August 1987; 17 February 1988).

The Supreme Court handed down its decision in the *Webster* case on July 3, 1989, opening the door to state laws that would restrict abortions in public hospitals or performed by public employees (albeit there was a narrow majority for this decision). As the Court announced its intention to hear additional cases, further restrictions by states seemed likely to prevail, and legislative battles were expected in states like New York that had supported abortions for poor clients out of state funds (*New York Times*, 10 July 1989).

States must offer voluntary sterilization as a family planning service, but some states impose limits on sterilization services (U.S. Department of Health and Human Services, 1986, table 4.8). States must offer nurse–midwife services to categorically needy recipients and must include direct reimbursement to nurse–midwives as a payment option.

Females of all ages account for 64.1 percent of the total number of recipients of all services under Medicaid (U.S. Department of Health and Human Services, 1989, table 4.11). Virtually all Medicaid-financed family planning services, however, are provided to women (one-third of them to women under 20), and almost all sterilizations are performed on women. In 1978, the last year for which a breakdown was available, 88.1 percent of sterilizations were tubal ligations, 2.0 percent were hysterectomies, 5.6 percent were other female procedures, and 4.2 percent were vasectomies (U.S. Department of Health and Human Services, 1983, table 2.20).

Coverage for prenatal service does not assure timely use. Many women who are eligible for service do not seek or obtain prenatal care until late in their pregnancies, and the problem is not confined to adolescents (Cronin, 1987). Although the sources of the behavior are complex, outreach programs that would take ethnic, cultural, and life-style factors into account would be a valuable component of prenatal services for the poor. For prevention of high-risk births, it is especially important to reach women with problems of drug or alcohol abuse and, where possible, integrate addiction treatment with maternity care and family planning.

The Elderly

Medicare benefits have been historically oriented toward acute care, leaving those in need of long-term care in a catastrophic financial position. In consequence, Medicaid has been used to finance long-term care for those who would not ordinarily be considered economically disadvantaged. Private insurance, although marketed by a number of companies, is not affordable by most elderly. The burden of long-term care is thus placed on the general taxpayer, rather than on the resources of the social insurance system, but the taxpayer constituency is not committed to preserving the previous standard of living of spouses and dependents of applicants under a means test program. The problem is not resolvable so long as Medicaid is providing virtually all of the public funds going toward nursing home care. In 1985 Medicaid paid $14.7 billion for nursing home care, Medicare only $.6 billion; private insurance paid $.3 billion (Lazenby et al., 1986).

It is impossible to determine how broad Medicaid eligibility should be without considering the gender issues in long-term care. Women's lifetime histories affect their need for nursing home care in old age. One factor is age differences at marriage. Butler and Newachek (1980) have noted that, in each age group among the elderly, married women are more likely to be institutionalized than married men. The difference is attributed to women's having older spouses who are not able to give needed care. Women also tend to survive their spouses because of their longevity advantage and spousal age differences. The life-cycle background of women (their division of time between home and work, their history of sex-typed jobs, their limited income sources in old age, etc.) is a source of the imbalance between need for care and financial resources. Only if this is recognized will a fair solution to long-term care financing be possible, including, in particular, what Medicaid should pay.

Federal standards do not prohibit nursing homes from refusing admission to Medicaid patients, and the homes, operating at a high occupancy rate (states having restricted expansion), are known to be selective in their choice of clients. In a recent study (Hochbaum and Galkin, 1987), proprietary homes in Nassau County, New York, were asked whether they would admit an aged infirm woman who had had a stroke and was eligible for Medicaid. They were generally unwilling, unless a substantial period of private payment (three months to two years) were guaranteed. Nursing homes with waiting lists are also known to have required substantial payments in advance to secure admission. Such practices are likely to delay initiation of rehabilitative care. It is important to note that this study was done in New York State, where regulations prohibit discrimination against Medicaid patients. Courts have, however, interpreted this to mean that an equal chance of admission is conditional on Medicaid's paying rates equal to fees charged to other patients. Other problems arise for the elderly when they make private payments to a nursing home, in order to spend down to Medicaid eligibility, and thus assure their continued residence, and the nursing home goes bankrupt or changes hands.

Medicaid eligibility standards particularly affect elderly women who are spouses of men requiring long-term care either at home or in institutions. The public became aware of the risk of rapid impoverishment of the spouse of a recipient before and after receiving Medicaid. It was estimated that, in Massachusetts, one-fourth of the married elderly could be impoverished within thirteen weeks of one spouse's institutionalization (U.S. Congress, 1986). These findings were subsequently confirmed on a national scale through a study commissioned by the Select Committee on Aging of the Congress (New York Times, 9 November 1987). Impoverishment occurred because a person entering a nursing home was required to use his or her income to pay the nursing home costs, and the income of the nondisabled spouse was "deemed" available for this. Only a small amount may be reserved for personal needs and for medical and remedial expenses not covered by third parties. A modest deduction for home maintenance for the noninstitutionalized spouse and dependents is also allowed. As an alternative, some states place a lien on the home but not if the spouse or dependent is living there. Limited amounts of liquid assets, personal effects, car equity, and burial reserve may be kept by the categorically needy without losing eligibility. In most states, spending down to 133 percent of the AFDC payment level qualifies elderly persons for Medicaid, even if there is no medically needy program, but in fourteen states this option is not available. Up to 1988, under the federal government's interpretation of Medicaid rules concerning income and assets, the amount of money available to the spouse not eligible for Medicaid was reduced, even if the asset was jointly held; in addition, states could prohibit transfer of assets within two years prior to application for Medicaid.

The financial position of spouses in Medicaid was changed by the Medicare Catastrophic Coverage Act of 1988. Under the new law, no income of the community spouse is considered available to the other spouse in determining eligibility, and the minimum monthly needs allowance is improved. The period for which the transfer of assets affects eligibility is specified at thirty months (U.S. Department of Health and Human Services, 1988).

It is easier to qualify for Medicaid if a person enters a nursing home. This promotes using institutional rather than community services as a source of long-term care. Tilly and Brunner (1987), reviewing the Medicaid provisions affecting the elderly, note that reforms that would help the disabled elderly and their spouses (especially more generous "deeming" rules) would also increase program outlays. Thus, the position of the disabled elderly remains vulnerable to fiscal pressures.

Like many other aspects of care for the poor, the nursing home problem is technically sex-neutral, yet it has a more extensive impact on elderly women. It also affects the well-being of children of the elderly, who are often middle-aged themselves and who carry responsibilities for their parents' care without suitable resources. Again, the children carrying the major responsibilities are more likely to be daughters.

Medicaid expenditures for older-women households (single women age 45+ living in the community or in institutions and married couples with a woman age 45+) were the subject of a 1986 study conducted for the American Association of Retired Persons by ICF, Incorporated (1986). The expenditures were estimated by means of a microsimulation model. The model's assumptions recognized that the proportion of women in single-person households increases as women age; that such households have lower incomes, compared with married couples; and that income falls sharply with age. Further, the study assumed that institutionalization is a significant and likely mode of delivering the cluster of long-term care services needed for those with serious functional limitations. The report estimated that 13 percent of all older-women households 45+ received Medicaid benefits, but 22 percent of the health care expenditures of nonwhite women came from Medicaid, versus 9 percent of those of white women (ICF, Incorporated, 1986). (The figures would have been higher if the analysis had focused on those 65 and older.) It was predicted that increasing longevity of women, operating within the foregoing assumptions, would make Medicaid an increasingly important source of health care for older women. However, unless Medicaid is able to provide community-based long-term care, the noninstitutional component may not grow. The ICF report does not spell out the relation between being an elderly woman and having restricted access to nonmarket sources of noninstitutional care. This relation is significant because widows may lack family members who would provide needed personal care. Home care services are underdeveloped, and this deprives many elderly women who are functionally disabled and live alone of the help needed for continued residence in the community. New York City, which has the largest home care program under Medicare in the United States and accepts anyone who qualifies for Medicaid, has a clientele made up chiefly of elderly women (Cronin, 1987). But nationally, only twenty-nine states have personal care (home attendant) programs under federal waivers, and they are very limited in size, because clients have to be at risk for institutionalization and total long-term care expenditures cannot be increased. Lacking community-based services, functionally limited women may enter the demand stream for nursing home care. Many of them, however, will face discrimination against Medicaid enrollees in securing admission.

Medicare home care benefits added in 1988 for "chronically dependent" individuals (limited in two ADLs) included homemaker and personal care services, as well as professional services and medical supplies and equipment. But, despite the language, the benefit was limited to eighty hours a year and applied only to those who met the cap for either catastrophic medical expenses or prescribed drug expenses (HCFA, 1988). It was, thus, inapplicable to a long-term clientele. This benefit was repealed in 1989. Therefore, for most elderly needing daily assistance, dependence on Medicaid or private resources will continue.

Impoverishment of spouses, chiefly wives, because of deeming rules concerning couples' economic resources, may have been relieved by recent legislation. Past barriers to admission of Medicaid clients to nursing homes and the absence of community-based long-term care that is not narrowly targeted remain special problems of the elderly with regard to Medicaid. These problems have particular significance for elderly women.

Health Status and Use of Care

Medicaid has the potential to improve access to health care for persons with major health problems, but program restrictions may interfere. A comparison of Medicaid-eligibles with poor persons who are not on Medicaid and the nonpoor (those with incomes above the poverty line) shows a difference in health. Adults who are Medicaid-eligible have poorer health status than the non-Medicaid poor or the nonpoor, as measured by several indicators: fair or poor health, activity limitation, functional limitation, and restricted activity days. In particular, AFDC cash recipients are four times more likely to have fair or poor health than the nonpoor of similar age (18–44) (Kasper, 1986).

Among those with fair or poor health, Medicaid has positive effects on access. This is shown when Medicaid-eligibles, under sixty-five and in fair or poor health, are compared with the non-Medicaid poor and with the nonpoor of similar age and health status. Those on Medicaid are at least as likely as persons not in poverty to see a doctor and to use one or more prescribed drugs. But this is not the case for the poor who are not on Medicaid; compared with the nonpoor, they are less likely to have at least one prescription, and, in the 45–64 age group, to see a doctor. These non-Medicaid poor have fewer doctor visits and prescribed drugs than those in similar health who are on Medicaid. Within Medicaid, the medically needy who are in fair or poor health use more care than those with comparable health on Supplemental Security Income. This is consistent with becoming eligible through spending down to a qualifying income, that is, the medically needy have high medical expenses before getting into Medicaid (Kasper, 1986). Among persons with functional limitations, the medically needy also have more probability of hospitalization. Overall, the medically needy number a little over one-fourth of the Medicaid population (U.S. Department of Health and Human Services, 1989, table 4.4.). That access to needed health care is provided by Medicaid is indicated in the higher use rates of the medically needy. However, Medicaid's high turnover rates may interrupt the flow of services to an individual (Blank, 1985). Furthermore, restrictions by state Medicaid programs on payment for medications have impaired access to drugs needed by patients receiving multiple drugs (predominantly female and elderly or disabled). This may be narrowing the difference between the non-Medicaid poor and those on Medicaid with regard to prescriptions (Soumerai et al., 1987). Medicare's prescription drug benefit passed in 1988 might have relieved this situation for the elderly poor, but was repealed in 1989.

CONCLUSION

Whether the situation of women on Medicaid is considered acceptable or not depends on the comparison group. Many employed women are not covered through their places of employment, or they have smaller employer contributions than men and, thus, shallow coverage, because of their weaker position in the labor market relative to men. For those with group coverage through their employment, access to care is jeopardized if they lose their jobs or if employers cut back on benefits, impose cost sharing, or use case management restrictively. These are problems of economic risk. Medicaid clients, however, face a political risk when federal or state legislatures and executives have other priorities. Some benefits may be less comprehensive under private insurance; for example, Medicaid covers drugs and ambulatory care, whereas private policies tend to cover these under major medical plans only (National Center for Health Services Research, 1986, p. 14). But owning private insurance is not strictly dependent on income level, family configuration, or other criteria used in Medicaid. So far, access to abortion under private insurance has not suffered the setbacks encountered by public funding of abortion, but inability to assure privacy in claims filing has effectively neutralized this insurance right for many, and the political assault on abortion may restrict local access even for the privately insured. Finally, the label of dependency carries with it a lessening of social status. We don't really know all the implications of using the health care system while bearing such a label, although we do know that clinic care often involves overcrowding, discontinuity of medical providers, and reduction of amenities.

Whether women, in addition to having a higher risk of becoming Medicaid clients through poverty, are also subject to a gender bias within the system of care for the poor is not known. It is conceivable that provider behavior toward individuals, one dimension of bias, is influenced by some ranking of the physically or mentally disabled, the single parent, and the elderly poor, and of men and women within these groups (except for the single parent group, which is almost exclusively female) that works to the disadvantage of one subgroup of clients among the poor.[1] Attitudes about out-of-wedlock births might be relevant to this; however, a provider's disinclination for economic reasons to accept the Medicaid client as a private patient may override all other considerations.

Employed men tend to have more nearly universal coverage and more adequate benefits than do employed women, owing to full-time employment, lower risk of unemployment, and other factors. As a result, Medicaid-eligible women as a class are generally less well-off with respect to health care access than employed men, who represent the vast majority of men under sixty-five.

Whether a uniform national benefit under Medicaid is worth aiming for depends on a critical assumption: the adequacy of the benefit scope (type of service) and level (number of service units covered) that would be presented in the national standard. A standard that would be politically feasible might be far less than what Medicaid-eligibles now receive in the more generous states. Also, a richer benefit content might be traded off against narrower eligibility or unrealistically low provider reimbursement levels. However, a decent national standard would help improve care in the states with the narrowest programs and might relieve financial burdens of the more generous states by reducing the incentive to move to states where benefits are more adequate and by cutting the states' costs if federal aid were increased.

---

[1]The spread of HIV infection has underscored the possibility of invidious ranking of patients by providers, affecting female and male patients.

For the near future, improving the situation of women Medicaid clients involves attention to the implications of the myriad details of current and proposed regulations, so that cost containment is not attained by sacrifice of needed care and deteriorated health status and so that promised improvements are actualized. It also means concern with assisting health insurance coverage during the transition to work. Ultimately (and soon, if possible) we must design a system of coverage that does not expose a large group in the population to the infelicitous combination of inferiority and uncertainty with regard to health care.

Note: An earlier version of Chapter Six appeared in *Women & Health*, vol. 14 (2), 1988.

References

Alan Guttmacher Institute. *Blessed Events and the Bottom Line: Financing Maternity Care in the United States.* New York, 1987.

Berk, Marc L., and Claudia L. Schur. *Nonphysician Health Care Providers: Use of Ambulatory Services, Expenditures and Sources of Payment.* Data Preview 22. DHHS Pub. No. (PHS) 86-3394. Rockville, MD: National Center for Health Services Research, October 1985.

Berk, Marc L., and Amy K. Taylor. *Women and Divorce: Health Insurance Coverage, Utilization and Health Care Expenditures.* Rockville, MD: National Center for Health Services Research, October 11, 1983.

Blank, Susan, with Thomas Brock. *Health, Health Care and Economic Self-Sufficiency.* Washington, DC: National Health Policy Forum, October 9, 1985.

Buczko, William. "Physician Utilization and Expenditures in a Medicaid Population." *Health Care Financing Review,* vol. 8, no. 2 (Winter 1986): 17–26.

Butler, Lewis H., and Paul W. Newachek. *Health and Social Factors Relevant to Long Term Care Policy.* San Francisco: University of California, Health Policy Program, June 11–13, 1980.

Children's Defense Fund. *Doctors and Dollars Are Not Enough.* Washington, DC, 1976.

Comptroller General of the United States. *Constraining National Health Care Expenditures.* GAO/HRD-85105. Washington, DC: General Accounting Office, September 30, 1985.

Cronin, Mark. Interview, September 10, 1987.

Feder, Judith, and John Holahan, eds. *HCFA Medicaid Program Evaluation: A Synthesis of Interim Findings.* MPE 9.1. Baltimore, MD: Office of Research and Demonstration, June 1986.

Gornick, Marian, Jay N. Greenberg, Paul W. Eggers, and Allen Dobson. "Twenty Years of Medicare and Medicaid: Covered Population, Use of Benefits, and Program Expenditures." *Health Care Financing Review,* 1985 Annual Supp., 13–59.

Hill, Ian T. *Broadening Medicaid Coverage of Pregnant Women and Children: State Policy Responses.* Washington, DC: National Governors' Association, February 1987.

Hochbaum, Martin, and Florence Galkin. "Medicaid Patients Need Not Apply." *Social Policy* (Spring 1987): 40–42.

ICF, Incorporated. *Medicaid's Role in Financing the Health Care of Older Women.* Prepared for the American Association of Retired Persons. Washington, DC, December 1986.

Kasper, Judith A. "Health Status and Utilization: Differences by Medicaid Coverage and Income." *Health Care Financing Review,* vol. 7, no. 4 (Summer 1986): 1–17.

Kasper, Judith A., Louis F. Rossiter, and Renate Wilson. *A Summary of Expenditures and Sources of Payment for Personal Health Services from the National Medical Care Expenditures Survey.* Data Preview 24. DHHS Pub. No. (PHS) 87-3411. Rockville, MD: Center for Health Services Research, May 1987.

Lazenby, Helen, Katherine R. Levit, and Daniel R. Waldo. *National Health Expenditures, 1985.* Health Care Financing Notes No. 6. HCFA Pub. No. 03232. U.S. Department of Health and Human Services, Health Care Financing Administration, September 1986.

Lurie, Nicole, N. Ward, M. Shapiro, et al. "Termination of Medi-Cal Benefits: A Followup Study One Year Later." *New England Journal of Medicine,* vol. 314, no. 19 (May 8, 1986): 1266–1268.

National Center for Health Services Research. *Inpatient Hospital Services: Use, Expenditures, and Sources of Payment.* National Health Care Expenditures Study, Data Preview 15. DHHS Pub. No. (PHS) 83-3360. Rockville, MD, May 1983.

———. *Private Health Insurance in the United States.* National Health Care Expenditures Study, Data Preview 23. DHHS Pub. No. (PHS) 86-3406. Rockville, MD, September 1986.

National Pharmaceutical Council, Inc. *Pharmaceutical Benefits under State Medical Assistance Programs.* Reston, VA, September 1986.

New York Times, 30 August 1987.

New York Times, 9 November 1987.

New York Times, 17 February 1988.

New York Times, 10 July 1989.

Pittman-Lindeman, Mary, Gale Berkowitz, and Tom Rundall. "Impact of the 1982 Medi-Cal Policy Reform on the Health Status and Health Care of the San Francisco Medically Indigent Adults." Paper presented at the annual meeting of the American Public Health Association, Washington, DC, November 17, 1985.

Rymer, Marilyn. *Short-Term Evaluation of Medicaid: Selected Issues.* Baltimore, MD: U.S. Department of Health and Human Services, Health Care Financing Administration, October 1984.

Soumerai, Stephen B., Jerry Avorn, Dennis Ross-Degan, and Steven Gortmaker. "Payment Restrictions for Prescription Drugs under Medicaid: Effects on Therapy, Cost and Equity." *New England Journal of Medicine,* vol. 317, no. 9 (August 27, 1987): 550–556.

Taylor, Amy K. *Contacts with Physicians in Ambulatory Settings: Rates of Use, Expenditures, and Source of Payment.* Data Preview 16. DHHS Pub. No. (PHS) 83-3361. Rockville, MD: National Center for Health Services Research, October 1983.

Texas Task Force on Indigent Health Care. Final Report. December 1984. Austin, TX: State of Texas, Governor's Office, 1984.

Tilly, Jane, and Debbie Brunner. *Medicaid Eligibility and Its Effect on the Elderly.* #8605. Washington, DC: American Association of Retired Persons, January 1987.

U.S. Congress. House. Select Committee on Aging. *Twentieth Anniversary of Medicare and Medicaid: Americans Still at Risk.* 99th Cong., 1st sess. Washington, DC: Government Printing Office, 1986.

U.S. Department of Commerce, Bureau of the Census. *Statistical Abstract of the United States. 1987* (107th ed.). Washington, DC, 1986.

——. *Statistical Abstract of the United States. 1988* (108th ed.). Washington, DC, 1987.

U.S. Department of Health and Human Services, Health Care Financing Administration. *Medicare and Medicaid Data Book, 1983.* Health Care Financing Program Statistics. HCFA Pub. No. 03156. Baltimore, MD, December 1983.

——. *Medicare and Medicaid Data Book, 1984.* Health Care Financing Program Statistics. HCFA Pub. No. 03210. Baltimore, MD, 1986.

——. *Medicare and Medicaid Data Book, 1988.* Health Care Financing Program Statistics. HCFA Pub. No. 03270. Baltimore, MD, 1989.

——. *The Medicare Catastrophic Coverage Act of 1988.* Legislative Summary. Baltimore, MD, November 7, 1988.

PART THREE

FERTILITY-RELATED SERVICES

CHAPTER SEVEN

Reproductive Care

BIOLOGY, WHICH DETERMINES THE technical possibilities of preventing conception and females' need for care for pregnancy and birth, is a major determinant of gender patterns of reproductive care. However, biology does not stand alone, for social norms, such as whether it is acceptable for a male to take responsibility for contraception, and economic factors, such as the market availability of contraceptive methods for males, are also influential. In addition, when a couple is faced with infertility or risk of genetic defect, decisions as to use of outside sperm donors and other options affect services used by each sex.

Overall, reproductive health care is largely utilized by women and is an important part of their total health care. Hence, its limitations and achievements should give some insights as to how well the health care system is functioning for women. Much time has passed since the Civil Rights Act of 1964 was passed and women's claims to equal treatment in social institutions began to be acknowledged. Health care, including fertility-related care, was a major part of women's critique. Yet much remains difficult or problematic in reproductive care.

Some of the issues potentially affect all women of reproductive age who are interested in either seeking or avoiding pregnancy. A persistent issue in pregnancy care is whether technology currently in use is appropriately employed. A related concern is whether prenatal care content is justified by scientific evidence. It is also argued that psychosocial aspects of pregnancy and childbirth are given too little weight in the care process, to the detriment of women and their families, because of a focus on biotechnical aspects of care.

Access-related issues have disproportionate impact on certain subgroups of women. These include low-income, black, and teenage clients or potential clients who may have unmet needs for contraceptive, prenatal, or maternity services and pregnant women needing programs addressing drug abuse, HIV infection, and other conditions. The connections between reproductive services and social expectations regarding women result in some special access problems. Abortion services are singled out for restrictions by the federal government. Newer infertility treatments are more likely to be available to those whose life-style, as well as economic ability, meets provider conditions. This may specifically affect single women and women in lesbian relationships who desire artificial insemination, in order to have children. Some of the ways in which individual characteristics may influence provider attitudes are difficult to document. They may be inferred, however, from controversies over ethical, legal, and economic aspects of reproductive services (abortion and surrogate motherhood). On the everyday level, teenage sexuality continues to be a hot potato, and, in the more exotic realm, decisions about selective survival in multiple pregnancies induced by fertility drugs or in vitro fertilization (IVF) trouble physicians (Bromwich et al., 1988).

These controversies may be seen as part of the disturbances of social equilibrium caused by changes in fertility-related technology and concurrent changes affecting women. Traditional assumptions as to family genesis and family structure, age-related norms of sexual and reproductive behavior, acceptable environments for child rearing, and other tenets have been challenged by both the behavior of younger cohorts and the expression of antitraditional views. Physicians serve as initiators of many new opportunities and, thus, have collaborated with the upset of previous norms. But they also serve as gatekeepers and, as such, are influenced by their own professional perspectives and by community acceptance of their patterns of decisions. This tends to make access variable insofar as it depends on individual providers' willingness to serve specific patients in a given hospital and community setting.

The activities of groups that would not give high priority to women's reproductive autonomy, a concept that includes a wide range of choices for women within a set of competing social goals, or would simply reject it as a goal are often in the press. They constrain the ability of women to use the market for services to satisfy their reproductive goals. Furthermore, subsidized care for reproductive needs falls within the class of services to the poor that are vulnerable to conservative fiscal ideologies (overriding conservative interest in population control). Other limitations may arise from resistance to services to minorities and to teenagers. Consequently, women's need for basic fertility-related care is not a guarantee of availability. Thus, insofar as reproduction is concerned, the health economy is much influenced by its political and social context.

A woman's demand for reproductive care is based on her desire for children in general and, specifically, her desire to determine the number and timing of births in harmony with her other present and planned activities. (Ideally, these desires reflect consensus with a loving partner.) Traditionally, demand has been channeled to particular services by professional dominance in decision making, but this influence has been lessened by consumer movements founded on beliefs concerning how birth should be experienced and what values should be paramount in choosing birth limitation methods.

Ability to avoid unwanted births was pictured by some feminists of the 1960s and 1970s as a halfway measure, because an ideal society would assure sustenance and development for all newborns and all needful supports for their parents. As things are now, however, the ability to avoid unwanted births is likely to remain a precious element in the personal autonomy of women.

The use of prenatal care and specific reproductive services varies between areas and by class and race, suggesting several problems. One of these is barriers to access: uneven distribution of supply, lack of third party sponsors, and limited ability to pay out of income. Another relates to technical processes, the excessive application of questionable technology or (the opposite problem) too slow diffusion of superior technology. Finally, cultural or educational problems in achieving utilization patterns considered optimal for health and for effective fertility planning may exist. Class and race differences in reproductive care indicate the impact of poverty and restricted educational and employment opportunities on women's ability to maximize their reproductive health. Only in part can the problems be solved by the health care system through special service programs and financial coverage (DHHS, 1985). Measures aimed at equality of opportunity are also needed.

FERTILITY LIMITATION

The fertility limitation market offers alternative methods, substitutes whose market share may be redistributed as choices of consumers change. This may happen as scientific information concerning health effects is produced and distributed, as users discover their individual preferences through trial and error, or as those preferences (notably for efficacy over reversibility) change with age and family circumstances. The history of the intrauterine device (IUD) involves not only a change in scientific knowledge but also the impact of court action and regulation on the market. The IUD became popular after women criticized the lack of sharing of information on health risks of oral contraceptives, which they claimed was motivated by population control and private economic interests, as careless disregard of their right to know (Boston Women's Health Book Collective, 1973). The tragic results of the use of the Dalkon shield (whose marketing success was based on misleading promotion) led to a wave of product liability suits and eventual discontinuance of all IUDs in the domestic market (Mintz, 1985).

The birth limitation market includes complements, two methods that are used together, especially abortion as a backup following failed contraception, and combinations of barrier and spermicidal methods for greater protection, as well as substitutes. Given the absence of perfect contraceptive methods, availability of abortion permits use of contraceptive methods that are safer (or more convenient) but not 100 percent effective. Desire for protection against disease also promotes use of more than one method.

Access to effective fertility control has economic implications. There are savings in health care costs from averting unwanted births and high-risk pregnancies. Use of health services becomes more rational, insofar as services are used to satisfy individual preferences for timing and number of births. Moreover, delayed childbearing and smaller families affect continuity of labor force participation, education, and earnings of women. Thus, gender equity and the status of women have been advanced by improved access to relatively effective fertility control services.

Nevertheless, despite use of contraception by the general population, unwanted and mistimed births are numerous. Deficiencies in the current array of products are believed to be a part of the problem. Development of methods that combine safety, efficiency, and acceptability requires continued research. The quality of evaluations is also beset with difficulties. Abortion, a backup method of birth limitation, is in chronic jeopardy because of public controversy, and contraceptive services are threatened because of linkages to abortion and direct attempts of the federal government to restrict availability of services to teenagers. These developments reduce the likelihood of a good match between preferences and actual births.

Family-planning Users

In 1987, 92 percent of sexually active women who would have been at risk of unintended pregnancy were using some form of contraception, including sterilization, and 8 percent were not. Exposure without protection was more common among black women. In all, 66 percent of American women 15–44 years of age were using contraception (Mishell, 1989).

Family planning visits for women aged 15–44 who had had some sexual experience and were not sterile numbered 1,077 per 1,000 women in 1982 (Horn and Mosher, 1984). The rate for blacks was 1,334; for whites, 1,033. The never-married and younger women (15–24) had higher rates than older and married women, some of whom were pregnant or trying to become pregnant, others of whom had been sterilized after completing their families.

The need for family planning services among sexually active women wishing to avoid pregnancy depends on the method of contraception selected. Age, race, and marital status differences in family planning visit rates to all types of providers reflect methods used by different subgroups of women. The pill, the leading method among young and never-married women, requires repeated visits, whereas sterilization, the leading method among older married women, does not. Black women tend to use methods requiring more visits and are less likely to use sterilization.

Clinics are a significant part of the supply of family planning services, providing over one-third of all family planning visits in 1982. They were especially important for blacks and teenagers. For black women, 56.5 percent of all family planning visits were to clinics, versus 31.3 percent for whites, and blacks were less likely to use private sources. Over half of all teenagers with family planning visits, and over three-quarters of black teenagers with visits, used clinics. However, by 1988, owing largely to a sharp rise in clinic use by white teenagers, there was no longer a significant difference between black and white teenagers in the percentage using clinics for family planning (Mosher, 1990).

Never-married women of all ages were more likely to use clinics than married women; over half did so. Clinic services tend to entail longer waits and fewer amenities than private family planning services, and overcrowding, making for dissatisfaction (Radecki and Bernstein, 1989).

Shortcomings in Product Menu and Information

A problem for all users is that, despite widespread use of contraception, the product menu and the quality of available information have serious shortcomings.

"There is no reversible method of contraception that is both highly efficacious in actual use, and acceptable to most women" (Trussell and Kost, 1987, p. 275). Paradoxically, "most methods work well if used consistently and correctly"; yet "failure rates in actual use are generally not low" (p. 273). Much of the failure is probably due to "user error" (engaging in some acts of unprotected intercourse). The frequency of such behavior cannot be estimated, but it is known that side effects and inconvenience contribute to lack of consistent use of theoretically efficacious methods. Inconsistent use and failure to become a user before initiating sexual activity must be widespread, because of the very large numbers of accidental pregnancies shown in the literature on trials of contraceptive methods and in survey data on unwanted births, confirmed by inference from out-of-wedlock births (Dunn, 1987).

For never-married women interviewed in 1982–1983, 24.8 percent of children ever born by 1982 were unwanted at conception: 18.4 percent for whites and 29.8 percent for blacks. For ever-married women, 9.6 percent of children ever born were unwanted (7.7 percent for whites and 21.8 percent for blacks). Failure of timing (a pregnancy occurred sooner than wanted) also caused a split between actual experience and women's desires or plans: 28.2 percent of births to the ever-married and 42.3 percent of births to the never-married were mistimed. Black–white differences were less on mistiming than on unwanted conceptions, and, for the never-married, the mistiming rates for blacks and whites were about equal.

If one combines the two types of undesired occurrences for ever-married women, 39.6 percent of all births were either not wanted at conception or came sooner than wanted. An increase in mistimed births among young women occurred that may have been due to shifting from the pill or the IUD, after health risks of these two methods were revealed, to less effective barrier methods. However, the proportion of births unwanted at conception declined between 1973 and 1982, by around 30 percent (Pratt and Horn, 1985). (Trend data are not available for unmarried women, who were interviewed for the first time in 1982.)

Mistiming for married women is usually a less serious outcome than unwantedness, and the decline in unwanted births is a substantial improvement for them. However, the broad use of abortion and sterilization (and the continuing occurrence of a considerable number of mistimed and unwanted births for both married and unmarried women) suggest that limitations of our present inventory of contraceptive products may be important. A method for women that would be used once a month, at the time the menses are expected, would be attractive, especially for teenagers.

Meanwhile, despite a host of research studies, the information they provide on efficacy is far from adequate to help users make informed decisions. Various limitations of the studies are responsible for this. The critical review of the research literature by Trussell and Kost cited above notes that randomized blind trials comparing methods are not possible, and, thus, women most motivated to avoid pregnancy will choose methods they view as most effective and will adhere to protocol. Hence, a ranking of methods by extent of user failure would be distorted. Clinicians' preferences can also steer patients to certain methods and affect the quality of instruction given to patients. The numbers of those who become pregnant may be underreported because of contraception researchers' peculiar conventions of counting subjects and lack of follow-up. Not controlling for recent use of the pill, which depresses fecundity temporarily after quitting, also biases failure rates downward. When a given method is studied, users of adjunctive (supplementary) methods may not be excluded, with similar effect: reported failure rates are lower than true rates. Misrepresentation, motivated by desire for profit or bias toward a particular method, regrettably has also been a factor. In the case of the Dalkon shield, Dr. Herbert Davis, the originator, did not reveal to the scientific world that the low pregnancy rate claimed for the first year later climbed or that women in the trial were instructed to use adjunctive methods.

Other problems arise from differences between research situations and ordinary practice: for example, a woman with an IUD would be seen more often if she were part of a study, and an expulsion would very likely be noted before an accidental pregnancy occurred.

Finally, concern over acquiring AIDS and other diseases through sexual contact is influencing condom use and may alter the rate of accidental pregnancies attributable to other methods, if condoms are used with other methods in order to prevent diseases (Cates et al., 1982).

The difference in perspective between medical innovators, who may consider that a new method of controlling fertility is safe and effective, and the individual consumer is illustrated by a female sterilization procedure. The results of a study of a certain method of tubal ligation in an ambulatory surgical center were used to recommend further use of the procedure (Kaali and Landesman, 1985). In this study, three hundred healthy patients received a thirty-minute counseling session, four-fifths requested and received general anesthesia, almost nine-tenths spent one to six hours in the recovery room, and fourteen had enough pain to require narcotics. There were four subsequent pregnancies including one ectopic pregnancy; seven patients had accidental tubal transection and three had uterine perforation; and there were twelve technical failures.

The authors called the procedure effective because the pregnancy rate was only 0.8 percent, which they compared favorably with the 1.8 percent reported in a series of 4,707 cases in which other techniques were used. They admitted, however, that 25 percent of the patients did not have an adequate follow-up. They warned that "great caution must be exercised" in patient selection and that there should be a hospital nearby in which the surgeon has operating privileges for emergencies. There is room for debate as to whether consumers would interpret these results as a good basis for selecting this procedure.

The different contraceptive methods vary widely in cost. A useful method of computing cost is to amortize initial cost over an appropriate period for each method and to apply a modest interest rate to the unamortized balance in a given period. Fuchs and Perreault (1985) assign a fifteen-year period of service for sterilization, based on the average age (thirty years) of women obtaining tubal ligations in 1979–1980, and a three-year period for the pill, the IUD, and the diaphragm. The pill, at $130 annual cost, including interest at 4 percent per annum, is the most expensive method; the diaphragm is next at $111; and female sterilization is third at $106. (By contrast, male sterilization costs only $22 when amortized and is the cheapest method.) Spermicides and IUDs cost about the same ($50 and $47 respectively), and condoms cost $30 per year. It is clear that relative cost alone is not responsible for the frequencies of the different methods, although it may affect some users, since the methods, in order of frequency of use (1987), are the pill, female sterilization, the condom, male sterilization, spermicidal foam, the diaphragm, and the IUD (Mishell, 1989).[1] But one should consider abortion (more expensive than even the most costly contraceptive, the pill) along with other birth limitation methods. There were 360.8 induced abortions per 1,000 live births in a thirteen-state reporting area of the United States in 1983 (Powell-Griner, 1986), nine-tenths of them in the first trimester. The rate was twice as high for blacks as for whites. As noted earlier, abortion is often used as a second method to avoid an unwanted birth after a first method has failed, for whatever reason. Therefore, selection of a method that would provide strong security against needing an abortion would make such a method a better buy at a given annual cost. However, flaws in available information as to efficacy of different methods applicable to actual conditions of use may result in less rational choices by consumers.

Consumers may also be ill informed as to certain benefits of a particular method, such as the pill's reducing the risk of iron deficiency anemia, benign breast disease, endometrial and ovarian cancer, and other conditions (Mishell, 1989), and as to the current state of knowledge about the health risks of each method.

Teenagers received one-quarter of the abortions performed in 1982–1983, and they had them at later gestational ages than older women. Social failure to inculcate and assure use of contraception, thus avert-

---

[1]The figures represent women 15–44 exposed to the risk of unwanted pregnancy.

ing unwanted pregnancy, during adolescents' transition to adult sexuality plays an important part in their demand for abortion. But limitations of the available methods of contraception may also be a factor.

New Product Slowdown

Lincoln and Kaeser (1988) remind us that, in the early 1970s, it was expected that a host of new contraceptive methods would soon become available in the United States, including methods applicable to men alone or to either sex. However, it appeared by 1988 that "contraceptive methods are disappearing faster than new ones can be introduced" (p. 20). Some methods distributed in other countries are not considered capable of passing Food and Drug Administration (FDA) review for marketing here. These include injectables, postcoital contraceptives, and devices for reversible sterilization.

The unsatisfactory rate of contraceptive development is attributed to several factors. Controlling population growth has ceased to be a priority goal of developed countries that have low birth rates and low infant and maternal mortality rates. This is not an exact description of the United States, for, although the birth rate is low, there is concern with infant mortality. (The U.S. rate in 1985, 10.6 deaths per 1,000 live births, was higher than the rate of sixteen other industrialized countries (U.S. Congress, 1988).) But this has stimulated legislative interest in prenatal and obstetrical services, rather than in fertility control. Both government and the pharmaceutical industry have reduced their spending for developing new products. Regulatory changes following the thalidomide disaster in the early 1960s made the FDA approval process a more difficult hurdle for manufacturers. Because of the abortion controversy, companies doing research on methods that work after fertilization risk boycott of all their pharmaceutical products by anti-abortion groups. Both the Agency for International Development and the National Institutes of Health are specifically barred, one by law and the other by policy, from funding any research related to abortion.

Manufacturers face other deterrents due to ever-present risks of side effects. Consumer concern about product safety has been expressed in political opposition to approval and marketing of certain methods and in liability suits. High premium costs for product liability insurance are thought to have particular impact on long-acting and low-profit contraceptives (such as implants), which do not yield enough revenues to finance self-insurance.

A panel convened by the National Academy of Sciences criticized the restricted range of currently available methods. In particular, lack of con-

venient methods for the young was said to result in "millions of unwanted pregnancies, unnecessary abortions, and avoidable sterilizations"
(Hilts, 1990). Other groups ill-served by the present menu of products
include nursing mothers and others who cannot risk taking the hormones used in oral contraceptives.

Representative Patricia Schroeder, co-author of a bill to support research on birth control and infertility, through five new centers, has
blamed "medical McCarthyism" in the federal government for the slowdown in discoveries (American Medical Association, 1990).

Recently, the Food and Drug Administration approved the cervical
cap, a barrier method that can be substituted for a diaphragm, after years
of lobbying by women's health groups. The label is required to warn that
women must have a Pap test with normal results before a cap is fitted
and must repeat the test after three months (New York Times, 24 May
1988). It may be presumed that the provider is motivated to do the tests
to protect the patient against progression of cervical cancer (and to avoid
later lawsuits). However, in the recent case of an anti-acne drug, Accutane, leaving it to the doctor–patient and pharmacist–patient relationship to assure avoidance or termination of pregnancy when using the
medication was not effective in preventing birth defects. Various reasons
for this were offered. Doctors do not necessarily take the time to instruct
patients carefully or respond to their questions; they do not ask parents
of a teenage girl to leave so that they can talk frankly to her; and they are
often indifferent to drug warnings in the Physicians Desk Reference.
Pharmacists do not necessarily call the patient's attention to the warning
against pregnancy on the Accutane bottle, as they are supposed to, and
they may fail to affix a warning label (New York Times, 27 May 1988). It
is an indication of the problems of the currently available methods that
women's groups favored the cap, although its effectiveness (85 percent) is
no better than that of the diaphragm. (Its merits are that it can be left in
place longer, is more comfortable for some women, and, like other barrier methods, avoids affecting body functions.)

Fragmentation and Access

The fertility limitation market has multiple connections with the maternity care market. Failures of contraception not followed by abortion result in need for maternity care and in more high-risk pregnancies, in
particular. Permanent suppression of fertility or successful use of temporary methods reduces the demand for maternity care and the number of
high-risk pregnancies. Side effects of birth limitation methods have produced infertility or temporarily reduced fertility. If childbearing is de-

layed, a woman is more likely, because of her age, to need prenatal genetic tests (amniocentesis or, possibly, chorionic villus sampling) and to have a cesarean delivery. Premature births are also more likely. All these add to resource use and costs.

However, birth control has been, to a large extent, organizationally separated from maternity care; abortion, from contraception. The fragmentation of reproductive health care, according to Aries (1985), initially facilitated the expansion of birth control services. The reason for fragmentation was that those services did not fit into the priorities of physicians. They preferred to deal with birth, rather than birth control, and they were seeking acceptance for obstetrics within medicine, where the disease model reigned. They succeeded in making birth the subject of medical ministrations. Doctors later began to play more of a role in family planning, when the technology changed so that medical skills were required (to fit a diaphragm, insert an IUD, or prescribe pills) and when federal funding was provided. Congress, however, followed the Planned Parenthood model of a distinct service organization separated from general health care even when physician services were involved. Aries contends that separation of family planning and abortion services into special organizations, locations, and funding programs made fertility control vulnerable to political attack. Since 1981 Medicaid has been paying for abortion only when the woman's life was endangered, and virtually no payments have been made.

The elimination of federal financial support led some states to finance abortions voluntarily, and others are doing so under court order.[2] However, abortions have been done at later gestational ages and with more complications, because of funding restrictions (or the pregnancy continued to term).[3]

In addition to funding changes, federal political objectives have singled out abortion services for restrictive regulations that would prohibit family planning clinics from doing abortions or providing referrals or counseling for abortion. Policymakers who support these initiatives are apparently willing to risk a shrinkage of family planning services to check abortion.

---

[2]Thirty-one states have policies as restrictive as the federal standard (abortion for life endangerment only), four have less restrictive policies (for rape, incest, imminent death, severe fetal deformity), five are under court order to provide funding, and nine plus the District of Columbia have full public funding of abortion for poor women (*NARAL News*, 1988).

[3]It is estimated that between 60,000 and 80,000 births occur annually that would have been averted had pre-1981 law applied (Torres et al., 1986). Mean duration of pregnancy is longer for abortions received by black women and out-of-state residents (Kochanek, 1990).

These efforts have been blocked only after legal struggles by family planning providers and advocates of reproductive freedom (*New York Times*, 17 February 1988), and similar battles are predictable for the coming years. Demonstrations, bogus clinics, and other actions by hostile groups intended to intimidate abortion users and providers succeed in preventing service at sources of mainstream care, at least temporarily (*New York Times*, 3 May 1988). These activities and restrictive federal policies may be mutually reinforcing. A recent Supreme Court decision, *Webster* v. *Reproductive Health Service, Inc.* (July 3, 1989), made it possible for individual states to restrict abortion services further, for example, by forbidding public hospitals to perform abortions, and this decision was regarded as a serious weakening of the constitutional right to abortion upheld in 1973 (*New York Times*, 4 July 1989).

Those who depend on clinics for fertility control services are vulnerable to fiscal constraints and politico-religious opposition to resource use for family planning and abortion. Users of private care have more security, for, while those obstetricians who have limited interest in fertility control may fail to provide optimal counseling or trial of methods best suited to an individual, the consumer may respond by seeking providers who offer more satisfactory service.

However, this is not always simple. A recent study gives insights into how doctors' attitudes may make obtaining an abortion a difficult process. It shows that private practice of obstetrics-gynecology becomes fragmented when elective abortion is viewed as unwelcome business. In an eastern city of 100,000 studied by Imber (1986), the social conditions of private practice allowed the city's twenty-six obstetricians to decide how they would spend their practice time and under what circumstances they would perform abortions or assist patients in getting them. Under two-fifths of the doctors were willing to do any abortions, and even they were generally reluctant to do second-trimester abortions. Doctors not doing abortions referred patients whom they did not know, through their appointments secretaries, to the abortion clinic in a nearby town (or simply had their offices say they did not do abortions). For a regular patient, however, they confirmed the pregnancy first. In group practices, certain members were understood to be willing to do an abortion, and the physician first approached by the patient would refer her directly to the performing doctor. Catholic influence not only prevented performance of abortions at the Catholic hospital, even by non-Catholic doctors, but also deterred the local Planned Parenthood chapter from offering either abortion service or referral.

Some doctors were sympathetic to abortion seekers because of their concern with poverty, overpopulation, or the medical system's responsibility for unplanned pregnancy. Others opposed abortion for religious reasons. Older doctors apparently avoided being involved because they had no training in abortion and use of the pill or the IUD and had made family planning in general the least important part of their practice. Doctors in this community felt that the stigma of being known to do abortions would affect their "obstetrical" practice. They were able to reconcile their responsibility to respond to patients' requests with their desire to avoid controversy because a clinic did exist. Indeed, non-Catholic doctors routinely recommended amniocentesis for women over thirty-five and, thus, were dependent on providers being available who would do second-trimester abortions. Obstetricians also did genetic counseling, which again implies that they relied on abortion providers.

After abortion was legalized in 1973, the courts held that it was the physician's responsibility to deliver information about abnormalities of fetal development to the pregnant patient, so that a decision about continuing the pregnancy could be made intelligently ("Father and Mother," 1978). Damages could be awarded for the physician's failure to diagnose rubella in early pregnancy or to inform a woman of the diagnosis (Lewis, 1986). Physicians' failure to do prenatal tests and to advise abortion has been legally recognized as a basis for parents' malpractice claims for "wrongful life" after the birth of infants with diagnosable hereditary defects (McCann, 1981). Thus, physicians have an incentive to facilitate patients' informed decisions about completing a pregnancy or having an induced abortion.

Private practitioners studied by Imber, however, were able to avoid actually providing the abortion. They were able to position themselves in that part of the reproductive services market that was convenient for them and in accord with their ideology. This study is not nationally representative, of course, but it suggests a problem, especially in smaller communities where anonymity is hard to come by. It is supported by a 1985 poll by the American College of Obstetricians and Gynecologists, which revealed that although 84 percent of respondents thought abortion should be legal and available, only one-third of these actually did any. Those who did perform abortions were harassed by hostile groups and often stigmatized by their medical peers (Kolata, 1990; Cousins, 1990). The absence of any abortion providers in 21 percent of metropolitan areas and 91 percent of nonmetropolitan counties, a significant limitation on access, reflects, at least in part, the attitudes and incentives affecting many physicians and hospitals.

However, today's (and tomorrow's) new abortifacient drugs may dilute the effect of physician attitudes toward serving as abortion providers. The possibility of using drugs to produce miscarriages in the first trimester as a substitute for surgical abortions is drawing nearer. In 1988 a World Health Organization panel "determined that a specific two-drug combination was safe and effective" for this purpose (*New York Times*, 16 February 1988). Clinical trials in the United Kingdom tested this combination (RU486, a drug developed in France by Roussel-Uclaf, plus prostaglandin) and found it successful in terminating 95 percent of early pregnancies (*Lancet*, 1989). Patients in studies where the drug combination was tested had to agree to a surgical abortion if the drugs failed, because it was known that there was an added risk of birth defects. Opposition of pro-life activists has blocked marketing of RU486 outside France, although it would provide more safety to patients in places where skilled personnel to perform abortions are scarce. If RU486 is ultimately approved for marketing in the United States, medical supervision will still be required, as the subjects who do not respond will need surgery. Doubt as to ability to enforce patients' commitment to a surgical abortion, plus lack of interest in doing the surgery themselves, may temper the interest of some providers. There could also be political opposition to an effective abortifacient.

MATERNITY CARE

The maternity care market has a structure of substitutes, organized around alternative models of delivery that have an ideological base. One model is based on maternity as a natural process and an experience in family bonding. The other is a systems approach characterized by risk classification, monitoring of deviations, and receptivity to technology (Arney, 1982).

This division is translated into alternative providers, settings, and levels of technical input. Consumers tend to go along with the medical model because of professional dominance and their desire for a perfect pregnancy outcome; that is, they share with medical authorities an interest in risk reduction and accept the provider's judgment about how to avert risk. The users of alternative settings and providers are a relatively small minority. The cohesion of the medical model is promoted by the effects of certain clinical decisions on later physiological states or events. For example, use of a certain birthing position may affect the probability of difficulties in labor and predispose to later interventions, and rupture of membranes predisposes to cesareans because of the risk of infection. Negotiated views of pain accepted by the physician and the patient also play a part in forming a cohesive medical model, affecting use of analgesia and anesthesia and decisions about continuing a trial of labor. In 1980 drugs or surgical procedures were used to induce or maintain labor in 48.1 percent of live births in hospitals; electronic fetal monitoring (EFM) was used in almost half of births (Heuser et al., 1984); and over one-fourth of births were cesareans (Placek, Taffel, and Moien, 1988). However, there are significant interstate differences in the use of these birth-related technologies (Heuser et al., 1984) (see pp. 197–198).[4] There are also differences between private and clinic patients, and between practices of individual doctors (Goyert et al., 1989), in the rate of cesareans that are not explained by obvious risk factors.

There is play within the medical model today, resulting from the challenge of alternative models and the women's health movement. Established institutions have coopted elements in the alternative model to preserve their status: they have installed birthing rooms, allowed a choice of birthing positions, and embraced the use of midwives within the hospital. Lamaze training has become quite popular, and participation of fathers and support from children have been incorporated into general norms for maternity care. However, when invited to sanction out-of-hospital births, medical organizations tend to draw the line. The New York Academy of Medicine rejected home births even for low-risk pregnancies on the grounds that a "no-risk" obstetrical population cannot be identified, even through careful screening; rapid emergency services cannot be provided in the home; and rapid transport to a hospital cannot be assured. The Academy did, however, recommend development of a homelike birthing environment in the hospital (New York Academy of Medicine, 1983). Advocates of birthing centers argue that using a birthing center at which midwives are responsible for care is a valid middle course between home and hospital settings. They also point out that superior safety of births in the hospital, in comparison with other settings, has not been demonstrated. Thus, the conflicting views of risk remain a critical obstacle to any major shift in birth setting.[5]

Midwife-attended births remain a small minority but do represent an active alternative provider group. Births attended by midwives increased during 1980–1984 by 51 percent. They accounted for 2.1 percent of all hospital births in 1984, or 78,040 births in hospitals, and 15,862 outside of hospitals. The recent increases were confined to white births (National Center for Health Statistics, 1986). For white women, they may represent the search for a holistic birth experience but, for some blacks, a form

---

[4]Statistical methods were used to derive synthetic estimates on obstetrical practices for individual states from the National Natality Survey of 1980. Variation for amniocentesis was also large, but the estimates are not statistically reliable because of the small numbers.

[5]Not only the evidence for the existence of risk and the amount of risk, but also whether a given amount of risk is tolerable, enter into the formation of attitudes about where births should take place.

of care they associate with previous poverty. Lay midwives, a group chiefly based on apprenticeship rather than on formal credentialed training, are reported to be "making a comeback" and attend home births where "women are virtually in charge" (Kay et al., 1988). The recent withdrawal of some obstetricians from the maternity market creates some space for midwife providers.[6]

Advances in medicine have made more diversity possible within the hospital. It is now feasible to avoid surgical intervention for some ectopic pregnancies (Ory, 1986; Frau et al., 1986). Also feasible is conservative management of Rh-sensitive pregnancies, aiming at longer gestation and better survival, based on intensive surveillance by ultrasound imaging and electronic monitoring of the fetal heart rate (Frigoletto et al., 1986). It may also be possible to decrease use of cesareans for complications of labor through active management of a first labor (Boylan, 1987). The comparative costs of such suggested approaches and traditional management have not been determined, although avoiding the neonatal intensive care unit (NICU) is generally economical.

Prenatal Care

Content of the Visit Protocol Prenatal visits can be used for detection and management of many conditions that could compromise fetal and maternal health and for identification of high-risk patients. They also promote general health maintenance and give emotional support. Therefore, despite questions as to the efficacy of prenatal care in low-risk, as opposed to multi-risk, populations, health professionals generally favor a protocol for regular prenatal care. The Institute of Medicine, for example, has defined a minimum of nine visits, starting in the first trimester, as adequate for a gestation of thirty-six weeks or more (Showstack, Budetti, and Minkler, 1984). The 1985 standards of the American College of Obstetricians and Gynecologists list seven tests to be done once and five others as possibly needed and twenty-three items suggested for risk assessment. The Canadian Task Force on the Periodic Health Examination lists about twenty conditions for which prenatal preventive services are recommended, the great majority of which are supported by very good evidence from one or more randomized clinical trials or other well-designed studies. The specific services include history taking, physical examination, tests, and counseling, and, in many of the conditions, repeated tests throughout pregnancy are advised (1979). The conditions

---

[6]Their existence provides a way of directly satisfying the preferences of some women. The midwife birth market, small as it is, is perhaps a reminder to physicians that the medical model, even after cooptations from alternative styles, should not be taken for granted.

include not only genetic disorders, infectious diseases, hypertension, diabetes, and blood group incompatibility but also parenting problems, postpartum depression, and alcohol use.

Hemminki (1988) questions the orientation of American prenatal care as compared with that of other countries. Our protocols focus on screening or biomedical problems at the expense of providing health education and support, which would oblige the physician to spend more time with each individual patient than the present average of eleven minutes. Furthermore, the efficacy of several elements in current prenatal care has been questioned. Some services that were once in wide use are now discontinued. Routine X-ray pelvimetry is now regarded as clearly harmful, for instance. Drugs widely advertised to medical, and specifically obstetrics-gynecology, audiences have been condemned for use in pregnancy.

Some practices continue despite the absence of strong evidence on their behalf. Recommendations concerning multivitamins, diuretics, and animal proteins are cited as examples. Others, such as ultrasound, have been introduced in advance of any good evidence from randomized trials and before their consequences when used in general populations were known.

Hemminki says these problems have several causes. Practitioners are poorly prepared to sift out evidence or to retain critical attitudes. Financial incentives of vendors and caregivers and a deficit in consumer influence also play a part. The content of care is thus influenced by nonscientific elements. Speert calls attention to educational and emotional support in pregnancy as the greatest gap in American obstetrics and states that providing emotional support "to the parturient in pregnancy and labor has been the distinctive function of midwives" (Speert, 1980, p. 20).

Much of the positive value of prenatal care as conventionally given by physicians inheres in the screening and monitoring functions. Yet only 77 percent of prenatal visits included blood pressure measurement in 1979–1980. Screening for old risks could be improved, and the offer of screening for new risks (such as HIV infection) needs to be added to protocols if shown to be useful. On the basis of a study showing that use of histories to select high-risk women for blood tests for hepatitis B misses almost half of cases, Jonas et al. (1987) conclude that all pregnant women should be screened before delivery. The cost of the screening would be similar to that of screening blood donors and is estimated at $10 per test, or $7,300 per case of neonatal hepatitis B prevented in a low-income population in Cleveland.

Even if information is collected, the use to which it is put is also a problem in prenatal care. Care for hypertension in pregnancy is important because of the possibility that preeclampsia will develop, but it is said to be often misdirected because of controversy over causes, processes, and treatment of the condition (Evans, Frigoletto, and Jewett, 1983). Presentation by authorities of "diametrically opposed approaches" (such as indications for use of diuretics in managing preeclampsia and whether women with chronic hypertension and mild blood pressure elevation should be treated) is bound to be unhelpful to some patients (Lindheimer and Katz, 1985). Increased distribution of prenatal care has, nevertheless, helped bring about a sharp decline in mortality from eclampsia. Research that will help resolve important controversies over treatment should be adequately supported, and the actual treatments in use in different types of practice and in different parts of the country should be compared with "best" protocols of the experts.

Assessing the Value of Prenatal Care   Little information on the value of prenatal care is available based on random assignment of subjects to treatment and nontreatment groups. For example, a study cited in a report on adolescent sexuality by the National Research Council showed a drop in the percentage of adolescents with preeclampsia after a prenatal clinic for teenagers was introduced. However, the editors of the National Research Council report note that it is impossible to evaluate these results, because the characteristics of teenagers using clinic services before and after the new program were not established, nor was the availability of the clinic to all teenagers discussed (Hofferth and Hayes, 1987).

In another example, prenatal care in a state-funded comprehensive care project in California was found to improve birth outcomes, compared with those for women with under three prenatal visits and similar maternal risk factors. The fetal, or birth, outcomes comprised premature rupture of membranes, preterm delivery, low birthweight, and admission to the intensive care unit. Maternal outcomes, cesarean section rate, and postpartum fever and hemorrhage, were no better for the group with care. Because of the improvement in fetal outcomes, there was considerably less inpatient hospital cost: the no-care group had costs 73.8 percent higher per mother–baby pair. However, self-selection into the group receiving care may have been a limitation of this study, for it is not clear that all the no-care patients (one hundred consecutive no-care deliveries at the University of California San Diego Medical Center) were an overflow (on a waiting list) from the comprehensive program. Moreover, there were more substance abusers proportionally in the no-care group (Moore et al., 1986).

Studies of the effect of participation in the WIC program, under which low-income pregnant women at high "nutritional risk" receive vouchers for food supplements, have shown improved pregnancy outcomes (Stockbauer, 1987) and more probability of receiving adequate prenatal care (Kotelchuck et al., 1984). But the scientific level of the research on WIC effects has been strongly questioned (Yankauer, 1984). Whether differences in motivation, personal habits, or amounts of prenatal care, rather than the program itself, account for good effects of WIC participation is hard to tell.

Careful research is needed to study the effect of prenatal services on infant mortality and low birthweight, because other factors are also at work. Absent or inadequate health care ("health care risks") is one of the categories used by the Institute of Medicine to classify the possible causal factors; the others include demographic factors, prepregnancy medical problems, pregnancy-related medical risk, and behavioral and environmental factors. Many of these are clustered in the same population group and are not easy to separate. In addition, prenatal care may affect another of the factors, such as current medical risks (McDonald and Coburn, 1986). However, a number of studies have found a positive relation between prenatal care and higher birthweight, which in turn is strongly related to better newborn survival (Showstack, Budetti, and Minkler, 1984). The effect of prenatal care on birthweight is supported for both white and black babies and is strengthened when length of gestation is taken into account, since this affects the number of prenatal visits that would meet a definition of "adequate" for a particular pregnancy. Joyce, Corman, and Grossman (1988) find the early initiation of prenatal care to be the most cost-effective means of reducing neonatal mortality for blacks and for whites, and it is far more cost-effective than neonatal intensive care, which has a very high cost per treated case.

Who Gets Prenatal Care   Most women start having babies when they are young and family income is less than it will be later in the work life of the parents. (And for some, poverty will be a chronic problem.) Four in ten pregnant women have incomes under $15,000. It is estimated that 27 percent of women of reproductive age do not have health insurance, and another 9 percent have insurance that does not include maternity care (Alan Guttmacher Institute, 1987). These economic facts inhibit receipt of care early in pregnancy for a substantial number of women. Only 77 percent of pregnancies started prenatal care in the first trimester in 1984. Dunn, speaking as a leader of the specialty of obstetrics-gynecology, regards the rate as unacceptable (Dunn, 1987). Eighty percent of white mothers and 62 percent of black mothers got first-trimester care; 5 percent and 10 percent, respectively, got no care until the third trimester (National Center for Health Statistics, 1986). These racial differences reflect economic access problems and other difficulties related to membership in a racial minority.[7]

The timing of conception in relation to marriage also affects when care is started. Teenage mothers who were married before conception were more likely to receive early prenatal care than those who married after conception, based on National Natality Survey data for 1980; and all married teenage mothers were more likely than unmarried ones to begin prenatal care in the first trimester.

The risk of low birthweight was substantially less for babies born to married, compared with unmarried, mothers and for those who married before, rather than after, conceiving (Ventura, 1987). Yet the percentage of teenagers, mothers for the first time, who marry before their children are born declined from 76 percent in 1964–1966 to 50 percent in 1980. White and black married women giving birth to a first child in 1980 were about equally likely to have conceived prior to marriage (17 percent and 14 percent respectively). The likelihood of having to depend on public programs for medical services and appropriate nutrition (or to do without) increased as single parenthood spread. Being "unmarried" does not exclude a stable partnership (really shading into common-law marriage), which may provide sufficient support for pregnancy needs in older women, but this is not likely to apply to teenagers. Furthermore, about half of teenagers who were married mothers in 1980 had less than a high school education, versus 7 percent of older mothers. They would too often be ill-equipped to take care of themselves properly during pregnancy or to pay for prenatal and obstetrical services.

Low-income Women   Medicaid provides maternity care to eligible low-income women. Before 1988, Medicaid coverage of pregnant women and children under age one, with incomes up to 100 percent of the poverty line, was optional for each state under federal law, and about three-fifths of the states adopted it. In the Medicare Catastrophic Coverage Act of 1988 this coverage was mandated. The law stated that a state could continue the eligibility of a pregnant woman, even if her income increased, through the postpartum period (U.S. Department of Health and Human Services, 1988).

The mandated coverage survived the repeal of most provisions of the 1988 act in 1989. However, for women between 100 percent and 185 percent of the poverty line, the federal government so far grants states only the option of covering maternity, infant, and family planning care,

---

[7]A 1984–1986 study shows that no care until the fifth month or later, or less than half the recommended number of visits, was received by 16 percent of women who gave birth (whites, 13 percent; Hispanics, 30 percent; blacks, 27 percent) (Lewin, 1989).

and very few states have picked up this option. In at least one state (New York), debate over including abortion (for which no federal aid would be received) in the state program delayed expansion of Medicaid to cover prenatal services up to 185 percent of the federal poverty line (*New York Times*, 17 May 1989).

In selected states that were studied by McDonald and Coburn (1986), Medicaid had a small, but definitely positive, effect on prenatal care: it increased the numbers receiving care early in pregnancy and the percentage of prescribed visits received, and it decreased the likelihood of inadequate care. The positive effect of Medicaid on timely utilization might be enhanced if the program were more generous as to population and specific benefits covered.

Medicaid finances 17 percent of all births each year, but reimbursement levels are usually less than in private care. Therefore the $1.8 billion outlay by Medicaid is only 10 percent of the nation's $16.5 billion bill for maternity and newborn care. Although Medicaid barriers based on family structure and employment have been modified since 1986, there are limits on mandated services, and women with complications could need services that Medicaid will not pay for. The income standard for coverage is severe, covering only 40 percent of women of reproductive age in poverty (Kenney et al., 1986). The low fee structure means that both hospital and physician providers have financial disincentives to accept Medicaid patients. Forty percent of obstetricians will not accept them (Alan Guttmacher Institute, 1987). Furthermore, as Medicaid pays a global fee that includes pre- and postnatal visits, we can't tell whether clients receive a full course of prenatal visits and a full range of services within visits (Kenney et al., 1986). Sixty percent of women with deliveries subsidized by Medicaid get their prenatal care at clinics (Alan Guttmacher Institute, 1987). Continuity of care is less probable in these settings, although many sponsors take pride in their efforts to provide comprehensive and caring services.

Nearly all states offer some prenatal care programs to low-income women under Title V of the Social Security Act (redesignated in 1985 as the Maternal and Child Health Block Grant program). But relatively few of those in need are reached by these programs (Rosenbaum, Hughes, and Johnson, 1988). These authors conclude that there is a "profound shortage of comprehensive maternity and pediatric services for low-income, uninsured women" (p. 321). Eligibility for maternity care may be restricted to those identified as high-risk before the start of labor, yet about one-quarter of prenatal risks do not emerge until the labor and delivery phase. "Only one state, Massachusetts, offered a truly statewide program to all uninsured pregnant women with incomes under 185% of the poverty level" (p. 315).[8] A report from the United Hospital Fund of New York indicates that a rising percentage of births was occurring in municipal hospitals, and these births had a higher rate of late or no prenatal care (1986).

The principle of fetal rights is being used as a basis for denying women the right to abortion and insisting that they undergo various procedures during pregnancy. Yet, at the same time, society has not conferred on childbearing an entitlement to the resources that may be required to assure a successful outcome. Entitlement is dependent on either status of self or spouse in an insured job or meeting a restrictive low-income standard. Protection of the primacy of the labor market and wage system in dispensing health care is given priority over universally adequate reproductive care. Protecting states' rights to set eligibility terms for programs for the poor (i.e., avoiding a federal standard) is another legislative priority that blocks a universal standard.

Restriction of the manner and timing of fertility control by laws against abortion is rendered a more serious constraint on women's lives when gaps in the provision of maternity care are tolerated. Consider, too, the implication of dropping women from Medicaid eligibility 60–90 days postpartum: it promotes discontinuity, separating reproductive from general health care, and suggests that help is available only if one is pregnant.

Health Maintenance Organizations With increasing enrollment in HMOs and a diversity of nonprofit and for-profit sponsors, the effect of HMOs on access to prenatal care is important. Despite social expectations about the preventive potential of HMOs, researchers from the Health Care Financing Administration in the 1970s concluded from a study of ten HMOs that HMOs were probably not providing more prenatal care than fee-for-service practitioners. However, a later study of 5,000 consecutive deliveries at a Boston hospital showed that 80 percent of the women with HMO deliveries had had eleven or more prenatal visits, significantly more than the fee patients (Wilner et al., 1982). In theory, prevention of adverse outcomes that will use more services for which the HMO is financially responsible creates the motivation for all HMOs, whether nonprofit or for-profit, to provide adequate prenatal care. But competitive pressures may interfere. Specifically, if an HMO is competing for market shares with other provider organizations in its geo-

---

[8]New Jersey recently announced a program for all pregnant women including the working poor, up to two and one-half times the poverty level. Comprehensive health and social services are to be offered under a case management approach. The announced object is to prevent low birthweight (Sullivan, 1989).

graphical area, it may wish to offer an attractive premium structure. Therefore, little attention may be paid to assuring utilization of prenatal services by patients at social or medical risk or to offering comprehensive prenatal services. The HMO may fail to respond quickly to new knowledge of risks such as hepatitis B, to invest in continuity, and to promote interspecialty consultations that would protect the pregnancy outcome. The prenatal care rendered by all providers, including HMOs, should be evaluated to help prevent slippage of preventive intentions. This could be done by professional bodies, through large public payers, or as regulations accompanying tax privileges of large group buyers.

MATERNITY TECHNOLOGY

Inappropriate use of technology is a general problem in health care today. It was encouraged by the reimbursement of all audited costs in the previous year or accounting period, a practice of both private and public insurers until fairly recently (Fuchs and Perreault, 1985). In a deeper sense, excessive use of technological aids is very likely related to an American tradition of medical activism, to popular worship of science, and to the appeal of instruments and gadgets. Technology also spreads because evaluations evolve more slowly than innovations and because, when decisions as to adopting new methods are made, possible long-term effects are often simply ignored. The use of technology in reproductive care has special roots. Doctors have strongly feared malpractice suits in obstetrics cases. Working in an era when childbearing is often delayed and each woman has fewer pregnancies, doctors believe that women patients highly value optimal birth outcomes. Moreover, diagnostic technology may provide information and reassurance to patients that they value, apart from the effect of the tests on medical decisions.

The merits of applying high-technology procedures to ordinary pregnancies that are not classified as high-risk continue to be debated by health researchers and the community, but such procedures are quite entrenched. Since medical and/or psychological gain to patients may result, continued evaluation including cost effects, rather than overall rejection or acceptance, is needed.

The evaluations of maternity procedures in the scientific literature fall short of being a satisfactory guide to provider behavior and resource allocation. Results may be ambiguous, and the initial premises may reflect professional biases. Providers may neither wait for objective evaluation before adopting procedures nor heed the inference that discontinuation would be rational. Third parties frequently pay for services that have weak scientific support, although they are more aware of the problem than in the past.

The problem of poor evidence was depicted in relation to diethylstilbestrol (DES) by Chalmers (1974). A younger generation was exposed in utero to later risk of cancer and fertility problems because DES had been prescribed for their mothers in pregnancy. Yet medical scientists eventually agreed that there was no benefit from DES in either normal or abnormal pregnancy. There were seven trials between 1946 and 1954 that reported DES to be effective in preventing intrauterine death and other serious "accidents of pregnancy," but they were all poorly controlled. Six trials of better quality between 1950 and 1955, using simultaneous rather than historical controls, showed uniformly negative results. Yet use of DES continued at ten out of twelve hospitals studied by Chalmers, albeit in a small percentage of pregnancies, until 1965. Analysis of drug sales suggests that in the decade 1960–1970 between twenty thousand and thirty-two thousand female children were exposed annually. Numbers do pile up in our large national market, but the issue was not so much numbers as the failure of major social institutions to prevent exposure of any pregnant women to the adverse effects with no probability of benefit. The Food and Drug Administration announced in 1971 that DES was contraindicated for use in pregnancy, but the *Physicians Desk Reference*, a publication widely consulted for drug information by physicians in practice, continued to describe the drug as useful. Chalmers notes that medical texts did not explain why the earlier trials were not valid, implying that the opportunity to reeducate physicians was lost.

Diethylstilbestrol has passed into history, although the effects on the daughters and sons of those for whom it was prescribed lingered on. These effects included not only actual cases of cancer and reproductive problems but also the necessity of repeated evaluations of those at risk over a period of years. The problem of evidence to support specific technologies in maternity care remains.

Electronic Fetal Monitoring

A major technological feature of pregnancy in the U.S. is electronic fetal monitoring. It is used in over one-half of U.S. births, but its appropriateness for routine use in low-risk pregnancies has not been demonstrated. Leveno et al. conducted a study of outcomes associated with EFM use by alternating between selective and universal monitoring in an obstetrical service each month over a thirty-six-month period. Aside from a higher rate of cesareans under universal EFM, there were no differences in intra partum stillbirths, Apgar scores, and other measures of fetal outcome (Leveno et al., 1986). Banta and Thacker (1979) and others had concluded that EFM increased the probability of having a cesarean section (regardless of medical need) because the monitor showed, or was interpreted to show, fetal distress when there was really none. This conclusion was questioned because of failure to control for use of analgesics and other alleged flaws in research on electronic fetal monitoring (Placek and Taffel, 1980). However, Placek et al. (1984) show that EFM does increase the probability of a cesarean delivery for a first birth. After that, the tradition of repeated use of cesareans in later births takes over; as EFM is not used for scheduled births, it is, thus, negatively associated with repeat cesareans. It has also been speculated that a false positive finding from EFM could lead to a decision to abort.

Women's groups that criticized EFM complained that it restricted the pregnant woman's mobility and its use caused loss of personal attention by nurses. However, the nursing shortage and obstetricians' fear of malpractice suits have helped sustain use of EFM. The American College of Obstetricians and Gynecologists, which long favored EFM, was reported to be moving toward a change in its policy, but it is doubtful that the use level will be affected (*New York Times*, 27 May 1988).

Cesareans

The rise in the rate of cesarean sections after 1965 was one of the most notable changes in American obstetrical practice. It affected all ages and marital statuses, and all hospital sizes, ownership types, and regions. Cesareans became the method of choice for breech deliveries, and this was an important factor in the trend.

Williams and Chen (1982) present evidence that suggests that increased use of cesareans was a significant factor in the decline of California's perinatal mortality rates in the 1970s. Breech presentations that had cesareans had lower neonatal mortality rates than vaginal breech births for all birthweight classes and overall. This was confirmed by a study based on a worldwide pool of birth records; the best effects were for women having their first birth and for "footling" breech births (Fortney et al., 1986).

Cesareans were also the preferred treatment for cephalopelvic disproportion and failed induction (Placek and Taffel, 1980). Fetal distress, as indicated by monitoring devices, became a stimulus to operative deliveries (see above), and a history of having a previous cesarean also influenced the growth rate. The American College of Obstetricians and Gynecologists issued guidelines encouraging vaginal birth after cesarean (VBAC) in 1982, but this action had little effect. In 1986, when 24.1

percent of all deliveries were by cesarean (according to the National Hospital Discharge Survey), the percentage of mothers with a previous cesarean who had a VBAC was only 8.5 percent, and repeat cesareans constituted 34 percent of the cesarean live births. Cesarean sections have double the length of stay of vaginal deliveries and, thus, have contributed to increasing the hospital costs of maternity care, as well as physician charges (Placek, Taffel, and Moien, 1988).

Cesareans were most likely for women with Blue Cross (27.1 percent) or other private insurance (26.3 percent), less so for government-paid (mostly Medicaid) deliveries (21.2 percent), and lowest for self-pay patients (18.7 percent). Older, married, and white women, who had a higher rate of cesareans, were more likely to have private insurance (Smith, 1983). Cesareans were more common in private hospitals.

Health Maintenance Organization patients, in a Boston study, had lower rates of cesareans, higher rates of admission for premature labor not resulting in deliveries, and fewer inductions of labor than fee-for-service patients (Wilner et al., 1982). The authors surmise that these findings are linked: fewer inductions mean more admissions for premature labor but also hold down the number of failed inductions that could lead to cesareans. Although these extra admissions added to cost, length of stay overall was less, because there were fewer cesareans. Birth outcomes were comparable for HMO and fee patients, despite these different input patterns. Thus, there was no gain from inclining toward induced labor or cesarean deliveries.

Goldfarb (1984) reports differences among hospitals in the use of cesareans depending on whether they are medical school affiliates and whether they have neonatal intensive care units. The highest percentage of births that were cesareans was in nonaffiliated hospitals with NICUs, and the effect of a NICU was stronger for insured women. However, hospitals could differ by reason of the medical complexity of a pregnancy, rather than by provider preferences. A doctor preparing for a high-risk birth that would require an NICU could decide that it was safest to perform a cesarean.

It is unfortunate that data bases do not always contain the information that would allow the researcher to hold constant all the relevant factors and help settle questions about appropriateness of obstetric technology. Nevertheless, it seems that the current use of cesareans is based on a blend of scientific, traditional, and other factors including ability to pay and organizational mode. In two states, Blue Cross and Blue Shield have removed the financial incentive for surgical births by paying the same fee for a cesarean and a vaginal delivery (New York Times, 10 January 1989). (In Rhode Island this applies to all physicians, and in Illinois to physicians participating in preferred provider organizations.)

Regional and Racial Differences

Regional and racial differences in use of obstetric technology have been documented by Kleinman et al. (1983) using National Natality Survey data for 1980. This was the first year in which a nationally representative sample survey of obstetrical practices for mothers of liveborn infants was done. They found the following:

1. Unless a woman enters the health care system for prenatal care, she does not receive prenatal technology. Women in southern states and nonmetropolitan areas are less likely to receive early prenatal care. Nationally, 65 percent of black women and 80 percent of whites did so.
2. Amniocentesis at around sixteen weeks is used for genetic assessment and counseling; when used later, it is to determine fetal maturity when a cesarean or induced labor is planned. In the survey, the purpose could not be identified. Only 20 percent of white mothers and 17 percent of black mothers thirty-five years of age and over received amniocentesis. For whites, the rate in the South was only half as high as in the North, and, in the North, metropolitan areas had higher rates.
3. Use of ultrasound expanded greatly in the 1970s as a substitute for diagnostic X ray in pregnancy, especially for determining fetal age. It has no known adverse side effects, although long-term effects cannot yet be determined. Nearly one-third of pregnant women received at least one sonographic examination. Among white mothers, this was more likely in metropolitan areas, but there were no regional differences. Among black mothers, rates were highest for metropolitan areas outside the South. There were no overall racial differences, because higher rates for white women in nonmetropolitan areas were offset by higher rates for blacks in metropolitan areas.
4. Exposure to medical X rays in pregnancy is contraindicated because of the potential for genetic damage, especially in the first three months. Nonetheless, 13 percent of the sample received a medical X ray. It is estimated from the stated diagnostic purpose in each case that one-third of them could have had ultrasound instead. Black mothers had much more interareal variation than other races: 10 percent of the black mothers in the rural South

received X rays that could have been replaced by sonograms, versus 3 percent in southern metropolises.

5. Electronic fetal monitoring during labor was used for 51 percent of white mothers in metropolitan areas and 41 percent in other areas. Black women had a rate similar to whites in metropolitan areas (55 percent), but in the rural South only 29 percent had EFM.

The overall conclusion of Kleinman et al. is that black women and women in rural areas had much less access than other women to newer obstetrical technologies, but the pattern varied by the specific technology. The welfare implication of unequal access also varies. True, there is concern over intrusion of technology into birthing, but some of the procedures clearly have medical utility under certain circumstances. They can reduce maternal anxiety over fetal abnormalities or increase bonding with the fetus (Fletcher and Evans, 1983). The geographical variation in continued use of medical X rays suggests that some women are receiving medically outmoded and questionable services. Further evaluation of all obstetric technologies is essential, especially in view of the cost they entail and the wide diffusion that has occurred. Unless scientifically grounded guidelines are developed and effectively implemented, nonrational factors will continue to influence diffusion. The socially disadvantaged woman and the well-financed, well-located woman may each receive questionable and wasteful services along with others that are safe and efficacious.

Studying Maternity Practices

The complexity of evaluation of maternity care practices is suggested by three studies of alternative approaches to the mode and setting of delivery. The first two of these indicate the problem of adequately conceptualizing the childbirth experience. The third study exemplifies the difficulty of dealing with variations in risk factors, self-selection, and procedures used in each setting.

The first example concerns the Leboyer method of delivery ("in a dark and quiet room, without sensory stimulation"). A scientific evaluation, based on randomization of low-risk women, is presented by Nelson et al. (1980). It shows no improvement in maternal or newborn morbidity or in infant behavior in the first hour of life and later, compared with "gentle conventional" delivery. Mothers' perception of the birth experience was not different either. The one difference was that labor was shorter. But the authors say this may have been due to a placebo effect, to the psychic benefits of being offered a new procedure. The Leboyer method did not lead to any serious morbidity, but the authors believe this may have been due to the clinical precautions taken in the study. This interpretation implies that it would be safer for a physician to stay with conventional methods.

Duff, however, in an accompanying editorial (1980), states that calling the psychological aspects of the "intervention" a placebo effect oversimplifies the situation of childbirth. Physicians ought to understand that women need "ample personal support in labor and delivery" and that family intimacy is important in providing that support and promoting adjustment to a birth.

The need to consider psychological aspects of pregnancy in analyzing the value of certain procedures and what sustains the demand for them is further suggested by a study of willingness to pay for ultrasound. Patients may attach value to information that has little medical significance. The study shows that one-fourth of the amounts people said they would be willing to pay was based on the "non-decisional value" of the information (Berwick and Weinstein, 1985). The "non" refers only to medical decisions, since knowledge about the normality of the fetus, the health of the mother, or even the due date would help prepare parents for changes in employment and other aspects of their lives.

The third example is a comparison of pregnancy outcomes at a birthing center, the Booth Maternity Center, and a tertiary hospital, Thomas Jefferson University Hospital. The study explored the relationship of outcomes to procedures used both within and between the two samples, while taking risk factors and demographic characteristics into account. The procedures studied were prenatal diagnostic procedures, oxytocin, anesthesia, analgesia, EFM, and method of delivery (spontaneous, outlet forceps, midforceps, breech, and cesarean).

The neonatal morbidity rate was higher and mean birthweights were lower at the tertiary hospital, but there were more infants with low 1-minute Apgar scores (an indicator of physical health) at the birthing center. The relation between use of procedures and outcomes differed for the two settings and for different outcome measures. A major block in interpretation was that procedures may have been used for patients with greater risks, rather than having been the cause of poor outcomes themselves. For instance, use of forceps and cesareans at the hospital was associated with higher birthweights there, but this may have been due to the difficulty of delivering a large fetus. Self-selection of low-risk women to maternity center care may have contributed to the "heavier and healthier babies born there." Therefore, say the authors, it cannot be concluded that care at the tertiary hospital following a medical model necessarily produces worse outcomes than birthing center care (Strobino et al.,

1988), nor can the contrary be proven. It is disappointing to have inconclusive results from serious work, and the problem is not solvable by randomization designs, since these are incompatible with voluntary choice of birth settings. However, a prospective design that ascertains risk status ex ante would be useful.

Traditional Practices and the Patient as Negotiator

A survey of Chicago hospitals that was reported in 1985 examined differences among the hospitals in obstetrical "customs." The list is a long one, including, among others, vaginal culture, intravenous infusions in the labor area, routine external and internal monitoring, allowing ice and liquids during labor, personnel doing vaginal examinations, analgesia during labor, position during pushing and delivery, episiotomy, birthing room, and birthing chair. Several items on the father's participation were also studied.

The study found that a given practice might be standard in one hospital, excluded in another, and left to the doctor's discretion in the third (Pasley, 1985). The birth experience, therefore, might be quite variable in different institutions. Furthermore, the individual doctor in attendance may have some influence on practices within a given hospital. If this is so, and the doctor is willing to negotiate with the patient, she may increase her control by an astute choice of doctor and hospital. She can also change her behavior as an obstetrical patient. Herzfeld, of the Harvard faculty, has written what is essentially a training and advice manual for pregnant patients. It aims to reverse the socialization that prepared many women to take a passive view of the environment and be concerned solely with their own performance in labor. The ideal proposed by Herzfeld is that the woman chooses her team and coaches it to play to her strengths. She is advised how to avoid a "medical delivery" with features such as rupture of membranes, drugs to stimulate contractions, episiotomy, forceps, and cesarean section. In particular, she is counseled to avoid pain medication, to prevent the need for labor stimulants and other aspects of medical delivery, and she is informed of the reasons why a "brisk schedule" of labor, which may be preferred by doctors, is not in itself a goal. The patient is advised on how to size up a hospital and how to choose, and negotiate with, a physician. This advice includes a written list of agreed-on items of supportive care related to labor; it may protect the physician legally and in dealing with hospital administration in carrying out the patient's wishes (Herzfeld, 1985). It is interesting to see a specific plan to set up countervailing power in obstetrics while remaining within the mainstream of providers (hospitals and physicians). It is similar to empowerment of the patient in breast cancer treatment while avoiding alternative therapies that are not accepted in medical circles.

Genetic Services

Genetic screening and counseling have become a part of the standard for adequate perinatal services; yet, according to a genetics committee of the American Public Health Association, access to services is unevenly distributed nationally. Several reasons for this are noted. Families are often referred by their provider of primary care, and low-income families outside the system do not get referred. Counseling by nonphysicians may not be covered by insurance. Genetic centers tend to be located in large tertiary care facilities that are geographically difficult to reach. Primary care providers are not necessarily up-to-date in their knowledge of genetics and genetic services. In addition to supply and finance factors, genetic services may not be culturally acceptable to minority ethnic groups (*Nation's Health*, 1987).

A New York City study examined the gap between actual services and what is needed for ten disorders considered to be significant for the city's maternal and child population (Medical and Health Research Association of New York, 1988). Carrier screening, involving provision of risk information and testing, for Tay-Sachs disease and the hemoglobinopathies was studied. Also examined were genetic counseling in the prenatal period, focusing on Down syndrome and open neural tube defects (NTDs), and assessment and counseling in the postnatal stage for these two conditions and six others. The perspective for an evaluation is the ability to assist the total fertility planning of a couple (current and future pregnancies), based on identification of genetic risks.

The study found that, for both Down syndrome and NTDs, but especially the latter, there were "fairly large unmet needs for screening and/or counseling" (p. 87). Sixty percent of the 11,000 women at risk for Down syndrome were counseled for amniocentesis, but only 10 percent of the 110,000 women at risk for open neural tube defects were screened by obstetrics departments in 1984. (Diagnosis is more complex and costly for NTDs than for Down syndrome, since a screening alphafetoprotein (AFP) test must be followed by amniocentesis if test results are positive.)

In the postnatal period, the unmet need for sickle cell disease counseling was marked. Even though screening for this condition is mandatory in New York State, a substantial portion of newborns who were carriers (65 percent) did not have even one parent counseled, and 80 percent did not have both parents counseled.

Several explanations are offered for the failure to reach all pregnant women age thirty-five or over with counseling for amniocentesis. Patients may be fearful of the procedures and not aware of their benefits. A certain percentage refuse the referral for counseling, and another group refuse the amniocentesis itself. Practitioners may lack knowledge about the procedures or the counseling; and they may be confused by disagreement among experts as to indications for AFP testing and the test values that would identify potential NTDs. Finally, reimbursement limitations hinder medical genetics units from serving all patients who would benefit.

Elias and Annas (1987) report that the American College of Obstetricians and Gynecologists will soon recommend offering AFP testing as part of prenatal care, and the FDA has approved a commercial kit for AFP testing. It seems likely that genetic testing will continue to spread, but whether counseling will accompany it, as Elias and Annas consider essential, is less certain.

Prenatal diagnostic methods, however, are still evolving. From a historical perspective, amniocentesis is a halfway technology. When there was no way of looking inside the uterus, doctors had to wait until 16 weeks of pregnancy had gone by in order to withdraw fluid safely. With ultrasound to guide the needle, earlier testing is feasible, and physicians at some centers have begun to do amniocentesis at 10 weeks. This has been responsive to patients' desire to have the information earlier and avoid the stress of not knowing whether a late abortion will be recommended. Also responsive to patients' interest in earlier testing is the development of chorionic villus sampling (CVS), initially done between 9-1/2 and 12 weeks. A major collaborative study comparing 2,278 women receiving CVS in the first trimester with 671 women receiving amniocentesis at 16 weeks showed CVS to be safe and effective for early diagnosis. It is more labor-intensive than amniocentesis, but a slightly higher cost might seem worth paying for earlier diagnostic information (Rhoades et al., 1989). First-trimester sampling may create a marketing problem: early miscarriages that might occur anyway might be blamed by patients and doctors on the procedure. A blood test applied to fetal cells in the pregnant woman's blood is an ideal not yet in view.

Patients and providers will probably be more receptive to genetic assessment and counseling if safe methods that are applicable early in pregnancy are perfected. As this happens, growth of the demand for pregnancy termination for genetic disorders can be anticipated, and with it the stress of current uncertainties as to legal and financial access to abortion. Some couples with genetic risks will be more willing to start new pregnancies if they know that fetuses with genetic defects can be identified, but only if abortion is available.

INFERTILITY AND THE NEW CONCEPTIONS

Impaired Fertility

Impaired fertility is a widespread problem. Mosher (1988) reports that 2.4 million married couples were infertile in 1982 and 4.5 million women or couples had impaired fecundity; this is a broad term referring to difficulty in either conceiving or carrying a fetus to term.

Such impairments generate demand for infertility services. Diagnostic and treatment techniques have proliferated, based on growing understanding of reproductive biology and medicine. Since many services are priced within the reach of large numbers of buyers and/or are insured, the market is substantial. It is estimated that, in 1982, 6.3 million ever-married women aged 15–44 had used infertility services at some time, and one million had done so in the previous year. The use rate was higher for whites, although the prevalence of infertility is higher among blacks (Mosher and Pratt, 1985), suggesting an access problem.

It is estimated that one-third of infertility is due to the male alone, 20 percent to both partners, and the rest, under half, to the female. Interest in the male factor has increased, and new tests for males have been created. Today's clinical standard calls for prompt screening of the male partner without waiting for a year of unprotected intercourse (Hammond and Talbert, 1985). When success in achieving pregnancy was measured on a life-table basis in a set of 409 cases of single-factor infertility, the success rate for the male factor was fairly similar to that for anovulation in females.

Studies have suggested that men may be the dominant partners in reproductive decisions of a couple to treat infertility (or to end pregnancies with genetic or developmental disabilities). The growing popularity of in vitro fertilization treatment (for male infertility) is explainable, according to Lorber, by men's interest in biological parenthood and women's willingness to carry the major physiological burden (Lorber, 1988).

Whether because infertility in males has been growing or because it was previously underrecognized, it has been noted that the percentage of infertility problems due to the male partner is rising. One author has argued that the level of spermotoxic substances in the environment has been increasing and that this could explain the rise (Castleman, 1983).

The prevalence of fertility impairments doubles after age 35 for women: it is 4.4 percent at 15–24, 13.4 percent at 25–34, and 28.0 percent after 35. The rise is due to the increase in both spontaneous pregnancy loss and infertility with the age of the woman. Both of these problems are associated with pelvic inflammatory disease, for which sexually transmitted disease and IUD use have been found to be risk factors. Prevention of this disease would reduce infertility and pregnancy loss (and of course, social costs of care and lost productive time). Preventive strategies should not be neglected because of the interesting scientific discoveries in infertility treatment, including the "new conceptions." Such strategies may be cost-effective if high-technology infertility treatments continue to grow.

The New Conceptions

Seibel (1988) describes 1978, the year in which the first baby conceived by in vitro fertilization was born, as the dawn of a new era of reproductive technology. In vitro fertilization was augmented by GIFT (gamete intrafallopian transfer) and embryo donation in 1984. The original indications for IVF included absent or badly damaged fallopian tubes. Later they were broadened to include several other conditions, plus unexplained infertility of two or more years' duration. The pool of possible beneficiaries now exceeds one million women. In the early days of IVF, a 2 percent success rate per laparoscopy was reported. Even today, although more than three thousand "test tube babies" have been born throughout the world since the success of Steptoe and Edwards in bringing about the birth of Louise Brown in 1978, five out of six couples undergoing IVF do not have a live birth (Lorber and Greenfield, 1987, p. 20). The success rate is estimated at 8 percent per cycle, which is low compared with other infertility treatments, but will doubtless be raised by technical improvements. Recent reports from Britain indicate that close to one-fourth of oocyte recoveries in women under 40 result in a clinical pregnancy, with over 70 percent of these continuing to term (or the third trimester if still in process) (Bromwich and Walker, 1989; Edwards et al., 1989). U.S. centers are having similar experiences. The IVF pregnancies may entail more risks: a comparison with spontaneous pregnancies showed a markedly higher incidence of arterial hypertension, breech presentations, and cesarean sections for the in vitro group (Frydman et al., 1986). But, despite the doubtful aspects, the interest of consumers, supported by the willingness of providers to supply services, has resulted in the establishment of 152 centers in 43 states and 8 in Canada, according to the American Fertility Society. The society, a provider organization, would like to see IVF included in all private health insurance as a nonexperimental procedure.

Infertility treatment costs depend on inputs required for different problems and success rates. In a Nova Scotia clinic, costs per pregnancy ranged from $31,841 (for tubal surgery) to $5,041 (for ovulation defects), and the overall average was $10,700 (Cooper, 1986). The expense of IVF is estimated at $6,000 per attempt, with a minimum of four attempts in some centers (Andrews, 1984). This makes IVF a possible substitute for microsurgery of the tubes. The cost may be reduced with retrieval of oocytes under guidance of ultrasonography as an outpatient procedure. GIFT is one-fourth less expensive than IVF and may be used as an alternative or a second method after one cycle of IVF.

Eleven experts on infertility express anxiety over the growing problem of exploitation of the infertile couple. They note that some obstetricians were forced by the "malpractice crisis" to enter the subspecialty without adequate training. They believe that the new technology is developing in an "ethical and regulatory vacuum" made worse by the entrance of for-profit organizations. Evaluations of couples are incomplete, and too little time is allowed after each step for pregnancy to occur. Claims of success far exceed true rates, because surgeons often do not quote their own experience and apply rates based on younger patients diagnosed as having tubal problems to older patients with other diagnoses (Blackwell and Garrison, 1987). A British estimate (described as generous) is that under 18 percent of the infertile population may conceive as a result of medical intervention, but this could be almost doubled (to 34 percent) if IVF and gamete intrafallopian transfer were made widely available (Lilford and Dalton, 1987). Thus, the balance between overuse and underuse is delicate and highly dependent on ethical and informed professional advice to patients.

Counseling is believed to be inadequate today, both for those who succeed in conceiving through IVF and those who fail. If centers offered adequate counseling, treatment costs would be increased. The burden this would bring to users or their financial sponsors might be offset by a reduced need for outside psychiatric help. The need for psychological services is understandable: the success rate is low, IVF outcomes are highly uncertain, and the situation does not exactly fit social norms with respect to traditional parenthood. Also, insensitivity of physicians is considered to be a common problem for patients undergoing infertility treatment (Andrews, 1984).

Consumers have other problems besides lack of counseling. Selecting a reliable source is one. The public could be helped by certification of centers. Criteria should include a minimum annual volume (as is done with deliveries and cardiac catheterizations, in approving facilities for graduate medical education or for reimbursement), a record of some definite successes, a qualified reproductive endocrinologist, laboratory standards, and counseling. Some insurance companies are willing to cover part or all of the costs of IVF. It is a fairly expensive obligation, for the possible extra risk of perinatal complications (or of multiple births) requiring delivery at tertiary centers adds to the cost of deliveries in successful cases. Also, since IVF babies are likely to be born to older women, cesareans may be more often involved.

The low-income woman or couple with infertility problems is unlikely to have financial access to the newer reproductive technology. Clinics do offer some infertility services but represent a less significant source of service for infertility treatment than for family planning (20 percent of ever-married women who received infertility services in 1982 got them at clinics) (Mosher and Pratt, 1985). Eventually we can expect, and should welcome, some cost-benefit analyses to guide resource allocation. Such study would compare social investment in prevention of infertility from occupational toxins (both sexes), pelvic inflammatory disease, deficient obstetrical care, and other causes with the new sophisticated treatments in terms of benefit to large groups of couples and the respective costs. However, the newer treatments do expand the choices available to currently infertile couples, and steps to improve the yield, bring the costs down, and prevent consumer exploitation would be welcomed. This would, in fact, provide a sounder basis for cost-benefit analysis, which can have misleading results if based on rapidly changing yields and costs per case. It is now being argued that artificial insemination procedures can be performed by nonphysicians, thus reducing costs. Too, IVF can probably be done effectively in small centers under proper management, and this may increase availability (Bromwich et al., 1988). New techniques of conception that could avoid genetic defects in fertile couples with high-risk histories would expand the group to which the new technology is attractive. The prevalence of sterilizations that are followed by remarriages or other changes in personal life still further expands the interested group.

COMPELLING TREATMENT

Women's autonomy in regard to reproductive care is under new challenges today. Medical interventions directed specifically to the fetus have increased, and the courts have been used in some cases to compel pregnant women to undergo treatments deemed necessary for fetal life and health. Some physicians have supported compulsion in specified circumstances or have thought they themselves were legally compelled to oblige women to acquiesce.

Kolder et al. did a national survey of obstetrical leaders that yielded detailed information on twenty-one cases in ten states in which courts ordered obstetrical procedures (including cesareans and intrauterine transfusions) to be performed after women's refusal. All were in teaching hospital clinics or public assistance cases, and most were black, Asian, or Hispanic women (Kolder, Gallagher, and Parsons, 1987). The court acted within a few hours in 88 percent of the cases, suggesting that deliberate consideration of risks and benefits for woman and fetus and the rights of the woman was unlikely and that adequate representation for the woman might be lacking. The authors think physicians tend to overemphasize the consequences of nonintervention. Court orders may result in driving groups most in need of prenatal care away from clinics and hospitals. Kolder et al. fear that compulsory treatment will spread to fetal surgery and interventions early in pregnancy, as the onset of fetal viability is pushed back by science.

Nelson and Milliken (1988) also oppose such compulsion. They point out in *JAMA* that the physician's obligation to promote fetal health is rooted in an ethical duty to the pregnant woman. She, in seeking prenatal care, has shown that she has chosen to work toward a successful pregnancy. No concept of the fetus as a "second patient" is necessary to establish the physician's responsibility. A woman who refuses to follow medical advice about her care should have the decision respected; the physician's value judgment should not be substituted for her own. For the doctor to seek a court order is ethically perilous: the precise legal status of the fetus and fetal rights is controversial, and interpretation of a standard of "serious harm" is bound to be arbitrary. Medical knowledge is not certain enough to deny women "the right to be wrong" while allowing physicians that right. Women are rarely unwilling to do anything within reason for the best interests of the fetus. The special problem of addictive behavior is better approached by offering rehabilitation programs than by coercion, and misinformation and fear can be countered by educational efforts over the months of prenatal care.

Medical innovations tend to gain popularity before full evaluations are feasible. Social pressure and women's fear that availability or quality of care will be affected if they withhold consent may be powerful coercers even if legal action is not used. Yet the intervention sought may turn out to have little potential value or to have a less intrusive but effective substitute. If reproductive medicine emphasizes a view of women as vehicles for fetal growth, autonomy is likely to be at risk.

The weakening of the constitutional right to abortion by the Supreme Court decision of July 5, 1989, is part of a major contest over women's rights over their reproductive capacity that is fueled in part by advances in fetal medicine and is matched by a contest for doctors' loyalties and sense of partnership.

CONCLUSION

Reproductive care for women shares with health care generally the problems of assuring care to low-income uninsured and minority groups, judicious use of technology to avoid resource waste, and seizing all opportunities for cost-effective prevention. One aspect in which it differs from general health care is the extreme vulnerability of abortion service availability to the politico-legal climate (legislatures and courts) and the specific debate over women's rights that is involved.

New fertility control technology may reduce some of the political difficulties surrounding access to abortion, but only if substitutable pharmaceutical approaches escape being restricted in the same manner as surgical abortions and if they do not have to depend on abortion as a backup.

The conflict over naturalistic versus medical models of birth is replicated in other domains of health care in critiques of invasive treatments. But in reproduction it has had extra weight as a gender issue because physician dominance was charged with depriving many women of a positive emotional experience. The opportunities provided by medical science to reverse infertility and improve pregnancy outcomes are interesting and exciting. In determining resource allocation for service and research in reproductive health, the interests of the mass of women in effective and user-friendly contraception that is safe over years of use and the access problems of disadvantaged and high-risk women should not be neglected.

Technology appears deeply entrenched today. Medical educators and leaders, and consumer groups, face the challenge of promoting scientific evaluation of reproductive technology and carrying its results into the marketplace, reimbursement, and both professional and consumer education. The financial incentives and sociopsychological factors that sustain use of services lacking firm scientific support should be examined.

References

Alan Guttmacher Institute. *Blessed Events and the Bottom Line: Financing Maternity Care in the United States.* New York, 1987.

American Medical Association, *American Medical News.* February 16, 1990.

Andrews, Lori B. *New Conceptions: A Consumer's Guide to the Newest Infertility Treatments, Including In Vitro Fertilization, Artificial Insemination, and Surrogate Motherhood.* New York: St. Martin's Press, 1984.

Aries, Nancy. *Fragmentation and Reproductive Freedom: The Evolution of Family Planning Services.* New York: City University of New York, Baruch College, May 1985.

Arney, William Ray. *Power and the Profession of Obstetrics.* Chicago: University of Chicago Press, 1982.

Banta, H. D., and S. B. Thacker. *Costs and Benefits of Electronic Fetal Monitoring: A Review of the Literature.* DHEW Pub. No. (PHS) 79-3245. Hyattsville, MD: National Center for Health Services Research, April 1979.

Berwick, Donald M., and Milton C. Weinstein. "What Do Patients Value? Willingness-to-pay for Ultrasound during Normal Pregnancy." *Medical Care,* vol. 23, no. 7 (July 1985): 881–893.

Blackwell, Richard E., and P. M. Garrison. "Are We Exploiting the Infertile Couple?" *Fertility and Sterility,* vol. 48, no. 5 (November 1987): 735–739.

Boston Women's Health Book Collective. *Our Bodies, Ourselves.* New York: Simon & Schuster, 1973.

Boylan, Peter C. Letter. *New England Journal of Medicine,* vol. 316, no. 8 (February 19, 1987): 480–481.

Bromwich, Peter, and Andy Walker. "Benefits of In-Vitro Fertilisation," *Lancet,* no. 8675 (December 2, 1989): 1327.

Bromwich, P., A. Walker, S. Kennedy, M. Wiley, et al. "In Vitro Fertilisation in a Small Unit in the NHS." *British Medical Journal,* vol. 296 (March 12, 1988): 759–781.

Canadian Task Force on the Periodic Health Examination. "The Periodic Health Examination." Reprinted from *CMA Journal,* vol. 121, November 3, 1979, by Health and Welfare Canada, Ottawa.

Castleman, Michael. "Toxics and Male Infertility." *Sierra* (March/April 1983): 49–52.

Cates, Willard Jr., Paul J. Weisner, and James W. Curran. "Sex and Spermicides: Preventing Unintended Pregnancy and Infection." *Journal of the American Medical Association,* vol. 248, no. 13 (October 1, 1982): 1636–1637.

Chalmers, Thomas C. "The Impact of Clinical Trials in Medical Practice." In *Principles and Techniques of Human Research and Therapeutics. Vol. 1,* edited by Gilbert McMahon. Mt. Kisco, NY: Futura Publishing Co., 1974, 193–203.

Cooper, Glinda S. "An Analysis of the Costs of Infertility Treatment." *American Journal of Public Health*, vol. 76, no. 8 (August 1986): 1018–1019.

Cousins, Amy. Letter. *New York Times*, 22 January 1990: I, 14.

Duff, Raymond S. "Care in Childbirth and Beyond." *New England Journal of Medicine*, vol. 302, no. 12 (March 20, 1980): 685–686.

Dunn, Leo J. "Responsibility, Obligation and Duty." *American Journal of Obstetrics & Gynecology*, vol. 157, no. 3 (September 1987): 521–530.

Edwards, R. G., P. Brinsden, K. Elder, et al. Letter, *Lancet*, no. 8675 (December 2, 1989): 1328.

Elias, Sherman, and George J. Annas. "Routine Prenatal Genetic Screening." Editorial. *New England Journal of Medicine*, vol. 317, no. 22 (November 16, 1987): 1407–1409.

Evans, Stephen, Frederic D. Frigoletto, and John Figgis Jewett. "Mortality of Eclampsia: A Case Report and the Experience of the Massachusetts Maternal Mortality Study, 1954–1982." *New England Journal of Medicine*, vol. 309, no. 26 (December 29, 1983): 1644–1647.

"Father and Mother Know Best: Defining the Liability of Physicians for Inadequate Genetic Counseling." *Yale Law Review*, vol. 87 (1978):1488.

Fletcher, John C., and Mark I. Evans. "Maternal Bonding in Early Fetal Ultrasound Examinations." *New England Journal of Medicine*, vol. 308, no. 7 (February 17, 1983): 392–393.

Fortney, Judith A., James E. Higgins, Kathy I. Kennedy, et al. "Delivery Type and Neonatal Mortality among 10,749 Breeches." *American Journal of Public Health*, vol. 76, no. 8 (August 1986): 980–985.

Frau, Lourdes M., H. Trent MacKay, Joyce M. Hughes, and Willard Cates, Jr. "Epidemiological Aspects of Ectopic Pregnancy." In *Extrauterine Pregnancy*, edited by Alvin Langer and Leslie Iffy. Littleton, MA: PSG Publishing Company, 1986.

Frigoletto, Frederic D., M. F. Greene, B. R. Benacerraf, V. A. Barss, and D. H. Saltzman. "Ultrasound Fetal Surveillance in the Management of the Isoimmunized Pregnancy." *New England Journal of Medicine*, vol. 315, no. 7 (August 14, 1986): 430–432.

Frydman, René, Joëlle Bellaisch-Allart, Nicolas Fries, André Hazout, et al. "An Obstetric Assessment of the First 100 Births from the In Vitro Fertilization Program at Clamart, France." *American Journal of Obstetrics and Gynecology* (1986): 550–555.

Fuchs, Victor R., and Leslie Perreault. *The Economics of Reproduction-Related Health Care*. Working Paper No. 1688. Cambridge, MA: National Bureau of Economic Research, August 1985.

Goldfarb, Marsha G. *Who Receives Cesareans: Patient and Hospital Characteristics*. NCHSR, Hospital Cost and Utilization Project. Research Note 4. DHHS Pub. No. (PHS) 84-3345. Rockville, MD: National Center for Health Services Research, September 1984.

Goyert, Gregory L., Sidney F. Bottoms, Marjorie C. Treadwell, and Paul C. Nehra. "The Physician Factor in Cesarean Birth Rates." *New England Journal of Medicine,* vol. 320, no. 11 (March 16, 1989): 706–709.

Hammond, Mary G., and Luther M. Talbert. *Infertility: A Practical Guide for the Physician,* 2nd ed. Oradell, NJ: Medical Economics, 1985.

Hemminki, Elina. "Content of Prenatal Care in the United States: A Historic Perspective." *Medical Care,* vol. 26, no. 2 (February 1988): 199–210.

Herzfeld, Judith. *Sense and Sensibility in Childbirth: A Guide to Supportive Obstetrical Care.* New York: W. W. Norton & Company, 1985.

Heuser, Robert L., Kenneth G. Keppel, Cecilie A. Witt, and Paul J. Placek. *Synthetic Estimation Applications from the 1980 National Natality Survey and the 1980 National Fetal Mortality Survey.* Hyattsville, MD: National Center for Health Statistics, 1984.

Hilts, Philip J. "U.S. Is Decades Behind Europe in Contraceptives, Experts Report." *New York Times,* 15 February 1990: I, 1; II, 18.

Hofferth, Sandra J., and Cheryl D. Hayes, eds. *Risking the Future: Adolescent Sexuality, Pregnancy, and Childbearing.* Washington, DC: National Research Council, National Academy Press, 1987.

Horn, Marjorie C., and William D. Mosher. *Use of Services for Family Planning and Infertility: United States, 1982.* Advance Data No. 103. Hyattsville, MD: National Center for Health Statistics, December 20, 1984.

Imber, Jonathan B. *Abortion and the Private Practice of Medicine.* New Haven, CT: Yale University Press, 1986.

Jonas, Maureen M., Eugene R. Schiff, Mary J. O'Sullivan, Maria De Medina, et al. "Failures of Centers for Disease Control Criteria to Identify Hepatitis B Infection in a Large Municipal Obstetrical Population." *Annals of Internal Medicine,* vol. 107, no. 3 (September 1987): 335–337.

Joyce, Theodore, Hope Corman, and Michael Grossman. "A Cost Effective Analysis of Strategies to Reduce Infant Mortality." *Medical Care,* vol. 26, no. 4 (April 1988): 348–360.

Kaali, S. G., and R. Landesman. "Tubal Sterilization with the Falopi Ring in an Ambulatory-Care Surgical Facility." *New York State Journal of Medicine,* vol. 85, no. 3 (1985): 98–100.

Kay, Bonnie J., Irene H. Butter, Deborah Chang, and Kathleen Houlihan. "Women's Health and Social Change: The Case of Lay Midwives." *International Journal of Health Services,* vol. 18, no. 2 (1988): 223–236.

Kenney, Asta M., Aida Torres, Nancy Dittes, and Jennifer Macias. "Medicaid Expenses for Maternity and Newborn Care in America." *Family Planning Perspectives,* vol. 18, no. 3 (May/June 1986): 103–110.

Kleinman, Joel C., Margaret Cooke, Steven Machlin, and Samuel S. Kessel. "Variation in Use of Obstetric Technology." *Health, United States, 1983.* DHHS Pub. No. (PHS) 84-1232. Hyattsville, MD: U.S. Department of Health and Human Services, Public Health Service, December 1983.

Kochanek, Kenneth D. "Induced Terminations of Pregnancy. Reporting States, 1987." *Monthly Vital Statistics Reports*, vol. 38, no. 9, Supp. January 5, 1990, 1–36.

Kolata, Gina. "Drug Combination Gains Support as Alternative to Surgical Abortion." *New York Times*, 16 February 1988, III, 3.

———. "Under Pressures and Stigma, More Doctors Shun Abortion." *New York Times*, 8 January 1990, I, 1; II, 8.

Kolder, Veronika E. B., Janet Gallagher, and Michael T. Parsons. "Court-Ordered Obstetrical Intervention." *New England Journal of Medicine*, vol. 316, no. 19 (May 7, 1987): 1192–1196.

Kotelchuck, Milton, Janet B. Schwartz, Marlene T. Anderka, and Karl S. Finison. "WIC Participation and Pregnancy Outcomes: Massachusetts Statewide Evaluation Project." *American Journal of Public Health*, vol. 74, no. 10 (October 1984): 1086–1092.

Lancet, November 4, 1989: 1112–1113 ("Mifepristone: Widening the Choice for Women").

Leveno, Kenneth J., Gary Cunningham, Sheryl Nelson, Micki Roark, et al. "A Prospective Comparison of Selective and Universal Electronic Fetal Monitoring in 34,995 Pregnancies." *New England Journal of Medicine*, vol. 315, no. 10 (September 4, 1986): 615–624.

Lewin, Tamar. "Study Cites Lack in Prenatal Care." *New York Times*, 2 November 1989, I, 25.

Lewis, Scott. *OB/GYN Malpractice*. New York: Wiley, 1986.

Lilford, Richard J., and Maureen E. Dalton. "Effectiveness of Treatment for Infertility." *British Medical Journal*, vol. 295, no. 6591 (July 18, 1987): 155–156.

Lincoln, Richard, and Lisa Kaeser. "Whatever Happened to the Contraceptive Revolution?" *Family Planning Perspectives*, vol. 20, no. 1 (January/February 1988): 20–24.

Lorber, Judith. "In Vitro Fertilization and Gender Politics." In *Embryos, Ethics, and Women's Rights*, edited by Elaine Hoffman Baruch, Amadeo S. D'Adamo, Jr., and Joni Seager. New York: Haworth Press, 1988, 117–133.

Lorber, Judith, and Dorothy Greenfield. "Test-Tube Babies and Sick Roles: Couples' Experiences with In Vitro Fertilization." Presented at the meeting of the Third International Interdisciplinary Congress on Women, Dublin, Ireland, July 1987.

McCann, Dennis J. "Liability for Negligent Prenatal Diagnosis: Parents' Right to a 'Perfect' Child." *Ohio State Law Journal*, vol. 42 (1981):551.

McDonald, Thomas P., and Andrew F. Coburn. *The Impact of Variations in AFDC and Medicaid Eligibility on Prenatal Care Utilization*. Final Report. Portland, ME: University of Southern Maine, Center for Research and Advanced Study, December 1986.

Medical and Health Research Association of New York City, Inc., and the City of New York Department of Health. *An Assessment of Unmet Needs for Genetic Services in New York City.* Final Report. New York, March 4, 1988.

Mintz, Morton. *At Any Cost: Corporate Greed, Women and the Dalkon Shield.* New York: Pantheon Books, 1985.

Mishell, Daniel P., Jr. "Contraception." *New England Journal of Medicine,* vol. 320, no. 12 (March 23, 1989): 777–787.

Moore, Thomas R., Willim Origel, Thomas C. Kay, and Robert Resnick. "The Perinatal and Economic Impact of Preterm Care in a Low-Socioeconomic Population." *American Journal of Obstetrics & Gynecology,* vol. 154, no. 1 (January 1986): 29–33.

Mosher, William D. "Fecundity and Infertility in the United States." *American Journal of Public Health,* vol. 78, no. 2 (February 1988): 181–182.

———. *Use of Family Planning Services in the United States: 1982 and 1988.* Advance Data No. 184. Hyattsville, MD: National Center for Health Statistics, April 11, 1990.

Mosher, William D., and William F. Pratt. *Fecundity and Infertility in the United States, 1965–82.* Advance Data No. 104. Hyattsville, MD: National Center for Health Statistics, February 11, 1985.

———. *Reproductive Impairments among Married Couples: United States.* Data from the National Survey of Family Growth, Series 23, No. 11. DHHS Pub. No. (PHS) 83-1967. Hyattsville, MD: National Center for Health Statistics. December 1982.

NARAL News, vol. 20, no. 2 (Spring 1988).

National Center for Health Statistics. *NCHS Monthly Vital Statistics Report,* vol. 35, no. 4, supp. (July 18, 1986), Hyattsville, MD.

The Nation's Health, vol. XVII, no. 9 (September 1987).

Nelson, Lawrence J., and Nancy Milliken. "Compelled Medical Treatment of Pregnant Women; Life, Liberty, and Law in Conflict." *Journal of the American Medical Association,* vol. 259 (February 19, 1988): 1060–1066.

Nelson, Nancy M., Murray W. Enkin, Saroj Saigal, Kathryn J. Bennett, et al. "A Randomized Clinical Trial of the Leboyer Approach to Childbirth." *New England Journal of Medicine,* vol. 302, no. 12 (March 20, 1980): 655–660.

New York Academy of Medicine. "Statement and Resolution on the Setting of Obstetrical Delivery." *Bulletin of the New York Academy of Medicine,* vol. 59, no. 4 (May 1983): 401–402.

New York Times, 17 February 1988, I, 10:1.

New York Times, 3 May 1988, III, 3.

New York Times, 24 May 1988, I, 1:1.

New York Times, 27 May 1988, I, 1:3.

New York Times, 10 January 1989, IV, 2:1.

New York Times, 17 May 1989, II, 3:4.

New York Times, 4 July 1989, I, 1:6.

Ory, Steven J. "Nonsurgical Treatment of Ectopic Pregnancy." *Fertility and Sterility*, vol. 46, no. 5 (November 1986): 767–769.

Pasley, Vickie. "Report on Maternity Practices in Chicago Hospitals." Paper presented at the annual meeting of the American Public Health Association, Washington, DC, November 1985.

Placek, Paul J., Kenneth G. Keppel, Selma M. Taffel, and Teri L. Liss. "Electronic Fetal Monitoring in Relation to Cesarean Section Delivery, for Live Births and Stillbirths in the U.S., 1980." *Public Health Reports*, vol. 99, no. 2 (March–April 1984): 173–183.

Placek, Paul J., and Selma Taffel. "Trends in Cesarean Section Rates for the United States, 1970–78." *Public Health Reports*, vol. 95, no. 6 (November–December 1980): 530–548.

Placek, Paul J., Selma Taffel, and Mary Moien. "1986 C-Sections Rise; VBACs Inch Upward." *American Journal of Public Health*, vol. 78, no. 5 (May 1988): 562–563.

Powell-Griner, Eve. "Induced Terminations of Pregnancy: Reporting States, 1982 and 1983." *NCHS Monthly Vital Statistics Report*, vol. 35, no. 3, supp. (July 14, 1986): 1–36.

Pratt, William F., and Marjorie C. Horn. *Wanted and Unwanted Childbearing: United States, 1973–82.* Advance Data No. 108. Hyattsville, MD: National Center for Health Statistics, May 9, 1985.

Radecki, Stephen E., and Gerald S. Bernstein. "Use of Clinic vs. Private Family Planning Care by Low-Income Women: Access, Cost and Patient Satisfaction." *American Journal of Public Health*, vol. 79, no. 6 (June 1989): 692–697.

Rhoades, George G., Laird G. Jackson, Sarah E. Schlesselman, et al. "The Safety and Efficacy of Chorionic Villus Sampling for Early Prenatal Diagnosis of Cytogenetic Abnormalities." *New England Journal of Medicine*, vol. 320, no. 10 (March 9, 1989): 610–617.

Rosenbaum, Sara, Dana C. Hughes, and Kay Johnson. "Maternal and Child Health Services for Medically Indigent Children and Pregnant Women." *Medical Care*, vol. 26, no. 4 (April 1988): 315–332.

Seibel, Michelle M. "A New Era in Reproductive Technology: In Vitro Fertilization, Gamete Intrafallopian Transfer and Donated Gametes and Embryos." *New England Journal of Medicine*, vol. 318, no. 13 (March 31, 1988): 828–834.

Showstack, Jonathan A., Peter P. Budetti, and Donald Minkler. "Factors Associated with Birthweight: An Exploration of the Roles of Prenatal Care and Length of Gestation." *American Journal of Public Health*, vol. 74. no. 9 (September 1984): 1003–1008.

Smith, Sandy. "Gravida with Insurance Is More Likely to Have Cesarean, Longer Stay in Hospital Than Self-Paying Patient." *Obs. Gyn. News*, vol. 18, no. 11 (June 1–14, 1983).

Speert, Harold. *Obstetrics and Gynecology in America: A History.* Chicago: American College of Obstetricians and Gynecologists, 1980.

Stockbauer, Joseph W. "WIC Prenatal Participation and Its Relation to Pregnancy Outcomes in Missouri: A Second Look." *American Journal of Public Health,* vol. 77, no. 7 (July 1987): 813–819.

Strobino, Donna M., Gigliola Baruffi, Woodrow S. Dellinger, Jr., and Alan Ross. "Variations in Pregnancy Outcomes and Use of Obstetric Procedures in Two Institutions with Divergent Philosophies of Maternity Care." *Medical Care,* vol. 26, no. 4 (April 1988): 333–347.

Sullivan, Joseph P. "Prenatal Care Offered to All in New Jersey." *New York Times,* 5 December 1989, I, 1; II, 8.

Torres, Aida, Patricia Donovan, Nancy Dittes, and Jacqueline Darroch Forrest. "Public Benefits and Costs of Government Funding for Abortion." *Family Planning Perspectives,* vol. 18, no. 3 (May/June 1986): 111–118.

Trussell, James, and Kathryn Kost. "Contraceptive Failure in the United States: A Critical Review of the Literature." *Studies in Family Planning,* vol. 18, no. 5 (September/October 1987): 237–283.

United Hospital Fund of New York. *The State of New York City's Municipal Hospital System: Report of the City Hospital Visiting Committee, Fiscal Years 1985 and 1986.* New York, 1986.

U.S. Congress, Office of Technology Assessment. *Healthy Children—Investing in the Future.* OTA-H-345. Washington, DC: Government Printing Office, February 1988.

U.S. Department of Health and Human Services, Health Care Financing Administration. *The Medicare Catastrophic Coverage Act of 1988.* Legislative Summary. Baltimore, MD, November 7, 1988.

U.S. Department of Health and Human Services, Public Health Service, Health Resources and Services Administration. *Health Status of Minorities and Low-Income Groups.* DHHS Pub. No. (HRSA) HRS-P-DV 85-1. Washington, DC, 1985.

Ventura, Stephanie J. "Trends in Marital Status of Mothers at Conception and Birth of First Child: United States, 1964–66, 1972, and 1980." *NCHS Monthly Vital Statistics Report,* vol. 36, no. 2 supp. (May 29, 1987): 1–16.

Webster v. *Reproductive Health Services,* 109 S. Ct. 3040.

Williams, Ronald L., and Peter M. Chen. "Identifying the Sources of the Recent Decline in Perinatal Mortality Rates in California." *New England Journal of Medicine,* vol. 306, no. 4 (January 28, 1982): 207–214.

Wilner, Susan, S. C. Schoenbaum, R. R. Monson, and R. N. Winickoff. "A Comparison of the Quality of Maternity Care between a Health Maintenance Organization and Fee-for-Service Practices." *New England Journal of Medicine,* vol. 304, no. 13 (March 26, 1982): 784–789.

Yankauer, Alfred. "Science and Social Policy." *American Journal of Public Health,* vol. 74, no. 10 (October 1984): 1148–1149.

PART FOUR

SUMMING UP
AND LOOKING AHEAD

CHAPTER EIGHT

How the Issues Have Changed

T HE HEALTH CARE SYSTEM figured in sociopolitical models advanced by feminist writers as an arena of expression of male power and inequitable treatment of women, a setting of activities that perpetuated the subordination of women. In the spirited campaign of the women's movement in the 1970s to reveal, define, and correct sexism in the health care system, a focal theme was that control over one's own body was part of autonomy dearly valued, captured by others but capable of being regained. Among the issues dissected were medicalization of normal childbirth, resistance of providers to the exercise of reproductive choice, labeling of women's discontent with social constraints and unequal sex role demands as mental illness, and overuse of radical surgery and psychotropic drugs. The women's movement also addressed itself to checking both excesses of sterilization imposed on low-income minority women without informed consent and, to a lesser extent, denial of sterilization to women who had not satisfied formulas of "age times parity" once standard at some hospitals. In addition, manufacturers and nonprofit agencies were charged with failure to inform women of the risks of contraceptive drugs; manufacturers, with using stereotypes of female personality to promote the sale of psychotropic drugs through advertising to physicians and marketing an unsafe contraceptive device (the Dalkon shield); and the federal government, with allowing the marketing of drugs with a poor benefit/risk ratio in pregnancy (e.g., DES). Fertility-related care, being a problem of younger women, fit into an expressive and goal-directed agenda covering education, industrial hiring practices, career development, and so forth.

The attitudes and behavior of male physicians with female patients also came under review. The medical encounter was depicted as an event

strongly influenced by male physicians' prior views on the ability of fe
male patients to produce valid information about their own health and
to receive information and on the right to, and meaning of, informed
consent. The adequacy of medical care received by women could be
affected. In addition, it was argued that physicians, who were important
authority figures in society, were prone to use their position to discour
age nontraditional behavior of women in their work life and their emo
tional life. The general tone of the complaints was in accord with a radi
cal epistemology in which the object of inquiry was to penetrate the
illusion of the humanity implicit in the doctor's role and in health care
institutions.

Another problem that attracted attention later was the shortfall of
insurance, initially a secondary concern because health care was viewed
politically, not economically. But insurance issues gained momentum in
connection with inequality in employment in the mid–1970s and pregnancy disability; later, with the resurgence of poverty.

Although certain issues (unnecessary hysterectomy and psychotropic
drug prescribing) involved older women, many of the complaints primarily affected younger women. Later, the health care problems of elderly
women attracted more concern, as their numbers increased and social
interest in aging developed. Women married older men, were less exposed to certain occupational risks than men, and lived to be widows and
the majority of the aged population. Their poor asset position and problems of access to unpaid help if disabled reflected past inequality and
current living arrangements. Ageism and sexism combined to deflect attention from them. The health care system was attuned to young healthy
males, the present and future breadwinners of traditional families. Doctors defined themselves in terms of curative procedures and use of magic
bullets and had a distaste for chronicity.

Some of the criticisms of health care depended more on appeal to personal experience than on formal research, but cogent evidence and argument as to the infiltration of society's psychological stereotypes into
medical care were produced by analysis of obstetrical textbooks, surveys
of therapists' attitudes toward normal behavior for each sex, and critiques of accepted psychiatric concepts.

Federal legislation in the 1970s outlawed discrimination against pregnancy benefits in group insurance. In this period, the raising of consciousness resulted in various activities that modified health care for
women. Women set up alternative sources of care, self-help groups, and
watchdog and lobbying organizations, and an articulate minority movement supported alternatives to medical childbirth. In the public forum,
the record of FDA performance in protecting women through its regula-

ion of drugs in pregnancy and of contraceptive drugs and devices was scrutinized. Practitioners and institutions coopted changes in maternity care, hospitals developed women's health centers, and voices within the medical profession acknowledged biases and neglect in previous training of physicians. Perhaps coincidentally, scientifically controlled trials were performed that upset the established preference of surgeons for radical mastectomy and altered women's readiness to accept such treatment. The entrance of many more women into medicine challenged the male doctor–female patient relationship, which was burdened with social cues to inequality. Gainful employment gave more women independent purchasing power including that provided by group insurance, and increased educational levels probably made more women confident of their rights. The health issues of women unfolded into a universalistic and wholesome consumerism that touched on the proper use of new technology, the right to information, and the diversity of human needs generated by different life-styles and choices in health care. Informed consent has been widely accepted as a standard for all patients and has been specifically implemented for breast cancer patients in some state laws. (Enforcement of truly informed consent remains difficult, and both cultural and situational factors continue to obstruct it.) The Dalkon shield and DES were withdrawn from distribution, and the courts decided that the manufacturers were liable for injuries caused.

While some important inequities were resolved, gender remained a factor in health care, but the nature of the issues changed. Inside the health care system, for conditions common to both sexes, there is a lack of firm evidence that gender affects care today. Once a patient enters the system, many functional requirements of the diagnostic and treatment process impose a pattern on the steps taken by physicians and hospitals and an ethical obligation to make the appropriate functional response to a given set of signs and symptoms, on behalf of the patient. Yet there are studies that keep the gender issue alive. They suggest the possibility that medical treatment, diagnostic steps, or the psychological dimensions of encounters are affected by the patient's gender or by the gender match of doctor and patient, with inequitable results. Overt gender bias is not a necessary assumption, but women may be treated differently if they present with a condition that is more common in men, for their test results may be harder to interpret and their anatomy may present more of a risk for surgeons. Also, medical educators are concerned about the faulty communication skills of many physicians. If they are not good at receiving and conveying information, this could affect women patients more for cultural reasons, with an impact on decision making, compliance, and treatment outcomes.

Prevention is somewhat different for the two sexes, but that does not necessarily imply inequities. Cancers of sex-specific sites are important for women as causes of mortality unless controlled, and both self-screening (breast self-examination) and professional screening (Pap test, mammography, and physical examination of the breast) are available as detection methods. The utility of screening depends on the natural course of the disease (probability and speed of transition to advanced states) and the possibility of preventing progression by early treatment. Analogous screening is not in general use for sex-specific sites in men, but for lung cancer, which has pronounced excess mortality in men, and for which smoking is a dominant risk factor, a major behavior change rather than screening seems to be the most effective approach. Part of the intervention for this purpose involves institutions outside the health care system (education against beginning to smoke and for quitting, prohibition of smoking in public places,[1] etc.). But smoking reversal is also a legitimate subject of physician counseling. Many women smokers or potential smokers are beneficiaries of these approaches. Yet it is possible that, when a condition is more common in men, program scheduling, incentives, and so on will not be tailored to women clients. Therefore, evaluations of smoking and hypertension-control programs should include utilization of the most effective known preventive services by each sex. For sex-specific conditions, evaluations that compare actual distribution of the most effective known preventive services with a desired goal or standard would reveal gaps in service for each sex.

The gender-related problems in health care that are most significant today lie in the socioeconomic and political context of health services. They derive from the economic status of women, the sex division of family roles, and the maladaptation of financial systems, both private and governmental, to women's needs. In addition, women in the fertile years may lack access to fertility-related services because of poverty and locality. Their problems are intensified by family planning program cuts and by official actions intended to prevent use of public funds for abortion and abortion counseling. These moves affect adolescents and adult women in poor and near-poor families and restrict the ability of family planning clinics to inform clients of their options if an unwanted pregnancy occurs. State legislatures are likely to see many attempts to reduce or eliminate recourse to abortion in the next few years, increasing women's dependence on the luck of geography and whether they have to turn to public funds. Inequality between classes of clients may be heightened,

---

[1]While the direct effect is to protect nonsmokers, the long-range effect is to reduce social tolerance of smoking.

)etween those with specific medical or genetic problems and those at risk
or socioeconomic reasons, for example.

GENDER AND THE HEALTH CARE MARKET

The Workplace

The current practice of financing health care through the workplace may
cause several difficulties for women. Those with the most marginal economic status (part-time workers and low-paid full-time workers) have no
coverage through private insurance. Insurance has not fully adapted to
marital breakup, single-parent families, and two-earner households. For a
policy to fit the needs of a two-earner family, a choice of benefits leading
to complementary coverage rather than duplication would be required.
Married women who are insured through a spouse are at risk of losing
the coverage if they are divorced, and legislation mandating continuation
of coverage tends to leave the financial burden of premiums with the
insured.

In addition, cost-sharing initiatives are more burdensome to those in
lower earnings brackets, where women are more often found, and requiring employee payment for dependent coverage may create difficulty for
single-parent families.

Nevertheless, employers do have a positive interest in retaining their
female labor force through family-centered benefits. They realize that, in
the coming years, a large proportion of the entrants into the labor force
will be female and that benefits enter into job choice by women with
marketable skills. The misfit of previous provisions with present and
emerging realities is seen as a disparity, and a constituency for its correction has been formed. This could mean that the difficulties of employed
women will diminish as future cohorts of women start to work and as
employers adjust benefit structures to them. Furthermore, the need for
arrangements to facilitate men's caregiving and parental roles as sex role
shifts occur in the community is increasingly recognized. Such arrangements would enable men, as well as women, to obtain parental leave
without losing health benefits.

Another positive outcome to be expected with the transition to a more
female labor force is that the job stress faced by women who are the first
of their sex, or one of a small number, in a given work group should
decrease.

Total optimism is not warranted, however. Health care and related
benefits, if dependent on individual employers, will be good for those in
the core labor force of a well-off firm and not necessarily for the rest,

which suggests that the government ought to serve as advocate for those women workers whose employers do the least for them. Women's occu-pational exposure to health hazards in the physical environment may increase if they enter previously male jobs and if the hazards on those jobs are not effectively controlled. (It has been a constant struggle for the labor movement to secure enforcement of existing laws.) Exposure is also increased by more continuous employment. Women's health and experi-ence of stress may be affected by the quality mix of the jobs being created throughout the economy. Jobs that are lacking in stimulation, respect, autonomy, and career possibilities are likely to be occupied by less ad-vantaged workers, a category often including women. Higher general education levels of women improve their job choices, but new waves of minority group females, young single parents, displaced homemakers, and other women who may have limited educational backgrounds tend to refill the ranks of those with low earnings, little insurance, and pre-cious little job satisfaction.

The adjustments needed in health care delivery to a more female labor force are suggested by the unequal treatment of women in Veterans Ad-ministration health facilities, as noted in a 1982 report of the General Accounting Office (New York Times, 30 September 1982). Despite the rapid growth of the proportion of women veterans, most veterans are male, and, whether or not discrimination has been deliberate, women may have remained invisible to the system. At one medical center (Syra-cuse) a minority of the women clients received pelvic examinations (27 percent) or breast examinations (40 percent); Pap smears were received by none. (Other centers did not monitor the completeness of the exami-nations, and no data were available.) At seven Veterans Administration centers, women were not eligible for outpatient treatment of gynecologi-cal problems, even if it was needed to avoid hospitalization, but men could receive outpatient care for all types of problems. Domiciliary and psychiatric programs did not accommodate women veterans because pri-vacy was not adequate for a mixed group. The administration acknowl-edged the need for change. The findings imply that various dimensions of a health care system—facilities, eligibility, service protocols, and mon-itoring—are involved in adapting the system to the needs of women.

The Elderly

The influence of gender on the health care of the elderly works through the survival of women as widows into high age groups in which a sig-nificant number face disability and/or income problems. Ageism as an obstacle to securing adequate care was challenged by economics (in alli-nce with legislative change), since effective demand generated by Medi-are increased the flow of health care services to the elderly. Providers vhose skills were useful to the elderly, such as those who could correct a ataract or a hip fracture, saw a dependable market in the Medicare-cov-red elderly. But Medicare had its limits and brought new problems: As osts rose, the benefits failed increasingly to give financial protection; loctors were not prevented from charging more than Medicare would ay; premiums were increased; Medicare embodied incentives for over-performance; and finally, Medicare failed to cover comprehensive geriat-ic assessment, the slower processing of an elderly patient, nonphysician services, and long-term care. The increased cost sharing for acute care hat was mandated in recent years has added to the out-of-pocket bur-lens of the elderly sick. Moreover, conspicuous gaps remained in provi-sion for outpatient drugs and, as was gradually recognized, cancer screening tests and other preventive services. Many of these shortcom-ings of the health care system offered to the elderly exist because the cost-effectiveness criteria that appeal to a money-driven economy are not easily satisfied by the elderly. (The repeal in 1989 of expanded coverage enacted in the previous year indicates that Congress is interested in cor-recting these omissions but has not devised an equitable and politically acceptable financing scheme for new benefits.[2])

The need for long-term care was based on the prevalence of functional limitations. This was, to a large extent, due to the increase in life expec-tancy at age sixty-five, to which the better standard of living for the elderly provided by government programs, including medical care, has contributed. Unfortunately, the task of reducing disability in old age is complex. It requires social investment in health care in earlier years of life, ample availability of assistive devices, and research into disabling conditions. Meanwhile, we do not yet have viable arrangements for the delivery of long-term care, most of which involves types of providers different from the physicians delivering acute care. Community-based care is unevenly and insufficiently developed, and nursing home care has been more or less left to proprietary interests whose service shortcomings are not always effectively disciplined. The market does not work well for consumers when the basis of the demand is dependence.

Elderly women have problems gaining access to health care because of their history of low labor force participation and low wage rates. They confront limitations in coverage supplementing Medicare through work-

---

[2]In March, 1990, a coalition of leaders in the House of Representatives proposed legisla-tion to restore several of the repealed benefits (respite, hospice, home health, and mammo-graphy), financed by a Part B premium increase (Tolchin, 1990).

place insurance groups either as retired workers or as dependents o
retirees and are not well situated economically to pay for care directly
Caregivers in both their maternal and their spousal roles, they may lack
informal sources of personal care when functionally limited. Additiona
problems may exist as to treatment. The rate of prescribing of minor
tranquilizers and other psychotropic drugs for elderly women has been
questioned, and studies have suggested that surgeons may be less (and
insufficiently) aggressive in their plans when the patient is elderly, for
diseases confined to women, and when the patient is female, for sex-
shared conditions of the elderly. Financial coverage does not assure access under such circumstances.

Market Demand and Poverty

Positive developments in health care such as shifts in preferred breast
cancer treatments, acceptance of family-centered birth arrangements, and
use of the physician's office to provide contraceptive services regardless
of marital status were influenced by women's market demand under conditions of rising expectations, as well as women's creation of alternative
sources of care. If physicians wish to adhere to previous styles and norms
of practice, doing so could cost them clientele and revenue. This powerful motive for change in a money economy is being reinforced through
reeducation by medical educators and writers in medical journals. Thus,
physicians have been alerted to the seriousness of spousal abuse as a
threat to women's health and as illegal behavior, and their responsibility
to call in appropriate social resources has been pointed out. Premenstrual
symptoms have been accepted within the set of legitimate medical problems. Although it has been acknowledged that understanding of PMS
is very incomplete, this admission itself could encourage well-designed
research.

The role of market demand, however, dramatizes the importance of
poverty as a gender problem in health. The demand of the economically
disempowered and disenfranchised is a weak force for influencing provider and system behavior.

One of the main objectives of Medicaid was to deal with the health
care aspects of the economic dependence of young women with minor
children. The state took over the financial role that had been filled in
traditional "intact" families by the responsible male for both income
support and health services, but a different track was used for the delivery of care, a track that had fewer amenities, relied on a different and
fluctuating subset of physicians (e.g., residents on a rotation in a teaching
hospital), and was separated from mainstream locations. Those clients

who depend on poverty health programs are dealing with either a provider system with little dedication to quality or one whose dedicated physicians may be treated in a hostile fashion by hospitals and private physicians fearing their competition and resisting indigent care. "Federal law requires hospitals with emergency rooms to accept critically ill patients and women in active labor," states a New York Times headline of July 25, 1988. The headline implies that there are some hospitals that would not do so voluntarily. Moreover, this requirement omits many other persons with medical needs who could be turned away for lack of funds, if they are uninsured and do not qualify for Medicaid. If indeed there were a gender bias in treatment, the clients would hardly be in a position to insist on changes in these circumstances. The person's overriding problem is how to be sure of getting care.

For poor elderly women with functional disabilities, ability to purchase assistance in activities of daily living from the market is income-related. Again, the economic dimension of women's health care problems stands out. But health care economics is closely connected with politics, because the funding for fertility control services, services for the poor, long-term care, and research on health, plus the tax treatment of employee health benefits, is determined in national and state politics.

FERTILITY-RELATED CARE AND GENDER

Much of the health care received by women is not comparable with that of men because of the functional dictates of care related to pregnancy and fertility. However, the sex distinction varies by type of service. Pregnancy care involves a protocol of periodic evaluation, counseling, education, and support for a normal biological process with a definite maximum termination date in view. In this respect it is unique. But it also embraces a repertoire of medical interventions to be used if the risk category changes. (Whether or not one approves of the criteria for a given intervention, that is how the system works.) Features of pregnancy-related care such as access, patient satisfaction, and scientific soundness could be compared with conditions restricted to men or affecting a great many men. Admittedly, analogies with illness care fall short, because most pregnancies are normal. Nevertheless, once the pregnant patient is in the care system, the monitoring of a pregnancy to detect changes in risk category is similar to care for a mild condition that has to be watched to see if a different level of care is necessary.

Contraceptive care involves prescribing, monitoring, and support over years of fertility, largely for women. It could become a unisex service if and when research yields one or more satisfactory contraceptive methods for men. Dependence on female methods could matter less for perceived equity if these methods attained very high levels of safety, efficacy, and convenience. Women do not necessarily resent responsibility for contraception, as they may prefer to retain direct control over fertility decisions.

One fertility-related service that is open to both sexes is contraceptive sterilization. The high proportion of tubal ligations, as compared with vasectomies, has been criticized by feminists as evidence of favoritism to men. The past frequency of female sterilization is probably related to the cultural attitudes that found the possible threat to men's quality of life if vasectomized intolerable. These did not arise from within the health care system, although providers perhaps accepted such attitudes more readily because they knew that the alternative procedure for women was available for couples choosing sterilization as their contraceptive method.

Another reproductive service that is used by both sexes today is infertility treatment. Although the person most directly involved in the newer infertility services such as IVF is usually the mother, the couple seeking parenthood have shared financial and emotional interests. It was not many decades ago that an infertility problem was assumed by providers and the public to be the woman's problem, but it has now been established that a large percentage of infertility is due to male factors. Evaluation and treatment of both members of a couple are now standard. The real desire of people to avail themselves of what science could offer changed behavior and attitudes, while providers had every reason to insist on including both partners, since they knew that the likelihood of success was increased thereby.

Within fertility-related care, then, there is a trend toward equal treatment of the two sexes where the biological potential for this exists, but the trend, being research-dependent in the case of contraception, is not complete.

An important difference between care for pregnancies and all other care is that expected effects of alternative decisions on the fetus are part of clinical decision making. Fetal rights controversies in society complicate this. Once a woman knows she is pregnant, she makes the important decision as to whether to accept and invest in the pregnancy. Fetal rights advocacy constrains this choice. It is used to support official initiatives, as well as illegal assaults and intimidation, that make voluntary termination more difficult to arrange. Furthermore, during the course of the pregnancy, medical situations may arise where fetal advocates would give priority to the fetus in clinical decisions. It has been observed that pregnant women, once committed to a pregnancy, generally give great weight to the welfare of the fetus they are carrying, as shown, for instance, by willingness to undergo tests, cesarean surgery, and other procedures and to change their diets and activities. But many obstetricians have conceptualized the fetus as a patient to whom they owe ethical duties, and some have drawn the conclusion that compelled treatment is justified in some cases. This issue will take new forms with the expansion of fetal diagnosis. Also, HIV seropositive fetuses pose special policy questions, because a proportion of infected pregnant women will have a limited life expectancy in which to care for the child. The administrative consequences of compulsion are complex and burdensome, because it is much easier to protect fetal health if the pregnant woman is a voluntary participant.

Since the criticism of obstetrical technology and a medical model of childbirth were first launched, there have been several competing trends in maternity care. Because of continued scientific discoveries relating to fertility and birth,[3] controversy over the role of obstetricians and hospitals has lost some of its importance. All but a small minority of births take place in hospitals. However, this environment has changed as hospitals have adapted their birthing practices to consumer preferences, especially for low-risk deliveries. The willingness of insurance companies to accept and even encourage use of birthing centers may have added an economic stimulus to hospitals to retain their market by accommodating diversity.

But fear that use of birth technology (ultrasound, EFM, cesareans, etc.) is expanding beyond valid indications associated with high-risk pregnancies is not confined to those who reject birth technology as part of an alienation of the birth experience. The rate of cesarean sections has been growing, and the American College of Obstetricians and Gynecologists' efforts to reduce the frequency of repeat cesareans have not been successful. Cesareans appear to owe their popularity to a combination of valid medical reasons, invalid or questionable interpretations of EFM as signifying fetal distress, convenience of physicians and patients, and fear of malpractice suits. First births at older maternal ages increase the probability of cesarean deliveries. Consumer demand sustains the use of high-technology care in obstetrics.

Consumer demand also supports the market for infertility care. Provider facilities seeking a clientele for combined clinical and research activities are said to be inflating expectations of success (Bonnicksen, 1986), whether out of hope of fame or desire for revenue. As for the patient, the service being bought is of undefined value, its estimated

---

[3] A newspaper headline reads, "Confident Obstetricians Discover New Frontiers of Prenatal Diagnosis" (*New York Times*, 12 May 1988).

probability of success having a huge standard error; and, although it is a discretionary purchase, the value clients place on what they may view as a last chance for parenthood wipes out usual standards of comparison and budgeting. The announcement of new techniques recruits fresh consumers prepared to face high cost and uncertainty of yield with high hopes, and it seems as though this situation will continue.

A SEX-SHARED PROBLEM: INNOVATION WITHOUT BENEFIT

The possibility of innovation without benefit is not limited to reproductive services. It applies to other health care and is a problem shared by both sexes as consumers and patients.

An imbalance between development of new medical technologies and scientific evaluation of their efficacy, toxicity, and cost appears to be a permanent feature of our health care system. Diagnostic and therapeutic innovations have quickly passed into common use on a wave of enthusiasm on the part of the innovators (Plum, 1985) and receptivity on the part of consumers. Later, calmer voices are heard, and evaluations appear showing whether the new approach is superior to the old or else showing that the comparison cannot be made as yet. Claims for a technology are then revised and its applications limited—after many patients have used it.

There were many reasons for the too rapid acceptance of new techniques in the past. The standards of clinical trials in use today are far more sophisticated than formerly. Neither physician nor patient is supposed to know which therapy is being received, what results are being observed as the trial goes along, and so forth (Chalmers et al., 1981). Previous trials that were not "blinded" in this way usually contained optimistic biases. Another problem was the comparison of present patients with "historical" rather than "simultaneous" controls. Historical controls are derived from past records of patients treated in the previous fashion; evaluation of a new method based on comparison with historical controls is sometimes too lenient, because the historical patients differ in some important respects from current patients who give informed consent (Chalmers et al., 1978).[4] In a trial, several different end points of treatment might be used by the investigator, who then might select only the favorable results for publication (Moskowitz et al., 1983). Furthermore, the recommendations might be far stronger than the findings warranted, and readers would interpret what they read accord-

---

[4]Patients in trials today may be screened to exclude those with comorbidities or advanced disease, for example.

ing to their own propensities. Surgeons were found to be more enthusiastic than nonsurgeons in interpreting articles on coronary bypass procedures (Chalmers et al., 1982). It was also observed that, because of the enthusiasm of the innovators, the grounds for support of bypass surgery were shifted to improved quality of life when there was no difference in mortality in trial results (Halperin and Levine, 1985). The procedure may, nonetheless, be worthwhile on the basis of quality-of-life effects for given medical indications.

The effect of poorly designed trials, paradoxically, was to hold back the diffusion of useful therapies while overpromoting others, meanwhile wasting the time of the experimental subjects.

Today the randomized controlled trial is considered the ideal method of determining the worth of therapies. But it is not always applicable or successful, for several reasons. For potentially life-saving procedures like the Pap test, it would be unethical to withhold service from a control group to run a test. In other instances, a trial cannot be done because a particular therapy has already been contraindicated for a certain risk group. In the case of trials of different modifications of breast cancer treatment (lumpectomy with and without radiation, compared with mastectomy), it proved impossible to recruit sufficient patients because the physicians knew that a previous therapy protocol was effective, and they feared both loss of their personal authority in individual cases and patient resistance (Taylor et al., 1984). For these and possibly other reasons, the proportion of eligible patients enrolled in clinical trials is well below what researchers would wish, delaying the process of attaining consensus on rational treatment. Moreover, doctors apparently try harder to obtain informed consent when they strongly believe in a new therapy, thus compromising random selection (Chalmers, 1976). Trials have been a hot issue in AIDS. The high case-fatality rate has made individuals eager to have new drugs without waiting for completion of conventional evaluation, and public attitudes have changed in regard to the necessity of FDA requirements in view of the seriousness of the disease. Furthermore, economic factors limiting access to clinical trials have been noted.

Accountability extends beyond researchers to physicians prescribing medication or advising surgery. They have an obligation to analyze critically the reported evidence for their choices, in order to protect the members of the general public from receiving useless therapy.

Health care financing systems have started to evaluate new technology but still pay for treatment costs in many instances where the value of the therapy has not been scientifically shown. Research could document whether the receipt of unjustified treatment and delay in receiving newer efficacious treatment are affected by gender and whether type of health plan, source of payment, and characteristics of the treating doctor influence these outcomes.

In the traditional belief that doctors are perfect agents of patients, doctors' desire to maximize revenue and free their own time for gainful work or for leisure is not conceded to be a factor in treatment decisions. This belief, which buttresses physician-dominant practice patterns, has been shaken by the alienation of patients from physicians caused by specialization and unshared secrets of high technology. A new equilibrium has not been reached. (Patients who do not hold the idealized view of physicians would still not be able to tell how individual doctors differed in their intention to be perfect agents or which decisions are most swayed by private considerations.) Malpractice litigation has added costs to the system, including those of self-defensive testing, whose value in reducing the volume of litigation has not been shown. Second-opinion programs put a curb on what doctors propose, but they do not supply what is not being done for the patient, and for the most part they have been limited to surgery (Mullan, 1985). Thus, a major cluster of problems affecting both sexes centers on technology and is related to the divergent objectives of the parties: researchers, practitioners, patients, and payment sources.

FUTURE ANALYTIC NEEDS

The tenacity of gender as a force determining one's position in the social structure and the damaging consequences of sex bias suggest that it is premature to withdraw attention from the fortunes of women in health care. Clearly, however, improving the performance of the system for women means resolving not only sex-specific but also shared problems such as research quality. Furthermore, the presentation of gender equity issues stimulates awareness of men's problems, specifically how male social roles, behavioral norms, and modal personalities interacting with the health care system may conflict with getting care and benefiting from it. Denial of illness is a culturally approved type of behavior for males, which may hinder seeking care and complying with a prescribed regimen. The deleterious effects of a chronic illness label on work relations and self-esteem for men diagnosed as having heart disease have been explored. Disapproval of, and hostility toward, male homosexuality have been an obstacle to access to needed care for individual AIDS patients, prevention efforts, design of care programs, and even research funding.

Health services research should specifically include attention to gender, because policies and practices, actual or proposed, that, on their face, are indifferent to gender in reality may have different implications for women and men that violate equity. This is made more likely by the many problems that beset the health care system today and that are often invested with urgency. One may choose to view gender effects as peripheral to some main theme or concern, but, if attention to them is regularly omitted, bias can accumulate in the system. The socioeconomic environment, affected as it is by a variety of governmental policies, contains many uncertainties as to gender equality in the workplace and disposable income in retirement years. It is also subject to waves of traditionalism regarding female sexuality and family roles, and it retains hierarchical features in important organizations. The net effects of such influences may be a precarious position for some women and chronic disadvantage for others. Their current health care may be affected, and they are vulnerable to specific retrenchments, reforms, and other changes in health care.

A key issue in the analysis of gender effects is understanding of clusters of variables that occur in association with each other. The same health care data that may be used to conclude that there is little or no gender difference after income, employment, age, or other factors are held constant can be interpreted to show that one sex has more difficulty because of economic weakness, age-related health problems, and the like. This may be quite important in assessing system performance and understanding reasons for unmet needs.

One of the major tasks of future health care research will be to examine the effects of different types of medical care organizations on access, quality, and cost; in this task, gender needs to be remembered, but often it is not. The adequacy of care of needs that are sex-specific and those that are more common for one sex should be explored, and protocols should be appraised to see if routine screening of demonstrated utility is offered for diseases restricted to one sex. For conditions affecting both sexes, volume of services used and visit content should be compared. A growing inventory of cost-effectiveness analyses for different treatments makes it possible to determine if the most desirable decision paths are followed equally often for patients of each sex.

There has been little research on gender differences, either in clinical decisions regarding evaluation and treatment of conditions common to both sexes or in the conduct of encounters. Methods of nonintrusive observation of encounters should be explored. Logs and other records would reveal information exchanges and the sequence and spacing of diagnostic steps and therapeutic actions and recommendations. For serious illness, the stage of the disease when it first comes under care is a potentially important measure of system performance if early detection is possible. Gender differences are not necessarily due to provider bias but may arise from patients' modes of relating to health care. They may also be due to biological sex differences (anatomical, hormonal, etc.) affecting what a physician thinks will be safest and most effective for a given patient. Hence, research design must be sensitive to covariates.

Incomplete communication has been noted as a problem in doctor–patient relations. Differences in communication based on doctor–patient gender combinations can be studied by interview surveys directed to patients and physicians. Failure to ask questions in sufficient detail or to evaluate symptoms compromises clinical decisions. Inattention to patient goals results in failure to ascertain them and attempt to advance them.

Vignettes describing hypothetical cases are useful in surveying attitudes of physicians. They have been used to study physician response to physical and psychological symptoms and prescribing. They are used in continuing medical education to test and teach clinical skills. Standard vignettes could be used to track changes in physician attitudes as new cohorts enter medicine. Specialty societies might incorporate other vignettes into their materials to test and teach gender neutrality where appropriate or gender sensitivity where it would maximize patient welfare. (A hypothetical example is a medication that, as a side effect, would affect sleep patterns of a single parent or working mother.)

Therapies in common use should be revisited to see if there was unsupported inference from research confined to one sex or a narrow age class. Financing of clinical trials should be examined to see if circumstances favor eligibility and continued participation of one sex over the other. Conditions for which one sex is distinctly in the minority should be studied to see if differential treatment flows from this fact; for instance, if the physician has little experience with the behavior of the disease in the minority sex.

Good capability to do gender analysis in health care studies depends on data systems set up to show the gender of the patient and, preferably, of the provider. Study samples need to be large enough to permit separation of subjects by gender, by socioeconomic attributes, and by clinical characteristics such as disease stage, where applicable. An important consideration in studies where income is a pertinent factor is to use a measure of income that recognizes different household circumstances. We need a measure, not only of family income, but also of per capita income, and an adjustment should be made for the fixed costs of running a household that make a small household less economical. Questions about household composition that would show whether rent is shared by unrelated individuals and family groups would help interpret income data so that ability to pay for health care or for insurance would be better understood.

In relation to distributional equity, gender is important, not statistically as a variable of classification, but as a factor in life situations that are associated with restricted access to care and greater financial risk.

In relation to respect for quality of life, autonomy, and utility of patient-provided information within the process of medical care, gender is a residual but potentially persistent element in care, because awareness of gender has biological and social roots and is hard to remove from personal service relationships. Any tendency to bias may be compensated for by deliberate protocols (such as modes of addressing patients) and gradually weakened by changing images of the competence, outlook, and needs of both adult women and adult men and by a more equal gender mix among physicians. Another factor that may change the place of gender in health care is use of more nonphysician services provided by professionals of both sexes. If these services are also associated with prevention, rather than treatment, the anxiety on the patient's side of the encounter, which may intensify dependence, may be less.

Reproductive health care is an important part of the health care system. Both older and newer advances in personal control of fertility have stirred up intense attitudinal divisions. These quite evidently affect resource allocation, use of public funds, and provider rationing of newer technologies where capacity is limited. Class, race, marital status, and life-style may affect access. Controversial or potentially controversial situations involving reproductive health care include contracts between a married couple and a surrogate mother; decisions about social investment in infertility prevention by control of pelvic inflammatory disease, versus support of sophisticated infertility treatments; decisions as to using resources for neonatology, versus primary prenatal care; and support of parenthood opportunities for single and lesbian women. These are not simple male–female conflicts of interest. Yet gender roles are involved as, for example, when biological fatherhood is dissociated from family roles of the male and when the biological roles of pregnancy are split between two women. Decisions about these evolving services may bring out latent differences of opinion about gender. Since success in meeting individual reproductive goals is part of the quality of life affected by medical care and, since reproductive care is an important part of women's health care, assessment of access to and effectiveness of such care and its relation to gender roles belongs in the future agenda for study.

FUTURE REFORMS

Gender equity is bound to be advanced by health care reforms that are universalistic in scope (apply to all) and humanistic in intent (provide all needed care without subjecting patients to unnecessary, especially invasive, procedures). They help assure that women will get a fair share of resources without discrimination based on their sex, age, income, lifestyle, or category of services needed. Promoting the delivery of a balanced spectrum of care encompasses, not only the conventional array of services for illness episodes (diagnosis, treatment, and rehabilitation), but also prevention, long-term care, and services that maximize the capacity to do activities of daily living. Promoting delivery of the entire range is favorable to equity with regard to the type of service a person needs. Assuring care to people living at or near poverty levels of income (e.g., by changes in eligibility and mandated services under Medicaid) will benefit many women, since women form the majority of the poor. Programs that address problems of old age, such as long-term care financing and home care, are important for gender equity because of the large numbers of women in the elderly population. All measures that improve consumer information and decision making and result in more efficient choices of health plan, individual provider, treatment strategies, and prevention strategies help both men and women get value for their dollar; but they are legitimate concerns of women because they have more marginal value to the groups with lower incomes and those needing more care either for illness or reproductive health.

Various specific reforms would be valuable to elderly women. Improved payment to providers for cognitive services will soon be in effect and should encourage careful and comprehensive evaluation of patients. Restoration of the Medicare mammography benefit would do more for prevention if accompanied by efforts to increase older women's acceptance of mammography. Elderly women would gain by competent diagnosis and treatment of depression, occurring alone and as a comorbid factor with physical illness or disability. Nonphysician services that are extremely necessary for adequate support of the elderly person's health should be financed, among them transportation to care facilities for the very old and social services. Provision of a package of services for chronic illness should be required for approval of HMOs for Medicare participation. Congregate housing options to assist the frail elderly should be expanded. For present and future elderly, protection of retiree benefits against financial convulsions within the corporate world would prevent some medical indigency.

Reform in reproductive care covers a wide range of situations. We live in the midst of unprecedented advances in reproductive medicine, yet there are still an unacceptable number of pregnant women who lack basic care or who use clinic facilities characterized by discontinuities, poor amenities, and limited budgets. Today there are special and urgent needs for designing and carrying out programs for treating drug abuse in pregnancy and delivering family planning services to women at high risk of AIDS. A set of prenatal screening services that would be paid by third-party sponsors, including government, and would help prevent diseases of the newborn should be developed. Laws and regulations that turn eligibility for Medicaid on and off depending on the existence of pregnancy are inimical to continuous care and to counseling and prevention opportunities. A reproductive care agenda should include investment in contraceptive research for both sexes. Aside from familiar reasons for increasing the number of available options, safe, acceptable, and effective contraceptive services will be even more important with the threat of new state laws restricting elective abortion. Hostility to abortion will no doubt create access problems in many communities, even where the procedure sought falls within legal limits. Abortion service availability needs to be protected by providing transportation funds, taking public and professional responsibility for referral to willing providers, and providing a direct source of service complete with family planning counseling and medical backup for complications and follow-up care. Compulsory fetal treatment should be avoided as a style of pregnancy management by providers, and it should be made difficult to order through the courts; again, this is more urgent if the woman's right to a decision as to whether to carry a pregnancy to term is not protected everywhere.[5]

The AIDS epidemic has compelled the public to accept more open discussion of sex but has not yet fully dislodged the attitudes that work against prevention. Behavior change can be promoted, however. Women and men need information about practicing safe sex and help in understanding how to get their partners to cooperate in this.

So long as health care is insured through the workplace, privacy in health care transactions must be protected through careful design of administrative procedures for claims filing. Women caregivers should be assisted by respite coverage programs and unisex parental leave. Part-time and contingent workers should receive health insurance coverage. This means not only that carriers be required to offer it to employers but also that employers be required to supply it to workers. In two-earner families, options for use of the premium should be provided to avoid demonetizing the wife's (or the husband's) wage supplement.

---

[5]In the 1989 elections, anti-abortion candidates fared poorly as their opponents appealed to public concern over the restrictive implications of the *Webster* decision in July. Republican leaders later softened their attitude toward a "litmus test" of candidates presaging that present restrictions might be politically costly (Toner, 1990).

Changes in the incentive structure of medical care would correct a long-standing problem in American medical practice. There should be no private financial reason for a practitioner to choose one diagnostic or treatment approach over another (present incentives are believed to be conducive to more invasive and resource-intensive procedures) or to intervene, rather than choose watchful waiting. There have recently been reports of changes in payment for deliveries, so that a doctor does not earn more for doing a cesarean than a vaginal delivery. Such change might spread to other services including those used by men. In view of the frequency of cesareans, hysterectomies, and breast operations, payment reform might improve the quality of care for many women and should be welcomed by them. Incentives are clearly at issue in current plans to enhance payment for cognitive services under Medicare, thus increasing rewards for deliberation and integrative case management, as against surgical intervention, and encouraging comprehensive care, rather than high case loads. Surgery may be just what the patient needs. But, with a more balanced payment method, clinical decisions would be more firmly attached to a floor of disinterest.

Most of the reforms discussed are directed at fairly intense problems associated with social deprivation, income limitations, or severe vulnerabilities based on reproductive needs or age-related health deficits, heightened by recent epidemiological trends and legal events. A research agenda to match the suggested reforms would include evaluation directed at means of identifying groups for targeted programs, alternative settings, and alternative reimbursement methods. It would also embrace monitoring of program effects once a program had been introduced. For example, we should study Medicare experience after the new payment system begins to operate to see if the care of elderly individuals with multiple problems is improved by better rewards for cognitive services. Retrospective, prospective, and simulation studies are all useful tools for such work.

Finally, the health care system would benefit from periodic review of the progress of gender equity, the opportunities available for the study of gender factors in health and service, and the redesign of data collection and analysis systems. The interplay of gender with class and ethnicity should be recognized in conceptualizing and modeling. The financial support of such research should be addressed. In the redesign of health care that may be a feature of the 1990s, it will be important to go beyond the egalitarian rhetoric of preambles. We need to ascertain whether gender has been prevented from directly or indirectly intruding into health care by intelligent policies of government, professional bodies, employers, unions, and others.

References

Bonnicksen, Andrea. "Consumer Awareness in High-Tech Births" (Letter to Editor). *New York Times,* 17 May 1986.

Chalmers, Thomas C. "Randomized Controlled Clinical Trials in Diseases of the Liver." In *Progress in Liver Diseases,* vol. V, edited by H. Popper and F. Shaffner. New York: Grune & Stratton, 1976, 450–456.

Chalmers, Thomas C., H. Smith, Jr., A. Ambroz, et al. "In Defense of the VA Randomized Control Trial in Coronary Artery Surgery." *Clinical Research,* vol. 26 (September 1978): 230–235.

Chalmers, Thomas C., H. Smith, Jr., B. Blackburn, et al. "A Method of Assessing the Quality of a Randomized Control Trial." *Controlled Clinical Trials,* vol. 2, no. 1 (May 1981): 31–49.

Chalmers, Thomas C., D. Reitman, A. Koffler, and H. Sacks. "Bias in the Interpretation of Clinical Trials." *Clinical Research,* vol. 30, no. 2 (April 1982): 549A.

"Confident Obstetricians Discover New Frontiers of Prenatal Diagnosis." *New York Times,* 12 May 1988.

"Federal Law Requires Hospitals with Emergency Room to Accept Critically Ill Patients and Women in Active Labor." *New York Times,* 25 July 1988.

Halperin, J. L., and R. Levine. *Bypass: A Cardiologist Reveals What Every Patient Needs to Know.* New York: Times Books, 1985.

Moskowitz, G., T. C. Chalmers, H. Sacks, R. Fegerstrom, et al. "Deficiencies of Clinical Trials of Alcohol Withdrawal." *Alcoholism: Clinical and Experimental Research* (Winter 1983): 42–46.

Mullan, Fitzhugh. "Seasons of Survival: Reflections of a Physician with Cancer." *New England Journal of Medicine,* vol. 313, no. 4 (July 25, 1985): 270–273.

New York Times, 30 September 1982, III, 2:3.

Plum, Fred. "Extracranial–Intracranial Arterial Bypass and Cerebral Vascular Disease." *New England Journal of Medicine,* vol. 313, no. 19 (November 1985): 1221–1223.

Taylor, K. M., R. G. Margolese, and C. L. Soskolne. "Physicians' Reasons for Not Entering Eligible Patients in a Randomized Clinical Trial of Surgery for Breast Cancer." *New England Journal of Medicine,* vol. 310 (1984): 1363–1367.

Tolchin, Martin. "House Moves to Restore Health Benefits for Elderly." *New York Times,* 4 March 1990, I, 23.

Toner, Robin. "Atwater Urges Softer Abortion Law." *New York Times,* 20 January 1990, I, 10: 1.

Name Index

Boldface numbers refer to tables.

Abbott, Robert D., 36, 51
Abrams, Herbert L., 36, 50
Adams, Patricia F., 5, 7, **18**, **19**, 20, 70, **93**, **95**
Administration on Aging agencies, 129
Advocates Senior Alert Process, 118, 138
Aetna Life and Casualty, 88, 99
AFDC. *See* Aid to Families with Dependent Children
Agency for Health Care Policy and Research, 8
Agency for International Development, 179
Aid to Families with Dependent Children (AFDC), 75, 147, 150, 151, 155–157, **160**, 162
Alan Guttmacher Institute, 156, 157, 165, 189, 191, 209
Albert Einstein College of Medicine, 36
Alcohol, Drug Abuse, and Mental Health Administration, 34
Allis-Chalmers Manufacturing Company, 89
Altman, Lawrence K., 116, 138
Ambroz, A., 239
American Association of Retired Persons, 106, 138, 161
American Cancer Society, 15, 136
American Civil Liberties Union, 60, 70
American College of Obstetricians and Gynecologists, 183, 186, 195, 196, 202, 229
American Fertility Society, 205
American Medical Association, 10, 180, 209
American Psychiatric Association, 44
American Public Health Association, 79, 99, 201
Anderka, Marlene T., 212

Andrews, Lori B., 205, 209
Annas, George J., 202, 210
Arie, Tom, 52
Aries, Nancy, 181, 209
Arling, Greg, 125, 145
Armitage, K.J., 29, 30, 49
Arney, William Ray, 184, 209
Arno, Peter S., 35, 54
Avorn, Jerry, 167

Bachman, Gerald G., 6, 20
Banta, H.D., 195, 209
Barnes, B.A., 53
Barry, F., 50
Barss, V.A., 210
Baruffi, Gigliola, 215
Bass, Martin J., 45, 49
Bass, Robert A., 29, 49
Bassett, Alan A., 14, 19
Batkin, Miriam, **93**, 99
Bauer, Madeline, 50
Bellaisch-Allart, Joëlle, 210
Belle, D., 44, 51
Benacerraf, B.R., 210
Benjamin, Fred, 42, 53, 63, 71
Bennett, Kathryn J., 213
Bergmann, Barbara, 59, 60, 70
Bergstahler, Janet Witte, 87, 99
Berk, Marc L., 76, 100, 101, 124, 151, 165
Berki, S.E., 52, 71
Berkowitz, Gale, 149, 166
Bernacki, Edward J., 90, 102
Bernstein, Amy, 124
Bernstein, Barbara, 137, 138
Bernstein, Gerald S., 175, 214
Berwick, Donald M., 199, 209
Bianchi, Suzanne M., 129, 138

Blackburn, B., 239
Blackwell, Richard E., 205, 209
Blanco, D.M., 140
Blank, Susan, 148, 156, 163, 165
Blatt, Charles M., 50
Bloom, Barbara, 6, 19
Bonnicksen, Andrea, 229, 239
Booth Maternity Center, 199
Boston Women's Health Book Collective, 174, 209
Bottoms, Sidney F., 211
Boylan, Peter C. Letter, 186, 209
Brabani, Carole, 71
Braham, Robert L., 129, 143
Brambilla, Donald, 120, 142
Brandwein, Ruth A., 60, 70
Brinsden, P., 210
Brock, Thomas, 165
Brody, Claire M., 44, 50
Brody, Elaine M., 127, 139
Bromwich, Peter, 172, 204, 206, 209
Brooks, Marie A., 35, 54
Broverman, Donald M., 44, 50
Broverman, Inge K., 44, 50
Brown, Byron, 50
Brown, John, 89, 102
Brown, Leahmae, 89, 100
Brown, Louise, 204
Brunner, Debbie, 161, 167
Brunt, Melanie, 66, 67, 70
Buczko, William, 153, 165
Budetti, Peter P., 186, 189, 214
Bundy, Darcie, 87, 100
Bureau of National Affairs, 65n, 70
Bush, George, 94
Butler, Lewis H., 159, 165
Butler, Robert N., 135, 139
Butter, Irene H., 211

Cafferata, Gail Lee, 118, 126, 128, 129, 139, 143
Campbell, William H., 119, 141
Canadian Task Force on the Periodic Health Examination, 186, 209
Carmen, Elaine Hilberman, 43, 50
Castleman, Michael, 204, 209
Cates, Willard, Jr., 177, 209, 210
Caton, Carol C., 34, 52
Census Bureau, 83
Centers for Disease Control, 39
Chalmers, Thomas C., 194, 209, 230, 231, 239
Chang, Deborah, 211
Charles D. Spencer and Associates, 88, 96, 100

Chen, Peter M., 195, 215
Chez, Ronald A., 27, 50
Children's Defense Fund, 149, 165
Christensen, Kathleen, 78
Clarkson, Frank E., 44, 50
Coburn, Andrew F., 189, 191, 212
Coleman, Daniel, 27, 50
Collins, James J., 51
Collins, John Gary, 51, 61, 70, 111, 139
Colon, Eduardo, 52
Commonwealth Fund Commission on Elderly People Living Alone, 109
Comptroller General of the United States, 165
Cooke, Margaret, 211
Cooney, Joan P., 74, 100
Cooper, Glinda S., 205, 210
Cooperstock, Ruth, 45, 50
Copeland, Paul M., 42, 51
Corder, Larry S., 110, 143
Corman, Hope, 189, 211
Cornoni-Huntley, Joan, 135, 139
Council of Economic Advisers, 60
Cousins, Amy, 183, 210
Cronin, Mark, 158, 162, 165
Croog, Sydney H., 33, 50
Cunningham, Gary, 212
Curran, James W., 209
Cypress, Beulah K., 8, 9, 11, 12, **14**, **15**, 19–20, 115, 116, 139

Dallosso, Helen, 52
Dalton, Maureen E., 205, 212
Davis, Herbert, 177
Dawson, Deborah A., 5, 7, **18**, **19**, 20, 70, **93**, **95**, 113, 139
Dellinger, Woodrow S., Jr., 215
DeLozier, James, 51, 142
De Medina, Maria, 211
Department of Agriculture, 151
DHHS. *See* U.S. Department of Health and Human Services
Diagnosis-Related Groups, 98
Dickerson, Vivian, 51
Dittes, Nancy, 211, 215
Dobson, Allen, 139, 166
Domenighetti, Gianfranco, 40, 50
Donovan, Patricia, 215
Doubilet, Peter, 36, 50
Drury, Thomas F., 114, 115, 141
Duff, Raymond S., 199, 210
Duffy, Brigitte M., 15, 20
Dunn, Leo J., 176, 189–190, 210
Durkel-Turnbull, J., 50

Ebrahim, Shah, 52
Edwards, R.G., 204, 210
Egdahl, Richard, 98, 100
Eggers, Paul W., 139, 166
Elashoff, R.M., 140
Elder, K., 210
Elias, Sherman, 202, 210
Enkin, Murray W., 213
Equitable HCA Corporation, 76, 78, 79, 82, 100, 131, 139
Evans, Mark I., 198, 210
Evans, Stephen, 188

Farley, Pamela J., 74, 86, 100, 101
Fahs, Marianne C., 142
Fay, Francesca C., 84, 100
FDA. See Food and Drug Administration
Feder, Judith, 155, 166
Fegerstrom, R., 239
Feldbaum, Paul J., 66, 71
Fentem, Peter H., 52
Finison, Karl S., 212
Fisher, Bernard, 32, 50
Fletcher, John C., 198, 210
Folmar, Steven J., 105, 140
Food and Drug Administration (FDA), 179, 180, 194, 202, 220, 231
Forbes, Daniel, 97, 98, 100
Forgy, Lawrence, 122
Forrest, Jacqueline Darroch, 215
Fortney, Judith A., 195, 210
Frau, Lourdes M., 186, 210
Freeman, C.P.L., 42, 50
Freeman, H.F., 140
Freud, Sigmund, 27, 43
Freudenheim, Milt, 79, 81, 100
Frey, Norma, 90, 100
Fries, Nicolas, 210
Frigoletto, Frederic D., 186, 188, 210
Frydman, René, 204, 210
Frye, Robert L., 50
Fuchs, Victor R., 178, 193, 210
Fulton, John, 113, 139

Gajda, Anthony J., 131
Galkin, Florence, 159, 166
Gallagher, Janet, 207, 212
Ganz, P.A., 140
Garnick, Deborah W., 121, 139
Garrison, P.M., 209
Gemson, Donald H. Letter, 62, 70
General Accounting Office (GAO), 35–36, 50, 94, 95, 100, 131, 139, 224
Gersh, Bernard J., 31, 50

Giammusso, Estelle, 90, 100
Gluck, Michael E., 15, 20
Goldberg, Robert J., 66, 71
Golden, Patricia M., 117, 143
Goldfarb, Marsha G., 196, 210
Goldin, Claudia, 59, 60, 70
Goldwyn, Robert M., 50
Gornick, Marian, 108, 122, 123, 139, 140, 142, 151, 155, 166
Gortmaker, Steven, 167
Goyert, Gregory L., 185, 211
Graboys, Thomas B., 38, 50
Graves, Edmund J., 16, 20, 121, 140
Greenberg, Jay N., 139, 166
Greene, M.F., 210
Greenfield, Dorothy, 204, 212
Greenfield, S., 136, 140
Greer, Steven, 30, 51
Griffin, M.R., 143
Grossman, Michael, 189, 211
Gruentzig, Andreas R., 38, 51
Gupta, Sudhir, 53
Guttentag, Marcia, 44, 51

Haddock, Cynthia Carter, 140
Hagan, Michael M., 101
Hall, Ferris M., 23, 51
Hall, Margaret Jean, 122
Halperin, J.L., 231, 239
Hamilton, Jean, 134, 140
Hammes, LaVon N., 53
Hammond, Mary G., 203, 211
Harwood, Henrick J., 34, 51
Haug, Marie R., 105, 136, 140
Havlik, Richard J., 114, 134, 135, 140
Hayes, Cheryl D., 188, 211
Hayward, R.A., 117, 140
Hazout, André, 210
HCFA. See Health Care Financing Administration
Headley, Adrienne, 50
Health Care Financing Administration (HCFA), 109, 122, 162, 192
Health Insurance Plan of Greater New York (HIP), 89
Health Maintenance Organization, 196
Hemminki, Elina, 187, 211
Hemminki, Karl, 65, 71
Hendershot, Gerry, 113, 139
Henderson, A., 50
Henshaw, Stanley K., 89, 101
Herold, Joan, 69, 70
Herzfeld, Judith, 200, 211
Herzog, David B., 42, 51
Heuser, Robert L., 185, 211

Hibbard, Judith, 132, 140
Higgins, James E., 210
Hill, Ian T., 155, 156, 166
Hilts, Philip J., 180, 211
Hing, Esther, 115, 122, 123, 140
Hirschfeld, Robert M.A., 141
Hochbaum, Martin, 159, 166
Hofferth, Sandra J., 188, 211
Holahan, John, 155, 166
Homan, Sharon M., 115, 140
Horn, Marjorie C., 59, 71, 175, 176, 211, 214
Horney, Karen, 43
Horowitz, Amy, 126, 140
Houlihan, Kathleen, 211
House of Representatives, 225n; Select Committee on Aging, 131, 132
Hricko, Andrea, 66, 67, 70
Hughes, Dana C., 191, 214
Hughes, Joyce M., 210

ICF, Incorporated, 161, 166
Imber, Jonathan B., 182, 183, 211
Institute of Medicine, 186, 189
Insurance Department, 85

Jack, Susan S., 6, 19
Jackson, Laird G., 214
Jewett, John Figgis, 188, 210
Johnsen, Pauline T., 139
Johnson and Higgins, 82, 83, 96, 97, 99, 101
Johnson, Dirk, 89, 101
Johnson, Kay, 191, 214
Johnston, Lloyd D., 6, 6, 20
Jonas, Maureen M., 187, 211
Jones, Denise Williams, 145
Joyce, Theodore, 189, 211

Kaali, S.G., 177, 211
Kaeser, Lisa, 179, 212
Kaiser-Permanente, 65n
Kane, Robert, 137, 138
Kannel, William B., 36, 51
Kaplan, Marci, 44, 51
Kaplan, Robert M., 145
Kapp, Daniel S., 52
Kasper, Judith A., 118, 125, 139, 140, 148, 151, **152, 154,** 155, 162, 163, 166
Kassirer, Jerome P., 31, 51
Katz, Adrian I., 188
Kay, Bonnie J., 186, 211
Kay, Thomas C., 213

Kennedy, Kathy I., 210
Kennedy, S., 209
Kenney, Asta M., 191, 211
Keppel, Kenneth G., 211, 214
Kessel, Samuel S., 211
King, M.B., 45, 52
King, Spencer B., III, 51
Kittner, Dorothy, 86, 101
Kleban, Morton H., 139
Kleinman, Joel C., 197, 198, 211
Knapp, Deanne E., 118, 141
Knickman, James R., 130, 141
Koch, Hugo, 83, 101, 118, 119, **119**
Kochanek, Kenneth D., 181n, 212
Koffler, A., 239
Kolata, Gina, 183, 212
Kolder, Veronika E.B., 207, 212
Kost, Kathryn, 175, 176, 215
Kotelchuck, Milton, 189, 212
Kovar, Mary Grace, 37, 51, 111, 114, 115, 124, 136, 140, 141
Kozak, Lola Jean, 16, 17, 20
Kristiansen, Patricia L., 51
Kronmal, Richard A., 50
Kuter, Irene, 54

LaCroix, Andrea Z., 111, 141
Lampert, Steven, 50
Landesman, R., 177, 211
Last, John M., 70
Latham, W. Bryan, 97, 101
Lazenby, Helen, 159, 166
Leveno, Kenneth J., 194–195, 212
Levin, Arthur A., 39, 51
Levine, R., 231, 239
Levine, Sol, 50
Levit, Katherine R., 166
Lewin, Tamar, 190n, 212
Lewis, Scott, 183, 212
Lichtenstein, Richard, 52, 71
Lilford, Richard J., 205, 212
Lincoln, Richard, 179, 212
Lindbohm, Marja-Liisa, 65, 71
Lindheimer, Marshall D., 188
Liss, Teri L., 214
Lobel, Brana, 120, 141
Lorber, Judith, 203, 204, 212
Lorenz, Gerda, 24, 52
Loring, Marti, 44, 51
Louis Harris and Associates, 106, 107, 141
Lown, Bernard, 50
Luft, Harold S., 41, 51
Luraschi, Pierangelo, 40, 50
Lurie, Nicole, 148, 166
Lyons, Barbara, 109, 143

McCall, Nelda, 130, 141
McCann, Dennis J., 183, 212
McDonald, Thomas P., 189, 191, 212
McDonald's, 77
Machlin, Steven, 211
MacKay, H. Trent, 210
McKinlay, John G., 120, 142
McKinlay, Sonja M., 120, 142
Macias, Jennifer, 211
McLemore, Thomas, 83, 101, 114
McMillan, Alma, 108, 142
Mandelblatt, Jeanne S., 117, 140, 142
Marazzi, Alfio, 40, 50
Margolese, Richard, 50, 239
Marriott, Ian A., 66, 70
Marshall, Elizabeth G., 66, 71
Mead, Diane, 21
Medical and Health Research Association
   of New York City, 201, 213
Meier, Diane, 116, 142
Mercer-Meidinger, Inc., 82, 101
Mergler, Donna, 66, 71
Messing, Karen, 71
Miller, Anthony B., 14, 20
Miller, Jean Baker, 43, 50, 51
Milliken, Nancy, 207, 213
Minkler, Donald, 186, 189, 214
Minkler, Meredith, 106, 142
Mintz, Morton, 174, 213
Mishell, Daniel R., Jr., 175, 178, 213
Mitchell, James E., 42, 52
Mogel, Wendy, 28, 54
Moien, Mary, 17, 20, 185, 196, 214
Monheit, Alan C., 75, 101
Monson, R.R., 215
Moore, Thomas R., 189, 213
Morgan, Kevin, 45, 52
Mosher, William D., 175, 203, 206, 211,
   213
Moskowitz, G., 230, 239
Mossey, J.M., 120, 142
Mt. Sinai Medical Center, New York City,
   37
Mount Sinai School of Medicine, 52, 142
Mullan, Fitzhugh, 232, 239
Muller, Charlotte, 5, 11, 20, 34, 52, 61,
   71, 74, 84, 101, 117, 142
Muller, James E., 53
Murt, Hilary A., 52, 71

Napolitano, Diane M., 51
Nathanson, Constance A., 24, 52, 66, 68,
   71
National Academy of Sciences, 180
National Cancer Institute (NCI), 11

National Center for Health Services Re-
   search (NCHSR), 7, 20, 34, 38, 52, 154
   163, 166
National Center for Health Statistics
   (NCHS), 5, 6, 8, 16, 21, 59, 61, 62, 64,
   71, 83, 101, 110, 112, 113, 116, 117n,
   121, 142, 186, 190, 213
National Institute on Alcohol Abuse and
   Alcoholism (NIAAA), 46, 52, 64, 68,
   71, 90, 99, 101
National Institute of Mental Health, 27,
   52, 134
National Institutes of Health, 179
National Pharmaceutical Council, 147,
   148, 166
National Research Council, 188
NCHS. See National Center for Health
   Statistics
NCHSR. See National Center for Health
   Services Research
Nehra, Paul C., 211
Nelson, Lawrence J., 207, 213
Nelson, Nancy M., 198, 213
Nelson, Sheryl, 212
Newachek, Paul W., 159, 165
New York Academy of Medicine, 185,
   213
New York Business Group on Health, 90,
   91, 92, 101, 130, 143
NIAAA. See National Institute on Alco-
   hol Abuse and Alcoholism

O'Malley, Patrick M., 6, 20
Origel, Willim, 213
Ory, Marcia G., 136, 140
Ory, Steven J., 186, 214
O'Sullivan, Mary J., 211

Parry, Barbara, 134, 140
Parsons, Michael T., 207, 212
Parsons, P. Ellen, 34, 52, 68, 69, 71
Pasko, Thomas, 21
Pasley, Vickie, 200, 214
Passanante, M.R.C., 66, 68, 71
Pechacek, Terry, 68, 72
Pederson, Linda L., 45, 49
Pego, Maria, 93, 102
Perman, Laurie, 76, 77, 102
Perreault, Leslie, 178, 193, 210
Physician Payment Review Commission,
   116, 143
Pilson, Judith, 89, 102
Pittman-Lindeman, Mary, 148, 149, 166
Pizer, Hank F., 54

acek, Paul J., 185, 195, 196, 211, 214
anned Parenthood, 181, 182
um, Fred, 230, 239
isson, Roger, 50
land, Ronald L., 33, 52
meroy, Claire, 52
pe, Clyde R., 132, 140
owell, Brian, 44, 51
owell-Griner, Eve, 89, 102, 178, 214
ratt, William F., 59, 71, 176, 203, 206, 213, 214
referred Provider Organizations, 81
rosnitz, Leonard R., 31, 52
ublic Health Service Task Force on Women's Health, 134

adecki, Stephen E., 175, 214
adloff, Lenore Sawyer, 43, 52
andolph, Lillian, 21
ay, W.A., 120, 143
eagan, Nancy, 33
eedy, Susan Miller, 90, 102
eimers, Cordelia D., 98, 102
eitman, D., 239
esnick, Robert, 213
hoades, George G., 202, 214
Rice, Dorothy P., 34, 52, 115, 140
Roark, Micki, 212
Roback, Gene, 10, 21
Rodrigo, E.K., 45, 52
Roos, Noralou P., 40, 53, 54
Rosenbaum, Sara, 191, 214
Rosenberg, Martin J., 65–66, 71
Rosenthal, Elaine, 116, 138
Rosenwaks, Zev, 42, 53, 63, 71
Ross, Alan, 215
Ross-Degan, Dennis, 167
Rossiter, Louis F., 80, 86, 102, **154**, 166
Roussel-Uclaf, 184
Rowland, Diane, 109, 143
Roybal, Edward R., 131
Ruchlin, Hirsch S., 129, 143
Rundall, Tom, 149, 166
Russell, Louise B., 33, 54
Russo, Nancy Felipe, 43, 50
Rymer, Marilyn, 153, 167

Sacks, H., 239
Sagan, Leonard A., 37, 53
Saigal, Saroj, 213
Salasin, S., 44, 51
Salkever, David H., 33, 53
Saltzman, D.H., 210
Samson, Suzanne, 27, 53

Sandberg, S.I., 39, 53
Sangl, Judith, 126, 143
Sawyer, Lenore, 53
Schaff, Hartzell V., 50
Schaffner, W., 143
Schechter, Clyde, 36, 53, 142
Schiff, Eugene R., 211
Schlenger, William E., 110, 143
Schlesinger, Mark, 132, 133, 143
Schlesselman, Sarah E., 214
Schlumpf, Maria, 51
Schneiderman, Lawrence J., 29, 49, 51
Schoen, Edgar J., 33, 53
Schoenbaum, S.C., 215
Schori, Alice, 54
Schroeder, Patricia, 180
Schur, Claudia L., **154**, 165
Schwartz, Janet B., 212
Scitovsky, Anne A., 127, 143
Scrimshaw, Susan C.M., 28, 54
Seibel, Michelle M., 204, 214
Seim, Harold C., 52
Sekscenski, Edward S., 122, 143
Select Committee on Aging, 160
Selikoff, Irving J., 65, 71
Shapiro, M., 140, 166
Short, Tobin, 121, 139
Showstack, Jonathan A., 186, 189, 214
Siegenthaler, Walter, 51
Silk, Leonard, 60, 71
Simons, Ronald L., 124, 136, 145
Smith, H., Jr., 239
Smith, Hugh C., 33
Smith, Kathy S., 84, 100
Smith, Mickey C., **119**, 141
Smith, Sandy, 196, 214
Social Security, 132
Social Service Employees Union Local 371, 74, 89, 102
Social Service Employees Union Welfare Fund, 89
Sola, Loredo, 54
Sorenson, Gloria, 68, 72
Soskolne, C.L., 239
Soumerai, Stephen B., 163, 167
Spain, Daphne, 129, 138
Speechley, Mark, 135, 144
Speert, Harold, 187, 215
Stark, Pete, 79
State Insurance Department, 79
Steingart, Richard M., 53
Steptoe, Patrick, 204
Stevens, Beth, 76, 77, 102
Stitt, Lawrence W., 66, 72
Stockbauer, Joseph W., 189, 215
Stoeckle, John D., 53

Stone, Martin L., 42, 53, 63, 71
Stone, Peter H., 53
Stone, Robyn, 106, 107, 108, 126, 142, 143
Strobino, Donna M., 200, 215
Stuckly, Maria A., 66, 70
Sullivan, Joseph P., 192n, 215
Supreme Court, 60, 88, 93, 158, 182, 208

Taffel, Selma M., 185, 195, 196, 214
Talbert, Luther M., 203, 211
Tannenbaum, Terry N., 66, 71
Taskinen, Helena, 65, 71
Taylor, Amy K., 76, 80, 86, 100, 102, 151, **154**, 165, 167
Taylor, K.M., 231, 239
Testa, Marcia A., 50
Texas Task Force on Indigent Health Care, 148, 156, 167
Thacker, S.B., 195, 209
Thomas Jefferson University Hospital, 199
Thompson, Clara, 43
Thornberry, Owen T., 61, 70, 117, 143
Tilly, Jane, 161, 167
Tinetti, Mary E., 135, 144
Tobin, Jonathan N., 36, 53
Toffler, Geoffrey H., 37, 53
Tolchin, Martin, 130, 144, 225n, 239
Toner, Robin, 237, 239
Torres, Aida, 181n, 211, 215
Tracy, Martin B., 106, 144
Treadwell, Marjorie C., 211
Trussell, James, 175, 176, 215
Tsai, Shan P., 90, 102

United Hospital Fund of New York, 104, 122n, 123, 144, 192, 215
University of California San Diego Medical Center, 188
U.S. Congress, 16, 32, 53, 80, 104, 109, 118, 120, 121, 129, 130, 131, 144, 160, 167, 181, 225; Office of Technology Assessment, 179, 215
U.S. Department of Commerce, 63–64, 67, 68, 75–77, 82, 104, 105, 151, **153**; Bureau of the Census, 72, **81**, 102, 144, 167
U.S. Department of Health and Human Services (DHHS), 13, 62–64, 107, 114, 121, 124, 127, 128, 131, 134, 173; Health Care Financing Administration, 144, 150, 151, 158, 160, 167, 190, 215; Public Health Service, 21, 62, 72, 215
U.S. Department of Labor, 87, 92, 102; Bureau of Labor Statistics, **78**

Venning, Penelope J., 66, 72
Ventura, Stephanie J., 190, 215
Verbrugge, Lois M., 23, 53, 104, 110, 111, 134, 145
Veterans Administration, 7, 224
Vezina, Nicole, 71
Vlietstra, Ronald E., 53

Wadman, William M., 110, 143
Wagner, Judith L., 15, 20
Waitzkin, Howard, 53
Waldo, Daniel R., 166
Waldron, Ingrid, 4, 21, **24**, 53, 69, 70
Walker, Andy, 204, 209
Walker, Stephen D., 66, 72
Wallach, Lynn S., 89, 101
Wallen, Jacqueline, 53
Wan, Thomas T., 125, 145
Ward, N., 166
Ward, Roxanne L., 106, 144
Warshaw, Leon M., 77, 102
Washington, A. Eugene, 35, 54
Wassertheil-Smoller, Sylvia, 53
Watkins, Linda M., 99, 102
Weinstein, Milton C., 53, 199, 209
Weisner, Paul J., 209
Weissberg, Joseph B., 52
Weitzman, Sigmund, 32, 54
Welfare Fund, 89
Wennberg, John E., 40, 41, 54
West, Candace, 28, 39, 54
West, Gale E., 124, 136, 145
Wexler, John P., 53
Wiley, M., 209
Williams, Judith, 122
Williams, P., 45, 52
Williams, Ronald L., 195, 215
Willich, Stefan N., 53
Willis, Judith, 32, 54
Wilner, Susan, 192, 196, 215
Wilson, Renate, **154**, 166
Wilson, Ronald W., 117, 143
Wingard, Deborah L., 123, 145
Winickoff, R.N., 215
Witt, Cecilie A., 211
World Health Organization, 184

Yankauer, Alfred, 189, 215

Zambrana, Ruth E., 28, 54
Zilboorg, Gregory, 43

Subject Index

Boldface numbers refer to tables.

abortion, 174, 176, 178–179, 181–184, 237; access to, 59, 180, 182–183, 203; as backup, 174; benefits for, 87, 89; coverage, 58, 88–90, 157–158, 191; epidemiological research in spontaneous, 65; funding, changes in, 181; opposition to, 88, 98, 183, 192; physician attitudes toward, 182–184; public funding of, 164, 222; right to, 192, 208; services, 59, 172, 181–182, 208, 237. *See also* physicians; teenagers; specific issues
Accutane, 180
activities of daily living (ADLs), 112, 114, 122; disabled elderly with limitations of, 125, 162
activity: days, restricted, 110; work-related, 111–112
activity limitation, 61–62, 64, 111–112; disabled elderly with, 125; due to chronic conditions, **95**, 104; self-report on, 111; women's severe, 122. *See also* functional limitations
ADLs. *See* activities of daily living
adolescents. *See* teenagers
affiliation, 124
AFP. *See* alphafetoprotein test
ageism, 135–137, 220, 224
AIDS, 47, 79, 177, 231, 237; men with, 89; patients, 232; women with, 47, 237
AIDS Action Now!, 47, 49
Alaska, 156
alcohol: abuse, 34, 46; 68; dependence, 17, 64; sex differences in use of, 6, **6**, 64
alcoholism, 46; among men, 63–64; insurance for, 89–90; treatment, 64, 99; treatment of women for, 45, 90
alphafetoprotein (AFP) test, 201–202
amniocentesis, 88, 181, 197, 201–202
anesthesiology, 10
anorexia, 42

arthritis, 114, 115
artificial insemination, 88, 206. *See also* in vitro fertilization
Asian women, 207
assets: Medicaid rules concerning, 160
acquired immune deficiency syndrome. *See* AIDS
autonomy, 206–208, 219, 235

balance billing, 131
Basic Health Plan, 79
battering, 27, 63
bed days, **94**, 110; sex differences for, 61
behavior: care-seeking, of women, 4–5; male, 232; of patients, 28; patterns, 26; risky, 68. *See also* physicians
benefit: content, 73; packages, 91, 96; plans, 82, 131
benefits, 58, 77, 106, 109, 236; flexible, 81; fringe, financed by employers, 79; mandated, 96; maternity, 84–88; nonuse of, 90; pregnancy, in group insurance, 220; quality of, 64; repealed, 225; for retirees, 131; Social Security disability, 132; uniform national, under Medicaid, 164; for women, 58, 81, 223. *See also* employed women; employers; Medicare; specific issues
benzodiazepines, 45
biases, 232–233, 235; age, 103; diagnostic, based on sex, 44; measurement, 34. *See also* physicians
biases, gender, 26, 63, 112, 164, 221, 232; in health care, 48, 49; in psychological theories, 43; in treatment, 227
birth, 171, 173, 200; arrangements, family centered, 226; limitation market, 174; limitation methods, 181; models of,

birth (continued)
208; outcomes, 188, 193, 196; rate in
the United States, 179. See also delivery
birthing centers, 88, 99, 185; acceptance
of, by insurances, 229; procedures used
at, 199–200
births, 185–186, 229; breech, 195; EFM
use in, 194; financed by Medicaid, 191;
first, 84, 105; high-risk, 158; home,
185, 186; mistimed, 176; unwanted, 59,
173, 174, 176. See also deliveries;
hospitals
birthweight, 189–190, 199
black males, 77
blacks, 77, 175–176, 178, 186, 203. See
also sex differences
black women, 198, 207; abortions received
by, 178, 181n; births to, 186; contraceptive methods used by, 174, 175; personality disorders in, 45; poverty rates for,
107; prenatal care received by, 197;
widowed, 129. See also mothers
blood pressure, 5, 14, 187
blood tests, 13; for Hepatitis B, 187
Blue Cross, 196
Blue plans, 84–86, 88, 96
Blue Shield, 196
Boston, 192, 196
breast: examinations, 14–15, 222, 224;
operations, 238
breast cancer, 10, 31–32, 221; older wom-
en with, 136; screening, 62–63, 97;
treatment, 62, 226, 231. See also laws
Britain, 45, 184, 204. See also England
bulimia, 41–42

"cafeteria" plans, 81
California, 93, 96, 97n, 148, 188, 195
Canada, 205
Canadian poultry slaughterhouses, 66
cancer, 39, 79, 222; death rates from, 62–
63; due to DES, 194; due to occupation,
65; screening, 97; screening tests for, 15,
117, 225; underuse of chemotheraphy
for, 35. See also breast cancer; lumpectomy; mastectomy
cardiac symptoms, 4–5
cardiovascular disease. See heart disease
cardiovascular operations, 16
care, 3–4, 6, 9, 74–77, 162; alternative
sources of, 226; ambulatory, 114, 115;
changes in incentive structure of, 238;
contraceptive, 227; for elderly, 108; fertility-related, 172; low-cost, 148; newborn, 191; personal, 112, 113, 162; for

poor, 161; pregnancy-related, 157, 228;
self-, 113. See also community-based
care; health care; long-term care; preventive care; specific issues
caregivers, 126–127, 130, 137, 226, 237
cataract surgery, 134–135, 225
catheterization, 36
Catholics, 182
cervical cap, 180
cesareans, 181, 185, 186, 195–197, 229,
238; coverage for, 86; under EFM, 195.
See also HMOs; hospital
changes, 82, 87, 131, 181; eligibility, affecting working poor, 155; in fertility-
related technology, 172; in health care,
233, 238; life, 136; in maternity care,
221; in Medicaid programs, 156. See
also specific issues
Chicago, 200
childbearing, delayed, 59, 91, 181
childbirth. See delivery
child-rearing issues, 91
children, 226; AFDC, 151; in caregiving
role, 122, 126–127, 161; unwanted, 176
cholesterol, 6, 63
chorionic villus sampling (CVS), 202
chronically dependent, 162
circumcision, 33
Civil Rights Act, 92, 171
class differences, 173
Cleveland, 188
clinical trials, 230–231
clinics, 149, 191; abortion, 89; family
planning, 158, 175, 222; for fertility
control services, 182
Commentary Report on State Legislation,
97n, 100
communication, 27–30, 221, 234
community-based care, 124–126, 129,
162, 225. See also services
compelling treatment, 206–207, 229
conditions: acute, 61, **94**, 111; chronic,
62, **93**, **95**, 111, 116, 133; female, 4, 17;
74; male, 4, 17, 33; newly perceived,
41–42; requiring prenatal preventive services, 186–187; responsible for ill
health, 23; services for, 186–187; sex-
specific, 222; subtle, 31
condom, 177, 178
congenital malformation, 65
Consolidated Omnibus Budget Reconciliation Act of 1985, 76, 82
contraception, 174–175, 177, 179, 208;
access to, 59; failures of, 176, 177, 180;
oral, 180; responsibility for, 171, 228.
See also services; specific issues

ntraceptive methods, 174–179, 180, 227–228. *See also* black women; tubal ligations; specific methods

ntraceptive products: menu short-comings in, 175–179; new, slowdown of, 179–180

payments, 82, 129, 131

ronary artery: bypass graft (CABG) surgery, 38; disease, 37, 115; disease, sex differences in prevalence of, 37. *See also* heart disease; surgery

st, 68–69, 83, 131, 178, 196; control, 57, 97; cutting, 98; -effectiveness, 12, 233; shifting, 70. *See also* health care costs; illness; infertility; specific issues

st sharing, 73, 74, 97, 223; for acute care, 225; Medicare, 109; by needy, 150; during pregnancy, 157; provisions, 83, 108; sex-neutral, 97

ounseling, 201–202, 205–206, 222

ourts, 160, 183, 207, 237

overage: of cancer screening services, 64; dual, 107–108; group, 163; for interrupted employment, 97; knowledge of, 129; loss of, through divorce, 76, 223; mandated, 190–191; of needy, by states, 149; percentages with, 75–76; for peripheral workers, 77–79; quality of, through employment, 79–82; services excluded from, 149–150; sex differences in rate of, 57; of women, 58, 73, 128–129, 190, 223. *See also* abortion; dependents; maternity; specific issues

rossover population, 107–108

CVS. *See* chorionic villus sampling

daily living, 112–113, 114

Dalkon shield, 174, 177, 219, 221

daughters, 126–127, 161

death rates, 24, 62, 67–68. *See also* mortality

decision making, 31

deductibles, 82, 83, 86; changes in, 131

Deficit Reduction Act (DEFRA), 155, 156

deliveries, 16, 238; HMO, 192; vaginal, 196, 197

delivery, 93, 199; alternative approaches to, 198; alternative models of, 184–185, 220; protection for, 86; vacation leave after, 94. *See also* labor; medical model of delivery

dependency, 120, 162, 164

dependents, coverage of, 82, 98, 223, 226

depression, 36, 43–45, 63; in old age, 119–120, 236

DES. *See* diethylstilbestrol

Detroit, 23

diagnoses, **14**, 17, 44, 69

diagnostic categories in health care, 69. *See also* services

diagnostic methods, prenatal, 202

diagnostic radiology, 10

Diagnostic and Statistical Manual of Mental Disorders (DSM-III), 44

diaphragm, 178

diethylstilbestrol (DES), 194, 219, 221

disability, 68, 113; acute, 110–111; days, 61; in old age, 225; in women, 112, 122, 224

disabled, 107, 125, 161

discharges, 4, 16–18, 108, 121, 122. *See also* hospital: discharge rates

discrimination, 60, 220

diseases, 3, 11; of both sexes, 35–39; causing death in women, 134; chronic, 64; fatal, 63; gender comparisons of, 4. *See also* conditions; heart disease; occupational disease; specific diseases

District of Columbia, 181n

divorce, 59, 223; loss of coverage through, 76, 223

doctor–patient encounters, 28–29

doctor–patient relationship, 9, 25, 48, 180, 221; conflicting expectations in, 29; in HMOs, 132; problems in, 234

doctors. *See* physicians

Donovan Act, 85n

Down syndrome, 201

drinkers, 34. *See also* alcoholism

drug: abuse, 34, 172, 237; addiction, 64; mentions, 118, 119; use, by elderly, 118–120, 134

drugs, 163; abortifacient, 184; analgesic, 118; contraceptive, 219, 221; outpatient, 225; used to induce labor, 185; used for pregnancy, 187, 219, 221. *See also* alcohol; psychotropic drugs; specific drugs

DSM-III. *See* Diagnostic and Statistical Manual of Mental Disorders

dual coverage, 107–108

dual enrollment, 153

duplication, 73, 81

eating disorders, 41–42, 63

ECG. *See* electrocardiogram

eclampsia, 188

Economist, 98, 100

Edinburgh, 42

education, 58–60; prenatal, 91

educational level, 105, 224
EFM. *See* electronic fetal monitoring
ELAs (elderly living alone), 106–108, 124–
    126; sex differences of, 124–125
elderly, 99, 103–105, 224–226, 236, 238;
    activity limitations of poor, 111; black,
    122n; community-dwelling, 126; differ-
    ences in health of, 110, 137; disabled,
    125, 161; economic status of, 103; func-
    tional limitations among, 112–114; gen-
    der comparisons, using public payment
    sources, 114; gender issues among, 133–
    134, 136, 137, 138; health care re-
    imbursement for, 130–133; low-income,
    108–109; married, 160; Medicaid eligi-
    bility of, 159–162; payment sources for,
    114; third-party payers for, 127–130;
    use of health services by, 114–126. *See
    also* crossover population; sex differ-
    ences; specific issues
elderly women, 105, 138, 220, 225–226,
    236; care received by, 134–135, 136,
    161; coverage of, 128–129; dependency
    problems among, 120; enrolled under
    Medicare, 127, **128**, 162; incomes of,
    123; life expectancy for, 104; poverty
    among, 106, 107, 161, 227; quality of
    life of, 105. *See also* mammography;
    specific issues
electrocardiogram (ECG), 4, 9, 13, 36
electronic fetal monitoring (EFM), 185,
    194–195, 198, 229
embryo donation, 204
employed women, 105, 223; married, 76,
    81; maternity benefits for, 86–87; occu-
    pations of, 80. *See also* health care; la-
    bor force participation; working women
employees, 77–80, 87, 92. *See also*
    workers
employer policies, 91
employers: benefits from, 81–82, 89, 132,
    223; contributions by, 57–58, 75–77,
    79–82, 163; cost cutting by, 98; cost
    shifting by, 70; and family needs, 90–
    96; health care coverage from, 73, 79,
    131, 138, 237; sex differences in cover-
    age through, 75–77, 164. *See also* laws;
    workplace
employment, 44, 80, 221; examinations
    required for, 13; full-time, 77, **78**; gen-
    der comparisons for, 59; inequality in,
    220; loss of, 34; part-time, 69, 77, **78**,
    79; part-year, 69, 77; without benefits,
    58. *See also* work
England, 39
estrogen therapy, 63

examinations, 9, 13–15, 224; breast, 14–
    15, 222, 224; sex differences in diagnos-
    tic and screening, 13
exercise, 33, 63, 112
expenses, 83, 154; of IVF, 205; of long-
    term care, 162; Medicaid, for older-
    women households, 161; medical, in old
    age, 106, 108; for personal health ser-
    vices, 153; sex differences in, 7–8, 127–
    128. *See also* out-of-pocket expenses

families: AFDC, 155; black and white, 105
family: leave, 95; needs, 90–91, 96. *See
    also* income; needs
family planning, 58, 183; counselors, 175;
    role of doctors in, 181; services, 91,
    158, 175, 182, 222, 237; users, 174;
    visits, 58, 175. *See also* clinics
fatality. *See* mortality
"Father and Mother Know Best," 183,
    210
Federal Employees Health Benefits
    Program, 88
federal policies, 181, 182
fee-for-service: patients, 196; practice, 48,
    74; providers, 130
female-headed family households, 151,
    153
feminists, 219, 228; critique of profession-
    al dominance by, 40; views of, 9–10,
    12, 32, 44, 173
fertility, 59, 172; control, 57, 63, 177,
    192, 235; control services, 174, 182,
    227; control technology, 208; impaired,
    203–204; limitation, 173–174, 180–
    181; planning, 173, 201; -related care,
    83–84, 219, 227–230. *See also*
    infertility
fetal development, abnormalities of, 183
fetal rights, 192, 207, 228–229
financing, 57–58, 73; health care, 96, 133,
    223; health care, for elderly, 137; long-
    care, 159; programs for health, 103. *See
    also* health care; payment
fractures, 135, 225
Framingham, 135; research project, 36
France, 184
functional limitations, 68, 112–113, 114,
    163, 225

gallbladder disease, 36
gender, 48, 57, 73, 137, 232–235; fertility-
    related care and, 227–230; and the
    health care market, 223–227; influence

of, on elderly, 103; issues, 26; and measurement of indirect costs of illness, 33–35; and physician attitudes, 136, 221; -related problems in health care, 222; roles, 235

gender comparisons, 3, 5; in death rates, 67–68; in drug use by elderly, 118–119; in employer or union contributions, 75–76; of full- and part-time workers, 77–81; in health care costs, 68–69, 83; NMCES, 8; of nursing home residents, 122, 126; of working women and men, 66–68, 77. *See also* hospital; illness; sex differences; specific issues

gender equality, 3, 49, 86, 90, 233, 235, 238

general checkup, 13. *See also* examinations

general and family practitioners (GFP): treatment of Medicaid patients by, 148; visits to, 7, **8**, 8, 9, 12, **15**; women, 10, 11

genetic defects, 171, 203, 206

genetic services, 201–203

GFP. *See* general and family practitioners

GIFT (gamete intrafallopian transfer), 204, 205

group health plans, 75–77

group insurance, 221; for elderly, 106, 138; inclusion of part-time workers in, 78; maternity benefits in, 84, 93; pregnancy benefits in, 220; privacy problems in connection with, 90; women with, 156

groups, 149; against women's reproductive autonomy, 172, 183; minority, 201, 208; special, 9, 155

Halsted method, 32

health: benefit programs, 58, 227; fetal, 229; issues of women, 221; levels, 5–6, 103–104; levels, cohort differences in, 105; sex differences in, 5, **5**, 61, 67, 110–114; status, 110, 148, 154, 162; status, self-reported, 5, 61, 110; variables, 154; work and, 64–68; of working-age adults, 60. *See also* risks; sex differences; specific issues

health care, 73, 208; costs, 57–58, 60, 68–70, 82, 127; criticisms of, 220–221; of employed women, 58, 59; financing, 231; gender-related problems in, 222; interaction between gender and, 57–58, 137, 221; market, 87, 223–227; for poor, 107; providers, nonphysician, **154**;

reforms, 235–236; research, 233; for women, 147. *See also* elderly; reproductive care; workplace; specific issues

health care system, 219–221, 224, 225, 238; economic problems of, 49; elderly in, 133; purposes of adaptations made by, 26; sexism in, 219

health centers, women's, 221

health maintenance organizations. *See* HMOs

health services, 114, 225; home, 124, 127, 128, 129; personal, 153, **154**; received under Medicaid, limitations on, 149; research, 232

heart disease, 16–17, 36–38, 62–63, 114, 232. *See also* coronary artery; myocardial infarction; surgery

hepatitis B, 187–188, 193

Hispanic women, 107, 207

historical controls, 230

HIV: infection, 47, 89, 164n, 172; seropositive, fetuses, 229. *See also* AIDS

HMOs, 29, 48, 81, 130–133, 236; cesareans for patients of, 196; effectiveness of, 97; needy enrollees in, 150; prenatal care, provisions of, 192–193; risk-sharing, 109; study of female and male physicians in, 30

home care, 106, 149, 161, 236

homemakers, 34, 58, 68, 74

homemaker services, 106, 162; value placed on, 34

home management, 112–113

homework, 78

homosexuality, 232

hormones, 24

hospital: admission, 121, 196; coverage, 86; days, 149; discharge rates, 120–121; gender comparisons for use of, 16, 83; services, inpatient, **154**; tertiary, 199; use, 3–5, 16–17, 83, 106, 120–121, 128; use of cesareans, 196

hospitalization, 74, 91, 121

hospitals, 221, 227; admission of Medicaid patients by, 148–149; births in, 185, 229; differences among, 200; early discharge from, 98; payment system for, 130

householders, 75–76, 113, 150–151

Human Immunodeficiency Virus. *See* HIV

husbands: as caregivers, 126; health care coverage through, 73, 76, 81, 106, 129; institutionalized, 123

hypertension, 74, 114, 115, 119; in pregnancy, 188

hypnotics, 45

hysterectomies, 32, 39–41, 220, 238

IADLs. *See* instrumental activities of daily living
Illinois, 197
illness: acute, 61, 64, 129; chronic, 57, 104, 106, 129, 132, 236; costs of, 34, 69; gender comparisons of acute, 61–62; indirect costs of, 33–35, 48; measures of, **94–95**; services for, 236; severity of, 122. *See also* diseases; occupational disease
impoverishment of spouses, 160, 162
IMs. *See* internists
income, 224, 234; and AFDC eligibility, 155; family, 59, 150–151; level, for Medicaid eligibility, 150, 157; Medicaid rules concerning, 160; of pregnant women, 189; protected, 123–124. *See also* retirement
Indiana, 87
indirect costs, 25, 33–35, 48
inequality, 43, 220–222, 224
infertility, 171, 181, 203–206, 208; care, market for, 229; services, 203; treatments, 172, 204, 206, 228; treatments, cost of, 205–206
informed choice, 33
informed consent, 32, 220, 221, 231
inguinal hernia, 40
injuries, 60, 69, **94**, 111; gender comparisons of work, 64–66
innovations, 230–232
inpatients, 16, 127, **128**, 130, **154**
Insight and Instatus, 88, 101
institutionalization, 123, 161, 162; gender comparisons for, of elderly, 159
instrumental activities of daily living (IADLs), 112, 113
insurance, 73–77, 79, 82, 220, 223; claims, underreporting on, 90; companies, 130, 206, 229; for employed adults, 57; hospital, 128; long-term care, 129–130; nonprofit, 85; policies, alternative, 133; for pregnancy, 87, 189; product liability, 179; services, unbundling of, 88; stop-loss, 130; use of, for abortions, 88–89. *See also* alcoholism; group insurance; private insurance; specific issues
interarea variation, 40–41
internists (IMs): visits to, 7, **8**, 8, 9, 12, **15**; women, 10, 11
intrauterine device (IUD), 173–174, 176–178, 183

in vitro fertilization (IVF), 88, 172, 203–206, 228
Iowa, 87
ischemic heart disease, 36
IUD. *See* intrauterine device
IVF. *See* in vitro fertilization

JAMA, 207
jobs, 58, 92, 223–224; equality in choice of, 90. *See also* employment

labeling, 42
labor, 198–199, 200, 227; complications of, 186; inducement of, 185, 196
labor force participation, of women; 34, 35, 57–60, 66–67, 69, 73
Lamaze training, 185
Lancet, 184, 212
laws, 32, 155, 160, 221; abortion, 88, 158, 192, 237; concerning Medicare, 109, 149; covering employers, 87; covering first-time pregnant women, 156; protecting women with breast cancer, 32–33; tax, 80. *See also* specific laws
leave, 91–96, 223. *See also* maternity
Leboyer method, 198–199
legislation, federal, 84, 220
length of stay, 121, 122
life expectancy, 104
longevity, 24–25, 104
long-term care, 129–130, 131, 132, 162; eligibility for, 147; financing, 236; gender issues in, 159; need for, 225; reasons for sex differences in, 123; services for, 227; use of Medicaid for, 159, 161. *See also* nursing homes
low-income women, 157, 189, 190–192, 206, 219
lumpectomy, 32, 33n, 231. *See also* mastectomy

Maine, 40, 41
male physicians, 30, 221; attitudes of, 219–220; attitudes of, toward older women, 136–137; behavioral tendencies of, 27–30
malignancies, 16. *See also* cancer
malpractice: claims, 183; suits, 193, 205, 229; litigation, 232
mammography, 14, 15, 97n, 222; benefit under Medicare, 16, 138, 236; for elderly women, 117–118
managed care systems, 79

anitoba, 40; Health Insurance, 41
anufacturers, 219
arital break-up. *See* divorce
arket demand, 226–227
arried women, 120, 190, 223; childless, 105; contraceptive methods used by, 175; coverage rates of, 76; institutionalization of, 159; in labor force, 59, 81; unwanted children for ever-, 176. *See also* unmarried women
aryland, 76
assachusetts, 97n, 160, 192
astectomy, 31–32, 63, 97n, 221
aternal and Child Health Block Grant program, 191
aternity, 83–88; care, 180, 184–186, 192, 221, 229; care, provided by Medicaid, 190–192; costs, changes in, 87; coverage, 57–58, 85–88, 99; coverage, for teenagers, 91; interpretation of, 43; leave, 58, 91–96, 98; practices, 198–201; services, 172. *See also* benefits; technology; specific issues
MCCA. *See* Medicare Catastrophic Coverage Act
Medicaid, 6, 107, 147–149, 163–165, 196, 226–227, 236; benefits for divorced women, 76; coverage, 108, 148, 156; coverage, loss of, 155; coverage for prenatal services, 158, 191; disabled elderly on, 125; for disabled husbands, 106; elderly on, 120, 122n; eligibility, 73, 75, 123–124, 129–130, 132, 162, 237; eligibility, of elderly, 159–162; eligibility standards, 150, 160; payment of abortion by, 181; presumptive eligibility, 156–157; preventive services under, 16; reform of, 156, 161; sources of variability within, 149–150; women on, 4, 114, 123, 163, 165; women, poverty, and, 150–154. *See also* elderly; long-term care; maternity; specific issues
medical decisions, 29–30
medical model of delivery, 184–185, 229
Medicare, 41, 82, 107–109, 127–128, 138; application of HMOs to, 132, 133; benefits, 109, 159, 162, 163; changes in, 131; cognitive services under, 238; coverage for preventive services, 117; discharges for enrollees, 121; eligibility for, 128, 131–132, 132n; home care under, 161, 162; increase of fees by, 116; payment of nursing home days by, 129; physician payment method, 130; preventive services under, 16; reimbursement by, 98, 127; value scale for, 29.

See also elderly women; laws; mammography; specific issues
Medicare Catastrophic Coverage Act (MCCA), 109, 118, 122–124, 156, 160; coverage of pregnant women in, 190–191
"Medigap," 107n, 108, 132
men, 42, 107, 223; activity limitations of, 111, 113; disease causing death in, 134; elderly, enrolled under Medicare, 127, **128**; infertility in, 203, 228; married, 76; occupational exposure of, 65–66; reproductive health of, 92; working, 74; use of, for clinical testing, 134. *See also* black males; gender comparisons; male physicians; sex differences
menopause, 120
mental health care, 43–47, 136; gender comparisons for, 44–45
mental illness, 119, 219; costs of, 34; insurance for, 89–90; in older patients, 120. *See also* depression; personality disorders
Michigan, 156
midwives, 88, 99, 158, 185, 187; lay, 186
military service, 13
Minnesota, 68, 97n
miscarriage, 65, 65n; risks of, 92
Missouri, 87
mistiming, 176
mobility, 113–114
modules used by National Ambulatory Medical Care Survey, 12–13, **15**
Monthly Labor Review, 94, 101
morbidity, 33, 35, 198, 199
"Morbidity Costs: National Estimates and Economic Determinants" (D.H. Salkever), 33
mortality: after bypass surgery, 38, 231; of crossovers, 108; diseases causing, 134; drop in, 104; gender comparisons, after myocardial infarction, 37; gender differences in adult, 24, 67–68; infant, 179, 189; rates, 24–25, 38–39, 41, 195; risks, 57
mothers, 126–127; care for black and white, 190; findings of obstetrical practices for black and white, 197–198; teenage, 190; working, 91; X rays received by black, 197–198
myocardial infarctions (MIs), 17, 36, 37

NAMCS. *See* National Ambulatory Medical Care Survey
NARAL News, 181n, 213

Nassau County, New York, 159
National Ambulatory Medical Care Survey
  (NAMCS), 116, 118, 119; of 1981, 8, 9,
  10, 12–13; of 1985, 114
National Health Care Expenditures Survey
  of 1977, 128
National Health Interview Survey, 6,
  121n; of 1978, 115; of 1986, 7, 60–61;
  Supplement on Aging (SoA) of 1984,
  111–114
National Hospital Discharge Survey
  (NHDS), 17, 37, 121, 121n, 196
National Long-Term Care Survey, 126
National Medical Care Expenditure Survey
  (NMCES), 7, 8, 74, 119, 129; of 1977,
  118, 124
National Medical Care Utilization and Expenditure Survey (NMCUES), 108, 110;
  of 1980, 153
National Natality Survey of 1980, 185n,
  190, 197
National Nursing Home Survey of 1985,
  122
The Nation's Health, 94, 101, 201, 213
NBER Digest, 59, 71, 101
needs: of elderly, 113; health care, 23, 63;
  family, 90–96; future analytic, 232–235;
  interaction between gender and health,
  57; of men, 33; of women, 8, 63. See
  also reproductive needs
needy. See poor
neonatal intensive care units (NICU), 196
neural tube defects (NTDs), 201, 202
never-married women, 175, 176
new conceptions, 204–206
New Hampshire, 78
New Jersey, 192n
New York City, 89, 122n, 161, 201;
  "Blue" plans, 84–85
New York law (L. 1985, ch. 203), 32
New York State, 32, 85n, 90, 126; abortion in, 158, 191; genetic services in,
  201; Medicaid patients in, 160
New York Times, 41, 52, 59, 71, 84, 101,
  118, 125, 136, 143, 158, 160, 166, 180,
  182, 184, 191, 195, 197, 213, 224, 227,
  229n, 239
NMCES. See National Medical Care Expenditure Survey
nonpoor, comparison of non-Medicaid
  poor and, 162–163
nonsurgical diagnostic procedures, 16
North, 197
Nova Scotia, 205
NTDs. See neural tube defects
nursing, 66

nursing home: care, 159, 162, 225; costs,
  160; expenditures, 127
nursing homes, 122–123, 126, 129; admission of Medicaid patients to, 162;
  payments for admission to, 159–160;
  problems for poor in, 160–161. See also
  gender comparisons

OBRA. See Omnibus Budget Reconciliation Act
obstetrician–gynecologists, 186, 207; and
  abortion, 182; attitude of, toward fetus,
  229; genetic counseling by, 183; sex
  differences in attitudes of, 28–29; treatment of Medicaid patients by, 148, 191;
  visits to, 8, 11, 12, 14, 15; women, 10–
  11, 29, 40
obstetrics–gynecology, 8–11, 17, 187,
  189–190; cases, 193; traditional practices in, 200–201. See also technology
occupational disease, 64–67
occupational exposure, 65–67
Oklahoma, 97n
Omnibus Budget Reconciliation Act
  (OBRA), 79; 155–156
Ontario, 45
ophthalmology, 8, 10
orthopedics, women, 10
out-of-pocket expenses, 4, 64, 83, 134;
  due to balance billing, 131; for elderly,
  109, 124, 127, 225; for women, 60
outpatient: department, visit of, 115;
  drugs, 225; insurance, 128; settings, 16,
  17, 98; surgery, 98; treatment, 224
overtreatment, 99, 137

Pap test, 14–16, 97, 180, 222, 224, 231;
  coverage of, 117; given by women doctors, 11; importance of, 13, 62; under
  Medicare, 16, 138
parents, 126–127
part-time employees, 77–79, 237
pathology, women in, 10
patients: conversations of physicians and,
  28; information supplied by, 27, 235; as
  negotiators, 200–201; women, 27–30,
  45, 219, 220. See also doctor–patient
  relationship; fee-for-service; inpatients;
  specific issues
payment, 116, 130, 150; AFDC, 157, 160;
  of home health visits, 124; reform, 238;
  source of, 3, 7, 154; for ultrasound,
  199. See also copayments
pediatrics, 8; women in, 10, 11

lvic inflammatory disease (PID), 35
nsion benefits, 106
ripheral vascular disease, 36
rsonality disorders, 44–45
armacists, 180
ysician contacts, 3, 114; gender comparisons for, 7, **18**, **19**
ysicians, 207, 220, 232; attitudes of,
   27–30, 38, 136, 220, 234; attitudes of,
   toward abortion, 182–184; behavior of,
   116, 119, 219; biases in training of,
   221; comparison of female and male,
   11; conversations of patients and, 28;
   economic self-interest of, 48; involvement with Medicaid of, 148; negotiating
   with patients, 200; personal outlooks of,
   31–32; prenatal care given by, 187; private, 148; sex differences in consulting
   of, 7, 12; sex differences in use of, 61;
   utilization of, 5–11, 23, 162–163; work-
   loads of, 16–17. See also doctor–patient
   relationship; male physicians; women
   doctors; specific specialists
hysicians Desk Reference, 180, 194
hysician services: ambulatory, **154**; use
   of, 83, 114–115, 153
ID. See pelvic inflammatory disease
ill, 175, 177, 178, 183
lacebo effect, 198–199
MS. See premenstrual syndrome
oor, 104, 147–149; cost-sharing by, 150;
   elderly, 111, 160; with Medicaid, 151,
   153, 155; near-, 108, 109, 155; non-
   Medicaid, 162, 163; programs for, 192;
   services for, 227
poverty, 73, 220, 236; level, definition of,
   151; market demand and, 226–227; in
   old age, 106–107, 109; vulnerability of
   women to, 103, 147; and women, and
   Medicaid, 150–154, 164, 191. See also
   elderly women
practitioners. See physicians
preeclampsia, 188
pregnancies: ectopic, 186; high-risk, 174,
   180, 181, 192; unwanted, 178n, 180
pregnancy, 84, 156, 171, 227, 228; benefits for, 57, 85–87; costs of, 69; disability, 220; drug abuse in, 237; educational and emotional support in, 187;
   failure of timing in, 176, leave, unpaid,
   93; Medicaid coverage for, 155–158;
   outcomes, 65, 65n, 189, 199; policies
   regarding, 147; psychological aspects of,
   199; rate after tubal ligation, 177;
   -related programs, 92; teenage, 84, 91,
   157; use of DES in, 194, 219; work dur-

ing, 83. See also drugs; prenatal care; X
   rays
Pregnancy Discrimination Act (PDA), 7n,
   87, 92
pregnant women, 172, 189, 228; coverage
   of, 75n, 190; low-income, 157, 189;
   manual for, 200; risk taking, 92; services for, 156
prejudice, 89
premenstrual syndrome (PMS), 26, 42, 63,
   99, 226
prenatal care, 171, 173, 186–187, 207;
   coverage for, 158; delayed use of, 58,
   156, 157, 189; early, 190, 191, 197; effect of HMOs on access to, 192–193;
   on-site, 91; problems in, 187–188; programs for low-income women, 190–192
prenatal services, 172, 186–187, 193; covered by Medicaid, 158, 191; effect of,
   on infant mortality, 189
prescribing, 118–120, 134, 226. See also
   drugs
prevention, 11–19, 132, 208, 222, 237;
   fall, 135; of heart disease, 63; opportunities, 57; separation of treatment from,
   85
preventive care, 4, 107, 116–118
preventive services, 11–16, 74, **116**, 116–
   118, 222, 225; effectiveness of, 14; prenatal, 186–187; use of, by women, 12
privacy, 88–90, 237; threats to, 98
private insurance, 4, 7, 163; access to
   abortion under, 164; coverage of cesareans by, 196; elderly with, 109, 114,
   128–129, 159; workers without, 155,
   223. See also "Medigap"
procedures: obstetrical, 207; relation between outcomes and use of, 199; sex
   differences in, 17, 121
proctosigmoidoscopy, 15
programs: for future elderly, 105, 236;
   home care, under Medicaid, 161; nutrition and health education, 156. See also
   specific programs and issues
pro-life activists, 172, 183, 184
prostate conditions, 4, 17, 33
prostatectomy, 40–41
psychiatrists, 44–45
psychiatry, 10, 119; women in, 10, 11.
   See also mental health care
psychotropic drugs, 118–120, 137; prescribing, 99, 134, 220, 226; use of, by
   women, 45, 219

quality of life, 25, 31–33, 231, 235; of
    elderly women, 105; improvement, 39

race, 44–45
racial differences, 197–198; in reproduc-
    tive care, 173, 190
RAD. See restricted activity days
random selection, 231
reforms, 156, 161, 235–238
regional differences, 197–198
reimbursement, 26, 30, 103, 121, 202;
    issues, vulnerability to, 130–133; under
    Medicare, 98, 127
relationships, subordinate, 39–40. See also
    doctor–patient relationship
reproductive care, 90, 171–173, 208, 235–
    237; fragmentation of, 180–182; use of
    technology in, 193; women's autonomy
    in, 206
reproductive impairments, 65–66
reproductive needs, women's, 3, 4, 97,
    172
reproductive services, 83, 98, 183, 228;
    connection between social expectations
    and, 172; differential treatment of, 84;
    problems related to, 173
research, 233–234, 237, 238
restricted activity days (RAD), 61, 65
retirees, 131, 226, 236; coverage of, 131,
    138
retirement, 131–132; income, 106, 150;
    independence after, 112. See also pen-
    sion benefits
Rhode Island, 88, 197
rights: abortion, 192, 208; patient, 26;
    women's, 207–208. See also fetal rights
risk: assumption of, 25n; attached to
    births, 185, 186; attached to surgery,
    41; exposure, 24, 48; factors, 135; nutri-
    tional, 189; political, 163; pools, 79; re-
    duction of, through prenatal education,
    91
risks: genetic, 201, 203; health, 24, 66;
    health, work-related, 68, 92, 224; pre-
    natal, 187, 192; to women, 66. See also
    workers
RU486, 184

San Francisco, 148
schizophrenia, 34
screening, 222, 233; genetic, 201; for risks
    in pregnancy, 187; services, 12–13, 64,
    237. See also breast cancer; cancer; Pap
    test

second opinion, 96; programs, 97, 232
self-interest, 48
sensory impairments, 113–114
services, 124, 129, 163, 236; ambulatory,
    127; clinic, 149; community-based, 149
    162; contraceptive, 172, 226, 237; diag-
    nostic, 9, 12–13; during pregnancy, 157
    fertility-related, 228; genetic, 201–203;
    home-based, 98, 106, 149; in-home,
    126; for needy, covered by states, 149–
    150; nonphysician, 235, 236; personal
    care, 162; sex differences in use of, by
    elderly, 125–126; use of, 5, 23, 233. See
    also health services; physician services;
    preventive services; reproductive ser-
    vices; specific issues
sex: ratios, 17; similarities, 96–99
sex differences, 5, 18, 23, 96–99, 137; for
    blacks and whites, 77, 122n; in cardio-
    vascular testing, 30; in caregiving, 126;
    in coverage of elderly, 128–129; in dis-
    charge rates for elderly, 120–121; for
    elderly, 103, 105, 106; of elderly need-
    ing help, 112–113; in incomes, 123; in
    limitations in usual activities for elderly
    111–112; of Medicaid and non-Medi-
    caid population, 152, 153; research on,
    233–234; in sensory impairments of eld
    erly, 114. See also expenses; health;
    visits; specific issues
sexism, 219, 220
sickle cell disease, 201
single parenthood, 150, 190
single-parent households, 91, 98, 223
single women, 76, 161
skilled nursing facility (SNF), 122, 128,
    128–129
SMI. See supplementary medical insurance
smoking, 24n; reversal, 62–63, 222; sex
    differences in, 6, 6, 68
social contacts, 125
Social Security Act, 191
Social Security Disability Insurance (SSDI),
    132n
Social Security system, 107
sons, 126
South, 197, 198
spending down, 157, 160, 163
spermicides, 178
spouses: financial position of, in Medicaid,
    160–161, 162. See also married women
states, 164, 226; abortion services by, 181,
    182; coverage of needy by, 149–150;
    need standards of, 155; personal care
    programs in, 162; prenatal care pro-
    grams in, 191; restrictions by, 158; ser-

vices for pregnant women offered by,
  156–157; spending down in, 160
ereotypes, 42, 89–90, 97, 99; age, 135;
  masculine, 44; psychological, 220; social, of women, 44, 59; about women,
  63, 134, 219
erilization, 175–178, 180, 219; access to,
  59; contraceptive, 174, 228; coverage of,
  88; voluntary, offered by states, 158
op-loss provisions, 83
ress, on-the-job, 67
roke, 62
upplement on Aging (SoA), 111–113
upplemental Security Income (SSI), 124,
  163
upplementary medical insurance (SMI)
  services, 127–128, **128**
urgery, 16, 17, 31–33, 238; coronary artery bypass, 37–38, 231; general, **8**, 8,
  10; heart, 16; overuse of radical, 219;
  prostate, 33, 40–41; unnecessary, 32,
  41; women in, 10. See also cataract surgery; specific issues
urgical procedures: gender comparisons
  of, 16
urvey of Income and Program Participation, 68
witzerland, 40
yracuse medical center, 224

Tax Equity and Fiscal Responsibility Act
  of 1982, 157
Tay-Sachs disease, 201
echnology, 30; birth-related, 185, 229;
  criticism of obstetric, 229; fertility-
  related, changes in, 172; findings on
  differences in use of obstetric, 197–198;
  maternity, 193–198, 201–203; new,
  221, 230–232; reproductive, 204, 206,
  208
eenagers: abortions for, 178–179; contraception for, 176; married, 190; pregnant, 84, 91, 157; services for, 174, 175;
  sexuality of, 172, 188. See also mothers
Tennessee, 150
tests, 9, 13, 15–16; for assessing risks of
  pregnancy, 186, 187; cardiovascular, 30;
  maternity, 88; of new treatments, 134;
  prenatal genetic, 181, 183, 201–202. See
  also blood tests; cancer; Pap test
"test tube babies," 204. See also in vitro
  fertilization
third-party payers, 127–130
tranquilizers, 45, 118, 120; use of minor,
  119, 226

transfer, 92
treatment, 23–26, 35, 74, 226; communication and, 27–28; compulsory, 207,
  237; decisions, 232; early, 11; heart disease, 38; gender bias in, 227; PMS, 42;
  process, gender within, 133–134, 231;
  programs, 90; separation of prevention
  from, 85; sex differences in, 25; unequal, 24, 25; women's, 24, 134. See
  also breast cancer; compelling treatment;
  infertility; undertreatment; specific issues
treatments, 9, 35–36; for AIDS, 47; alternative, 38; for bulimia and anorexia, 42;
  preferred, 31
tubal ligations, 177, 178, 228
two-earner couples, 58, 59
two-earner families, 91, 98, 223, 237

ultrasound, 197, 199, 202, 229
undertreatment, 35, 99, 137; of women,
  135, 136
underutilization: of mammography, 117;
  of therapies, 35–36
undervaluation of quality of life, 31–32
uninsured, 75, 82; Basic Health Plan for,
  79
unions, 67, 91; sex differences in coverage
  through, 75–77, 164
United Kingdom. See Britain
unmarried women, 105, 190
urinalyses, 13
utilization, 23, 83, 97, 98; of crossovers,
  108; gender comparisons of, 8–9, 74;
  importance of, 13; physician's sex and,
  10. See also physicians; underutilization

vaginal birth after cesarean (VBAC), 196
variables, 154, 233. See also Medicaid
Vermont, 150
veterans, 114, 224; women, 224
Virginia, 125
Virgin Islands, 151
visits: causes of, 115; comparisons for,
  162–163; content of, 3, 4, 233; drug,
  117; home health, 122, 124; increase of,
  with insurance, 74; number of, 3–4,
  132, 154; office, by elderly, 114–116;
  paid by Medicaid, 191; prenatal, 186,
  192; preventive, 64, 116; probability of,
  153; sex differences for office, 7, 8, 12–
  13, 114–115. See also family planning;
  specific physicians

wage: determination, 79; ratio,
    female–male, 59–60
wages, 34, 57, 60
Wales, 39
Wall Street Journal, 92, 95, 102
Washington: Basic Health Plan, 79
Webster v. Reproductive Health Service,
    Inc., 158, 182, 237n
wellness programs, 67
West Coast, 127
white men, 45
whites, 77, 175–176, 178, 203. See also
    sex differences
white women, 45, 186, 197. See also
    mothers
WIC (Women-Infants-Children) program,
    156, 189
widowed persons, 116, 118, 122
widowers, 115
widowhood, 116, 128, 150
widows, 115, 128–129, 161, 224; pension
    payments for, 106
Wisconsin, 67
wives, 105, 123, 137; impoverishment of,
    160, 162
women: AFDC clients, 155, 156; autono-
    my of, 206–208, 219; body integrity of,
    32; differences between older and youn-
    ger, 60, 84; discontent of, 219; divorced,
    76; exploitation of, 26; output values
    for, 34; perceptions of, 42; physical lim-
    itations of, 58–59; and poverty, and
    Medicaid, 150–154, 164; in rural areas,

198; valuation of, 34, 48, 67, 86; with-
    out private insurance, 74–75. See also
    black women; married women; mothers;
    white women; specific groups and issues
women doctors, 3–4, 10–11, 28–30, 40
women's movement, 219
work, 64–68; home-based, 78; part-time,
    69, 77, 78; part-year, 77. See also activi-
    ty; employment; jobs; risks
workers: contingent, 237; covered by
    group health plan, socioeconomic char-
    acteristic of, 76–77; full-time, 80–81;
    indemnity plan for federal, 88; low-
    income, 80, 82, 83; maternity benefits
    for, 86; occupational hazards for, 65–
    68; part-time, 80–81, 237; peripheral,
    77–79. See also gender comparisons; oc-
    cupational exposure
working women, 74, 98; government help
    for, 224; health care coverage, problems
    of, 73, 77; health risks of, 68; protec-
    tion for, 66–67. See also gender com-
    parisons
work-loss days (WLD), 61, 94–95
workplace, 57–58, 73, 223–224; coverage,
    97; financing health care through, 96,
    225–226; injury at, 66, 67; sex discrimi-
    nation in, 60
World War II, 59, 105

X rays, 9, 13, 187; exposure to medical, in
    pregnancy, 197–198